T0306301

AMERICAN DEMENTIA

AMERICAN DEMENTIA

Brain Health in an Unhealthy Society

Daniel R. George, PhD, MSc

Peter J. Whitehouse, MD, PhD

JOHNS HOPKINS UNIVERSITY PRESS

Baltimore

© 2021 Johns Hopkins University Press
All rights reserved. Published 2021
Printed in the United States of America on acid-free paper
2 4 6 8 9 7 5 3 1

Johns Hopkins University Press
2715 North Charles Street
Baltimore, Maryland 21218-4363
www.press.jhu.edu

Library of Congress Cataloging-in-Publication Data

Names: George, Daniel (Daniel R.), 1982– author. | Whitehouse, Peter J. author.
Title: American dementia : brain health in an unhealthy society /
Daniel R. George, PhD, and Peter J. Whitehouse, MD, PhD.
Description: Baltimore : Johns Hopkins University Press, [2021] |
Includes bibliographical references and index.
Identifiers: LCCN 2020022479 | ISBN 9781421440477 (hardcover) |
ISBN 9781421440484 (ebook)
Subjects: LCSH: Alzheimer's disease—Government policy—United States. |
Alzheimer's disease—Economic aspects—United States. | Alzheimer's
disease—Social aspects—United States. | Right to health—
United States.
Classification: LCC RC523 .G464 2021 | DDC 362.1968/31100973—dc23
LC record available at https://lccn.loc.gov/2020022479

A catalog record for this book is available from the British Library.

Special discounts are available for bulk purchases of this book. For more information, please contact Special Sales at specialsales@jh.edu.

Johns Hopkins University Press uses environmentally friendly book materials, including recycled text paper that is composed of at least 30 percent post-consumer waste, whenever possible.

To our families, to those affected by and at risk for dementia, and to the prospect of a more humane, hopeful, and sustainable future for all the species on our planet

Contents

Preface

The idea for this book emerged in 2017 while pondering a simple question about a complicated but rather exciting finding: Why have dementia rates appeared to *decline* in the United States and other Western countries over the last decade? Given the failures of big pharma, which has "achieved" a 99.9% fail rate for Alzheimer's drugs since the turn of the century, this phenomenon ostensibly had little to do with biotechnology or free market innovation. So what the heck was going on to reduce dementia?

As we began investigating the question, delving into the recent studies and reaching out to our network of Alzheimer's experts around the world, the answer became clear: the emerging trend we were studying was strongly linked with particular historical and political-economic circumstances realized after the Great Depression and World War II that brought about widespread access to brain-healthy resources like education, quality health care, and cleaner air, soil, and water. At a historical juncture when the world had been mired in deep crisis, the international postwar social democratic consensus—which took the form of the New Deal in the United States—had transformed public institutions in more egalitarian ways for tens of millions of citizens, while investing heavily in public health. In improving the material conditions that shaped the biological destinies of countless bodies and brains, the active interventions of Western states seemingly helped reduce long-term risk for dementia for those now in their graying years.

Unfortunately, as a society we have abandoned this wisdom. Over the last four decades, our political-economic system has once again been thrown badly out of balance. Just as in the Gilded Age that preceded the Great Depression, corporations and the ultra-wealthy have amassed unprecedented levels of riches, effectively capturing the government and using it to upwardly transfer wealth, roll back social protections, and turn unfettered free markets loose in the United States and around the world. Gradually, our political class—strongly co-opted by moneyed interests—has undone many of the egalitarian societal gains made during the postwar social democratic period, which created a robust, thriving, and healthy middle class; extended collective life expectancy; and created the material conditions for the improved lifespan brain health we are witnessing in our current elders. We now live in a society marked by historic income and wealth inequality, stagnant wages, falling lifespans, failing public and private institutions, deep-seated individualism, and general precariousness, anxiety, and despair. New Deal–era safety nets have been frayed by austerity policies that have limited access to brain-protective resources and have left the average person's well-being increasingly susceptible to the whims of free markets. Environmental protections and public health regulations that have safeguarded the health of our brains and bodies but limited profit have been dismantled or removed as market inefficiencies.

In short, the political-economic reordering of our society over the past several decades around hyper-capitalist principles has reduced our shared commitment to one another and made us less healthy in every sense.

In this volume we put forward a relatively simple thesis based on the current evidence: that winning the struggle for a fairer political-economic order where prosperity is more inclusively shared and the public's health and well-being is once again aggressively protected will provide the conditions for *everyone* to build greater resilience to brain aging. Our message is that we, as a society thrown badly out of balance over the last forty years of runaway capitalism, have become so intellectually deficient, so behaviorally unmoored, and so functionally impaired that it represents a long-term case of American dementia. At present, our country—and the globalized world's—political economy is rigged to benefit the very few to the detriment of our collective health. It urgently needs to be leveled again—more sanely and democratically reorganized around an enlightened collectivism that reduces unnecessary large-scale suffering, which is damaging our bodies and brains, and improves the failing institutions, structures, and policies that shape our collective destinies.

What we are talking about when we talk about addressing our American dementia, then, is *making life better for people*—creating healthier and more equitable material conditions for our neighbors (and their brains) to exist and age in across their lives. This world is one where everyone has a right to nutritious food and uncontaminated water, health care, an enriching education, housing, a secure job that pays a living wage, a humane retirement, and basic environmental security—a world that eradicates random senseless cruelty, where no one is denied a dignified life, and where no one is too poor to live. Simply, what we have learned in pursuing the question we originally posed at the outset of this project is that moving in the direction of a healthier society and restoring our shared commitments to one another will protect our brains, allow us to better care for the aging and vulnerable, and heal our broad societal derangement.

It is a story at odds with our dominant cultural understanding of Alzheimer's. In our hyper-capitalist era, we have "medicalized" illness as a discrete pathology and thus cast dementia as a problem of the individual to be solved through technological innovation and enlightened consumption. The depoliticizing tendencies of this reductive approach have, in effect, blinkered us to the political-economic conditions that affect brain health at the population level, and existing power structures have largely gone unchallenged in the Alzheimer's field. But other ways of looking at brain health are possible, especially if we make a stronger effort to break from a more aggressively individualistic, medicalized, market-based model of "disease" and regard brain health as a collective undertaking that is entangled with material forces. Such a reconceptualization demands that we reframe our efforts at prevention not in terms of individuals acting within ever-innovating free markets but in terms of banding together to improve population health and rectify structures of societal power that have been increasingly thrown out of balance since the 1970s.

We believe that our argument within the Alzheimer's field mirrors a larger stirring in our species right now—a broader and necessary awakening within modern societies beset by constant crisis, instability, inequality, alienation, despair, and erosion of our living and natural environments. We are recognizing that we need to respond to crisis by deepening our empathy for one another, building a sense of common purpose beyond mere individualism, and feeling broader and deeper connections in our lives with the natural world. But to stabilize our imbalanced society and pursue a more humane agenda that materially improves brain health across populations, we will need to think beyond the many narratives that currently imprison us and stifle our thinking. This means questioning everything from the stories we tell about capitalism and socialism to the dominant belief that unleashed free markets and biotechnology will solve our most pressing social problems, including Alzheimer's. New stories, such as the ones we share here, invite new forms of solidarity and bold collective actions that can guide us in building a healthier and more compassionate society that is materially better for our bodies and brains. As president, Dwight D. Eisenhower articulated a problem-solving tactic now referred to as the Eisenhower Principle. In his words: "Whenever I run into a problem I can't solve, I always make it bigger. I can never solve it by trying to make it smaller, but if I make it big enough, I can begin to see the outlines of a solution."[1]

This book on brain health is thus an invitation to *enlarge* the problem of Alzheimer's disease in ways that help us think about the type of society we want and how to get there. It is, in this way, somewhat unique in that we have written not merely a conventional self-help book for readers concerned about their own brain health, but an *other-help* book with a higher moral charge that looks *outward* at society and our collective destiny. By making the Alzheimer's problem "bigger," as Eisenhower advised, we will invariably begin to "see the outlines" of a social democratic platform aiming at a healthier and more dignified human society as the most effective and efficient intervention for our brain health.

In 2008, we published a provocatively titled book: *The Myth of Alzheimer's*. The word *myth* drew attention to several key misapprehensions that have powerfully shaped the Alzheimer's field over the last several decades, while sowing enormous fear and stigma in the public. Among the myths we addressed were that Alzheimer's

1. is unrelated to aging,
2. is one discrete disease,
3. is likely curable by biomedical science,
4. causes an irretrievable loss of self in those affected, and
5. imposes an inevitable despair on caregivers.

These mythical beliefs have suppressed the emerging evidence that Alzheimer's is heterogeneous and intimately linked to aging, and that we can lower risk for dementia and improve quality of life for those affected and their caregivers without relying on the unbridled free market to produce a technical fix. While we critiqued the "Alzheimer's empire"—the multibillion-dollar corporate-political infrastructure that has promoted these myths since the 1980s while largely subordinating the importance of public health, prevention, psychosocial interventions, and caregiving—our book was largely apolitical and aimed more at colleagues within the purview of our field.

Just after we published it, however, the Great Recession destabilized the country and world and threw us into a societal crisis that we continue to feel every day. Our lives are inherently political now, and the dangers and consequences of hyper-capitalism have been exposed. Any serious book about Alzheimer's and brain health must deal with the deteriorating material circumstances we and our public institutions find ourselves in during this era of American dementia and reckon with the "forgotten" lessons of the past that we share in this book.

Understanding the social, political, and economic forces at play in the Alzheimer's field is a gateway into larger questions about the organization of our society and how we are governed. What does it mean to be a member of a local, national, and international human community? What responsibilities do we have to one another, to the aging and vulnerable, to future generations, and what are the critical lessons of the past we must heed? What role should corporate power and technology play in structuring our lives and hopes? What collective investments ought we make to reduce poverty and suffering, give people a chance to flourish with healthy bodies and brains, and provide care and security for the cognitively frail and their caregivers? What should the role of the state be in tempering the excesses of the free market and providing for all citizens?

In our current moment, people are hungry for transformative change and want to organize and act in local communities that have been degraded—materially and spiritually—by decades of hyper-capitalist and austerity policies, which have left us feeling more atomized, precarious, and alienated from one another. This book is one voice within a larger movement that is seeking regeneration and revitalization from within the malaise of late capitalism. In the chapters to come, we show how winning the struggle for a more humane, equitable society will multiply our collective brain health. A successful response to Alzheimer's—a moral commitment to protecting those at risk (all of us) and compassionately supporting those living with dementia—will embolden us with the necessary tools, mindset, and ethos to resist other major societal challenges of our time.

Speaking of those living with dementia, we walk arm in arm with persons already affected by aging-associated cognitive challenges and their family and professional carers on an intellectual and ethical journey to pursue the goal of "curing" what ails us culturally. Dementia is an issue that provides us space to find the imagination, passion, and moral grounding that will make all our lives better.

In this moment of cultural tumult, let us venture forward together, in solidarity, exploring our American dementia as a means of fostering collective action in service of better brain health, more compassionate treatment of those with memory loss, and, most importantly, the realization of a more just and humane world.

Authors' note: As we were working with our editors to finalize the manuscript in Spring 2020, the "moment of cultural tumult" we described in what was to be our concluding paragraph above accelerated quite dramatically as the SARS-CoV-2 virus (coronavirus) began spreading around the world. The resulting COVID-19 pandemic has not only been deadly on a mass scale, it has also acted as a magnifying glass, bringing into focus all the cracks in the failing social, political, and economic systems of the neoliberal era that we interrogate in this book through the lens of Alzheimer's disease. Unsurprisingly, people living with dementia—not to mention low-wage caregivers who often work without full benefits—in long-term care facilities have been most vulnerable to coronavirus. So too has the virus disproportionately exposed other members of the working-class with "essential" jobs (grocery clerks, bus drivers, nurses, mail carriers and delivery workers, gig economy contractors lacking health insurance or benefit structures, and so on), many of whom have continued laboring at below a living wage without hazard pay and at great personal risk. Our poorest citizens will feel the worst effects of the economic contraction, mass unemployment, and precariousness that follow in the virus's wake. How much worse will depend not only on epidemiology, but on whether we can effectively progress toward a fairer and more equitable society, as we advocate in this book.

Indeed, the crisis has grown exponentially, largely because of the "demented" social organization we interrogate above and will continue to explore throughout the book. Poorly funded public health and disease surveillance programs; weakened social safety nets; vast amounts of people with preexisting conditions due to being un- or underinsured and without consistent health care; the absence of policies that could have helped mitigate the crisis (such as universal health care, universal basic income, a jobs guarantee, rent controls); critical policy decisions driven by a commitment to preserving a neoliberal economic system, rather than offering sustained help to vulnerable citizens; markets aimed at short-term profit and unprepared to rise to the emergent needs of an epidemic; vast poverty, homelessness, and disparities in wealth; diminished domestic production capacity due to procorporate free-trade deals that have shipped millions of manufacturing jobs offshore; badly weakened labor unions; and a deep and abiding greed, individualism, and anomie that permeate our society and its structures have all played a role in sowing conditions for the virus to spread out of control. From our highest levels of leadership on down, COVID-19 is a crisis defined by failed institutions and the deranged political-economic organization of our hyper-capitalist era. As we write this in May 2020, we are only beginning to see the suffering—physically, mentally, economically, and spiritually—that will continue unfolding into the future.

In many ways, the conflagration of COVID-19 is rapidly exposing what is structurally amiss in our society in a manner the slower burn of dementia has only recently begun to do. As with the lessons imparted by brain aging that we share in this book, the crisis of the virus can point us toward a material reorganization of our society around more life-affirming values, which our "American dementia" has caused us to forget—greater fairness, equitability, compassion, solidarity, fellow feeling, mutual care, collective prosperity, and responsible stewardship of our natural and built environments. A pandemic reveals in depth how interconnected we are as human beings and how interwoven (and fragile) our shared destinies are. Can we use this moment of flux to begin moving toward the "revolution of values" that Martin Luther King championed a half-century ago? Can we develop a collective wisdom that will not only help us safely navigate the COVID crisis and address the challenges of dementia, but also allow the human species to flourish on the only planet we have? In the chapters to come, let us join together in thinking about how to push our society in a healthier direction—one that bridges beyond the many crises that define our current moment.

Acknowledgments

We would like to thank our respective institutions—Penn State College of Medicine and Case Western Reserve University—for providing us the time and resources to undertake this project. Our family and friends have been a highly valued and loving source of support, and we'd like to specifically thank Debra Rex, George M. George, Emily George, and Cathy Whitehouse for their ongoing encouragement and constructive feedback. We would also like to offer special thanks to our colleagues Bob Whitaker and Rick Moody, both of whom believed in this project and helped give it life when we weren't sure it would see the light of day. Danny would like to thank the Rodale Institute in Kutztown, Pennsylvania, for kindly providing space in its guest house in 2019 for the final writing push. We both extend major gratitude to our John Hopkins University Press editors Robin Coleman and Kimberly Johnson, catalog copy writer Hilary Jacqmin, and freelance copyeditor Melanie Mallon for their expert guidance in helping shape and refine our book's message.

Many colleagues made this book possible, and while it is impossible to properly recognize them all, we'd like to offer special thanks to Ken Langa, Bill Thomas, Mona Hanna-Attisha, Margaret Lock, Carol Brayne, Peter Rabins, Stephen Katz, Kimberly Myers, Cheryl Dellasega, Bernice Hausman, Wade Edris, Jesse Ballenger, Anne Basting, Simon D'Alton, Darryl Wilkinson, Eric Larson, George Perry, Tomi Dreibelbis, Jim Gruber, Heather Snyder, Lori Snyder, Kavan Peterson, Joel Kroft, Shannon Harvey, Stephanie Walter, Ryan and Katie Hanson, Elizabeth Lokon, Al Power, Lin Bartle, Ian Kremer, Stephanie Fallcreek, Sylvia Kruger, Matt Kaplan, Maria Valenti, Ted Schettler, Jill Stein, Sarah Jaffe, Jeremy Bendik-Keymer, Kerstin Langenberger, Arthur Kleinman, Oliver Sacks, Rachel Remen, Roland Griffiths, Albert Garcia-Romeu, Richard Geer, Kristin Bodiford, Mariano Sanchez, Patrik Standar, Maria Genne, and many others. Peter would also like to thank other species for their inspiration, especially majestic long-lived trees.

This book would also not be in existence were it not for Bernie Sanders and the movement he helped launch with his presidential campaign in 2015. Others who have inspired us in the popular culture include Noam Chomsky, Glenn Greenwald, Naomi Klein, Cornel West, Adolph Reed, Cedric Johnson, Bill McKibben, David Orr, Paul Hawken, Aimee Terese, Benjamin Studebaker,

Amber Frost, Angela Nagle, Anna Khachiyan, Dasha Nekrasova, Michael Tracey, Matt Christman, Fredrik deBoer, Zaid Jilani, Russell Brand, and Joe Rogan, just to name a few. Peter wishes to dedicate this book to his children and grandchildren in hopes that this volume constitutes—even in some minuscule way—a path to a brighter future for them and all future generations of every living creature everywhere.

AMERICAN DEMENTIA

1

Occupy Alzheimer's!

Setting the Scene for Resistance

On September 17, 2011, hundreds of people began gathering in lower Manhattan's Zuccotti Park. Brought together by the rallying cry "We are the 99%!," they set up tents, public kitchens, and peaceful barricades in the epicenter of the global financial services industry, providing free food and health care for all protestors. The mainstream media questioned the Occupiers' purpose. It quickly became clear, however, that they hadn't just built this ramshackle village to protest the recent use of trillions of dollars from the Federal Reserve to bail out Wall Street institutions, whose reckless "casino capitalism" had helped drive the global economy into the Great Recession of 2008. There were also larger issues of deep economic inequality; austerity cuts to social services in federal, state, and local budgets; the disappearance of good jobs, political corruption, and excessive corporate power.[1] Their presence represented a scant but surprising resistance to the global elite—the largely faceless legion of 36 million millionaires and 2,400 billionaires (that is, the 1%) who exercise disproportionate power over the rest of us (the 99%).[2] This plucky, leaderless movement soon became known as Occupy Wall Street.

Later that fall, I (Danny) visited Zuccotti Park, which the Occupiers had renamed Liberty Plaza, and spoke to some of the protesters as they staved off the bracing cold (figure 1.1). While morale remained high, the encampment was feeling mounting pressure from the FBI, the Department of Homeland Security, local police, local politicians, mainstream media, and the world-spanning corporate forces on whose turf they were squatting.[3] Occupy came to a semiofficial close on New Year's Day 2012. Even so, the animating force of the movement didn't go away: the raw

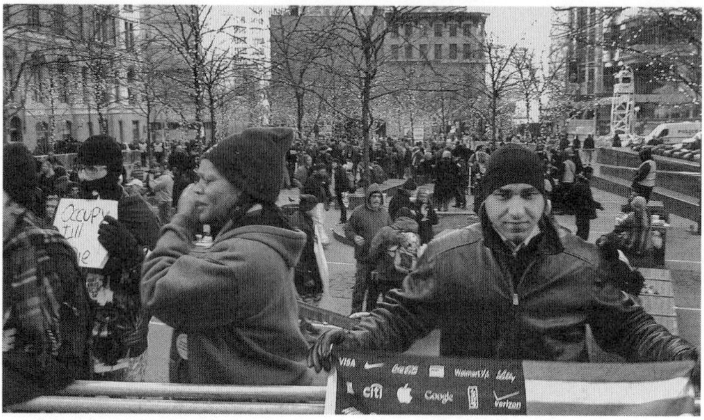

Figure 1.1. Occupy Wall Street protestors in Liberty Plaza, December 2011.
Source: Photograph by Daniel George.

upwelling of anger and injustice at the elites hoarding immense wealth and the venal political establishment and Wall Street financiers doing their bidding,[4] coupled with a powerful, if nebulous, vision of a more fair, humane, and healthy society that would provide mutual aid, support, and dignity for all citizens. Indeed, Occupy diffused into hundreds of protests and encampments across the country in banks, in foreclosed homes, on college campuses, and even amid the 2012 Superstorm Sandy, where volunteers mobilized into disaster response teams to clear damaged homes, serve meals, and provide supplies and medical care to thousands of people in need.[5]

More recently, the movement found expression in electoral politics as part of Senator Bernie Sanders' 2016 and 2020 presidential campaigns, which adopted Occupy's inclusive vernacular of the "99% vs. the 1%." So too has it manifested in emergent movements like Black Lives Matter, the Sunrise Movement and Extinction Rebellion for political action on climate change, the Fight for $15 (for a living wage), the Poor Peoples' Campaign, Medicare for All, and the historic wave of teachers' strikes.

Thanks to Occupy Wall Street, the very notion of *occupying* has come to serve as shorthand for collectively resisting establishment power through acts of civil disobedience. It is in that spirit that we launch the book by asking what it might mean to "occupy Alzheimer's"—in other words, to interrogate how a "disease" we've come to so deeply fear as an abstract biological entity might be interwoven with our current political-economic order and the struggles, grievances, and material privations of those who occupied Zuccotti Park. To understand how Alzheimer's fits into this story, and to realign our efforts at achieving brain health in a society that has become deeply imbalanced and decidedly *un*healthy, we must first appreciate the changing political and economic tides that sent the Occupy protestors flooding into Zuccotti Park and unleashed a decade of popular mobilization around the world.

While our age of scientific reductionism has biased us to conceive of disease at the level of biology alone, this book argues for a broader picture. In doing so, we draw on the perspective of political economy—a social science built around the study of political policies and economic processes and their effects on power relations—to examine the role of societal organization in materially affecting the raw biology of our brains and bodies, and thus shaping our *brain health*. In this chapter, we set the table for an understanding of Alzheimer's disease as inextricably entangled with the material conditions mediated by structures, institutions, and policies that have been engineered to favor the individual good of a few over the greater good for the many across the last four decades—a span of time we define as the era of *American dementia*. Not only has increasingly "demented" political-economic organization led to the unhealthy society we find ourselves in, it has caused an amnesia whereby we've collectively "forgotten" important lessons about brain health from the past and narrowed our creative thinking about scientific approaches to Alzheimer's disease and myriad other social problems.

Let's begin examining this proposition, starting in Zuccotti Park.

THE ONSET OF AMERICAN DEMENTIA: NEOLIBERALISM'S VICTORY OVER SOCIAL DEMOCRACY

When the Occupy tent village defiantly entrenched itself amid Wall Street's steel-and-glass skyscrapers, it revived public debate about the moral responsibility of Western governments to regulate capitalism, reverse deep inequality, and represent the interests of ordinary citizens rather than society's elite. In doing so, Occupy has gradually exposed a deep tension between two theories of governance: neoliberal capitalism (or *neoliberalism*) and social democracy. These two systems, born of the 20th century, play an important, if underappreciated, role in the story of

Alzheimer's disease, which will become clear as you read this book. Let's examine each system more carefully.

The Birth of Neoliberalism

Neoliberalism is a form of extreme capitalism that merges the long tradition of individualism (*liberalism*) in Western thought, associated with philosophers like Adam Smith and John Locke, with more modern (*neo*) efforts to use government as a tool for expanding free enterprise, deregulating markets, and globalizing national and world economies. Drawing on the laissez-faire liberalism of the 17th and 18th centuries, the neoliberal political movement has sought to expand unfettered free markets into social and economic territory previously controlled by the state. Viewing markets as the most efficient means of organizing society and meeting the needs of individuals, its proponents have pursued policies to retrench the state from social and economic affairs, reduce public spending, and let free markets function autonomously and rationally, fueled by profit and competition. Such conditions inevitably create inequality but also generate enormous wealth and theoretically maximize individual liberty by reducing the influence of the state over individuals.

The intellectual movement that plotted a course for neoliberalism in current establishment politics emerged in the 1930s and ascended in the 1950s and '60s as networks of academics, politicians, think tanks, and others built a coherent suite of political-economic policies organized around the general concept that a modern government's role in solving societal problems like education, hunger, health care, and poverty ought to be reduced, and that solutions would be best delivered by an unleashed free market. Neoliberal proponents, including Mont Pelerin Society founders Friedrich Hayek, Milton Friedman, Karl Popper, and others, attacked the then-dominant political-economic theory associated with John Maynard Keynes, which in the mid-20th century—after the devastation of the Great Depression and two world wars—had established a more *active* role for the state in the management of a mixed public-private economy.[6]

The Keynesian postwar consensus in Western countries had succeeded in correcting wealth concentration and gross inequities produced by the unrestrained monopolistic free markets of the Gilded Age and had fostered rapid economic growth to rejuvenate ailing national economies. In the United States, this tightly managed capitalism took the form of the New Deal, which aimed numerous state institutions, programs, actions, regulatory protections, and experiments at a broad spectrum of problems in the country (social security, financial reform and Wall Street regulation, public housing, housing finance, conservation, jobs and the right to unionize, civil infrastructure, commissioned art and literature, and so on). The state effectively recaptured swaths of social and economic territory that had been overrun by private interests in the free-market extravaganza of the Gilded Age. As the mid-20th century progressed, however, neoliberal critics persistently argued that such a model was antithetical to the natural law of economic growth through untrammeled markets and ought to be replaced.

Unleashing the "Beast" of the Free Market

Whereas the Keynesian approach to the crisis of capitalism sparked by the Great Depression had amounted to placing the "beast of the free market" on a tight regulatory leash after 1945, neoliberals envisioned a world with the regulatory shackles of the free market shaken off. To emancipate markets, proponents pursued a policy framework organized around what we might call *the four D's*[7]:

1. Deregulated markets
2. Decreased taxation of the wealthy
3. Decreased funding of social programs and increased privatization
4. Deunionized labor

When numerous financial perturbations disrupted the global economy in the seventies and created an international economic climate that become known as *stagflation* (simultaneous high inflation and high unemployment), champions of neoliberalism sensed an opportunity to respond to crisis by profoundly reordering the political economy around new principles. In this era, which scholars refer to as "the Pivotal Decade,"[8] the political elite began implementing the four D's as formal policies in Western governments in ways that began laying the foundation for the acceleration of modern globalization. In the United States, the Democratic Party began distancing itself from its Keynesian New Deal roots and its traditional role as a staunch advocate for the working class.

To jumpstart a lagging economy beset by falling profit rates and the strongest recessionary forces since World War II, President Jimmy Carter's administration initiated in the late seventies the deregulation of airline, railroad, trucking, banking, electric power, and natural gas industries; eliminated rules against financial concentration; enacted large tax cuts for the rich; and imposed strict austerity measures under neoliberal Federal Reserve chair Paul Volcker to control inflation (rather than attacking unemployment) and promote a balanced budget (rather than stimulating growth).[9,10] As a result, significant unemployment marked the late seventies—particularly in mining, construction, and manufacturing, which absorbed 90% of job losses—and in places like Flint, Michigan, more than one in five workers were unemployed.[11] But for Volcker this was by design, as neoliberalism regarded unemployment as "natural" for a functioning free-market economy.[12]

In the eighties, US president Ronald Reagan and British prime minister Margaret Thatcher, under the direct advisement of prominent academic neoliberal economists Milton Friedman and Friedrich Hayek, more aggressively embraced free market-fundamentalist policies, cutting taxes on capital, scaling back social protections, freezing minimum wage, tolerating high unemployment, dismantling business regulation across sectors, landing major blows to weaken organized labor in both countries, eliminating New Deal–era antitrust rules, and generally pursuing an unshackled market-based vision that Thatcher described as "roll[ing] back the frontiers of the state,"[13] and that Reagan described in a speech to Wall Street as "Turn[ing] the bull loose."[14] Such reforms by Thatcher and Reagan—both of whom, somewhat ironically, went on to develop dementia in later decades—limited the state's capacity to rein in the worst excesses of the free market, as had been its role since the disaster of the Depression. Reagan famously gave voice to this inversion in his 1981 inaugural address, proclaiming, "Government is not the solution to our problem, government *is* the problem."

Whereas the political-economic order of Keynesian managerial capitalism had managed to keep the "beast" in check, the new paradigm of neoliberalism viewed its role as freeing businesses solely to concentrate on increasing shareholder profit, unmoored from any questions about corporate responsibility to society. Friedman's essay in the *New York Times* titled "The Social Responsibility of Business Is to Increase Its Profits"[15] asserted the neoliberal ethos quite bluntly. A powerfully resurgent Wall Street guided shareholders and boards in a deregulated landscape. This growing era of *financialization*—wherein financial actors and institutions began acquiring disproportionate power and influence in the domestic and increasingly global economy—more and more led to cost-cutting decisions to offshore more and more jobs in the manufacturing industries, which had employed millions of middle-class Americans in places like Flint, to developing countries with cheaper labor forces.

In the United States, the dominance of neoliberal policies and retrenchment of public welfare services continued under Reagan's vice president George H. W. Bush in the nineties. It gained further momentum with Bill Clinton's "ideologically ambidextrous"[16] administration, which accepted the premise of the neoliberal political-economic order, supporting the passage of global free trade deals (NAFTA, for one), dramatically cutting the welfare benefit system for the poor,[17] and repealing protective New Deal–era regulations in the finance[18] and housing markets (at the behest of multinational investment bank Citigroup),[19] which laid the groundwork for the Great Recession that rocked the world just as George W. Bush's Wall Street–dominated administration was handing off to Barack Obama's team in 2008.

As we've all felt in our own lives, the effects of the Great Recession were devastating. The Dow Jones shed half its value; 8.7 million people lost their jobs as unemployment climbed to double digits; 10 million people lost their homes; and we confronted a rippling crisis of capitalism that hadn't been felt since Keynesians macroeconomics were marshaled to stabilize a shocked global economic system after the Great Depression and two world wars.

Obama responded not by nationalizing banks or prosecuting Wall Street leaders who squandered $10 trillion but rather by maintaining most of Bush's Wall Street–backed neoliberal economic team (appointing as director of his National Economic Council the neoliberal Larry Summers, who famously proclaimed, "We are now all [Milton] Friedmanites"[20]) and administering $16 trillion of bailouts. By 2011, the cumulative failure of these "demented" neoliberal policies, which had, with central direction from Wall Street financial institutions, bottomed out global economies and increased concentrations of wealth at the very top of the economic scale while devastating the working class, brought the restive masses into the streets in Zuccotti Park and around the world. Popular anger at a political-economic establishment that had visited such harms across the heartland helped bring Donald Trump to power in 2016, and neoliberal efforts continue apace today, with finance still representing a nearly $18 trillion industry as of 2020.

RISE OF THE ZOMBIE ECONOMY: CONTEMPORARY NEOLIBERAL SHOCK POLITICS

Even with the damage neoliberalism's dogmatic free-marketeering policies have caused since the dramatic reordering of the seventies, it remains an admittedly perplexing term since the word *liberal* evokes associations with what people imagine to be to the left of the political spectrum. It has been suggested that less confusing terminologies like *hyper-capitalism* or *market fundamentalism* would more accurately describe the ideology,[21] and we use these terms interchangeably with *neoliberalism* in this book as we explore the effects of the unfettered market on Alzheimer's disease and brain health during the four-decade era of American dementia.

While the ongoing confusion around the term *neoliberalism* has made the incremental dominance of its policies in our lives relatively inconspicuous, on occasion, the whole nation has borne witness in real time to the specific cultural formation it has ushered in. For instance, in the wake of 2005's Hurricane Katrina, when all eyes were on the damage and devastation of New Orleans, George W. Bush's administration responded to the crisis by turning the city's public spaces and services into what Republican representative Paul Ryan called a "free-enterprise zone"[22]—employing private security firms to patrol the city, privatizing utilities, replacing public schools with private charters (and firing thousands of teachers), bulldozing housing projects and building condo and hotel developments, removing regulatory barriers, and, as is the wont of hyper-capitalist politics, generally leaving the city's fate in the hands of the unshackled free market. In Naomi Klein's book *The Shock Doctrine*,[23] she has identified how this strategy of *shock politics*—that is, seizing on moments of crisis and confusion caused by natural disasters or by capitalism itself as opportunities to implement the four D's and fundamentally reorder reeling societies around vertiginous free-market principles—has been the dominant power-grabbing strategy of the neoliberal era.

Simply put, a neoliberal vision for the world embeds market logic in all dimensions of our lives, and, like New Orleans, *everything* (health care, education, housing, food, water, police) becomes a potential commodity. From this vantage point, proponents generally reject any notion of solidarity, collective responsibility, and pursuing shared prosperity through public institutions. Individuals are exalted as independent monads with rights who act rationally within markets to optimize self-interest.

Without a doubt, the hyper-capitalist "freeing of the beast" has succeeded in opening domestic and global markets integrated around American-driven economic principles and liberating powerful financial institutions on Wall Street—the central axis on which the financial world turns. This has generated vast sums of wealth and economic growth, spurred profit-driven technological innovation, and to some degree helped reduce poverty, illiteracy rates, and low life expectancy in the developing world. But like a rabid animal frothing at the mouth, the unleashed free market rabidly serves *its* interests, generating wealth but largely blind to where the wealth goes and inconsiderate of what is good for humanity or the world. As MIT professor Noam Chomsky has written, neoliberalism represents a peculiar arrangement where "the economy is doing fine but the people aren't."[24]

Indeed, the beast we raised from the crisis of the seventies to create a system that better served us is now controlling us, widening the rift between economic "winners" and "losers" and again driving our capitalist system to the precipice of crisis. This has led some to characterize neoliberalism as effectively giving rise to a modern dynamic known as the *zombie economy*—an economic order that, like the shambling monster, lurches forward in a relentless single-minded pursuit of short-term profit, trampling on ecological habitats, social structures, traditional values, communities, and workers that stand in the way of free-market capitalist logic and sowing vast inequalities and societal traumas in its wake.[25,26]

Consequently, as zombie capitalism has advanced in its rapacious mission of profit maximization in our era of American dementia, it has demonstrably drained the life out of other areas of society, playing a substantial role in creating historic levels of income and wealth inequality, stagnating wages, generating insecurity in modern jobs, driving up poverty rates and debt, destabilizing global markets, damaging and warming the environment, transferring excessive power to multinational corporations and a ruling class of political and business elites, and—as we witnessed in New Orleans—weakening the collective commitments of our public institutions to citizens in favor of private markets and individual choice. So too has this deranged political-economic system selected for our most base tendencies. Today, a widespread ethos of crass individualism, personal responsibility, meritocracy, atomization, consumerism, and competitiveness prevail as dominant organizing principles in our society—a shift that we all viscerally feel in our societal fabric.

Thatcher is often remembered for the famous remark, "There is no such thing as society. There are individual men and women and there are families. And no government can do anything except through people, and people must look after themselves first."[27] In proclaiming this, she gave voice to the market-fundamentalist contempt for the very idea that human communities exist, much less share a collective bond or material interests with one another above and beyond isolated individuals and families. In this hyper-liberalized worldview, governments exist to protect property rights, free markets, and free trade, thereby fostering conditions for private interests—so-called job- and wealth-creating entrepreneurs—to maximize profit and then have their riches "trickle down" to the rest of society.

Even with its outsized impact on modern life, neoliberalism, being a rather dry liturgy of economic policies (deregulate, decrease taxes on the wealthy, defund social programs, deunionize labor) rather than a graspable "thing," remains an inscrutable, zombie-like force in our lives that is only now working its way into our modern lexicon. In many ways, this dynamic is reminiscent of the famous 2005 commencement address at Kenyon College by David Foster Wallace in which the late author relayed a parable about two younger fishes encountering an older fish who asks them how the water feels. After swimming downstream, one of the younger fishes looks quizzically at the other and asks: "What is water?"

In the 21st century, neoliberalism is our water—it surrounds us, touching nearly every aspect of our lives even as most citizens are hard pressed to define what "it" is.[28]

Indeed, as American-driven neoliberalism has surreptitiously become the global architecture in which we all exist, Democratic and Republican political elites have gradually assimilated its core tenets into a nearly indistinguishable economic centrism. Democrats, once the party of the working-class post–New Deal, have capitulated to the market-fundamentalist consensus and become the party of the professional and managerial classes (including corporate America), with little interest in challenging imbalanced structural power or delivering material benefits for ordinary workers and the poor. Both parties, despite *performative* opposition around culture war issues, are largely funded, lobbied, and legislatively directed by Wall Street financiers, big banks, Silicon Valley tech elites, and other influential industries (defense, health insurance, big pharma, big agriculture, fossil fuels, and so forth) that invest excess wealth generated by their minimally regulated enterprises in the continuation of the neoliberal political-economic order. Gradually, the concentration of wealth at the very top has allowed a societal elite to capture democratic institutions, which pass laws and policies that advance their interest. As the late comedian George Carlin darkly teased his average joe audience about our modern political-economic predicament, "It's a big club, and you ain't in it!"[29]

The end of the Cold War and the ostensible triumph of capitalism—not to mention a badly weakened labor movement and a public increasingly fragmented through suburban sprawl and corporate media—has often precluded deep cultural conversation about the effects of neoliberalism in our lives. But the 2007-2008 Great Recession effectively burst the balloon of hyper-capitalism, exposing it as a deeply flawed and demented political-economic order. Movements like Occupy Wall Street, with its populist rallying cry assailing the wealth and income inequality and structural corruption worsening life for the 99%, have empowered us to take stock of our American dementia. Like the fish in the parable, we have begun questioning the very water we've been swimming in for four decades.

OUR CRISIS OF CAPITALISM: DISPARITY, AUSTERITY, AND PRECARITY

What that meditation has revealed is that a world dogmatically (and dementedly) structured around hyper-capitalism is failing to deliver meaningful livelihoods for the bulk of the population. Absent the buffering force of the state in providing a structure to enable human flourishing, ordinary people are finding the trappings of even a *basic* secure life—reliable jobs and careers, pensions, medical care, housing, and education—elusive. While the 1% are thriving, for normal people in the 99%, the zombie economy has wrought a crisis-ridden landscape—one materially defined by *disparity*, *austerity*, and *precarity*.

Disparity is clear and present in a societal landscape where the richest 1% own about 40% of the country's wealth.[30] According to the Federal Reserve, while the country's super rich have grown $21 trillion richer since the eighties, the bottom half of the wealth distribution has grown $900 billion poorer,[31] with real earnings actually falling for middle- and low-paid workers for forty years and costs of living rising dramatically.[32] While 45 million Americans (15 million children) live in poverty, with 40 million on federal food stamps and almost half of US workers between the ages of 18 and 64 employed in low-wage jobs,[33] the zombie economy has churned out 585 billionaires. In 2019, the United States hit its highest levels of income inequality since the Census Bureau started tracking it 50 years ago.[34]

As individuals and communities, we *feel* these widening disparities in the millions of jobs lost to globalization and free trade deals; in the wage stagnation that has afflicted 90% of Americans over the last four decades despite rising worker productivity;[35] and in the federal minimum wage that has been frozen at $7.25 since July 2009 (becoming in 2019 the longest stretch in US history with no minimum wage increase). Sixty-two million people scratch out a living for under $15 an hour, and an unconceivable 34 million American adults are among the world's poorest 10%.[36] Such a maniacal political-economic ordering has imposed massive strains on the working poor, which we explore throughout the book, especially in chapters 5 and 6 when we consider poverty and its material effects on the brain. Tellingly, gaps in life expectancy between the rich and poor are large and expanding in the United States—with the wealthiest American men living 15 years longer than the poorest men.[37,38] Ultimately these disparities are the inevitable culmination of restructuring the political economy around neoliberal principles in the seventies that, rather than making us freer and more prosperous, have in reality pushed us toward oligarchy, with a wealthy minority of elites ruling over a disempowered majority.

So too do the *austerity* measures embraced as part of the market-fundamentalist turn mark our lives. As the forces of globalization have created intense domestic and international competition to keep tax bases low to encourage business investment, both parties have cut public spending, gradually attacking the welfare state and reducing equitable access to services affecting health, such as high-quality education, health care, public transportation, nutrition, and environmental protection. Bipartisan austerity policies passed in the wake of the Great Recession effectively transferred the failures of Wall Street investors and politicians to welfare recipients, pensioners, and public sector workers, echoing Martin Luther King's observation that the United States has "socialism for the rich, rugged individualism for the poor."[39] Compared to the rest of the world, we feel austerity more acutely in America, where social spending represents only 18% of the GDP compared with an average of 20% elsewhere in the world, including 31% in France.[40] Tellingly, in 2019, the US senate passed a fiscal budget allocating $738 billion for the military and just $638 billion for everything else.

Indeed, the disparities and austerity policies of zombie capitalism have suffused the lives of the 99% with a growing sense of *precarity*. More than two-thirds of Americans live paycheck to paycheck, struggling to pay bills.[41] An astounding 60% of middle-income families do not have enough savings to cover three months of expenses, leaving them financially vulnerable to a layoff or other economic shock, such as the one imposed by the COVID-19 epidemic.[42] Many carry massive amounts of debt from soaring tuition, housing, health care, food, transportation, and other costs of living, and they possess so little savings that—according to a Federal Reserve study—*40% of adults* don't feel they could cover a $400 hospital bill without going into debt or selling something[43] (or crowd funding their medical fees).[44] Tragically, 44 million Americans lack health care altogether, with tens of millions more underinsured.[45] As a result, medical or other unforeseen emergencies can send people into rapid downward spirals, and annually, the United States sees tens of thousands of deaths from lack of health insurance,[46] with 137 million adults reporting medical financial hardship.[47] The lethal consequences of such cuts has led scholars like Michael Marmot to refer to austerity as "death by politics."[48]

Precariousness defines workplaces as well. Less than 10% of workers are represented by unions, and Americans thus enjoy fewer labor protections than workers in other wealthy countries. Many have lost traditional benefit, wage-ladder, collective bargaining, and workplace safety structures and are forced to work multiple jobs to survive, including as independent contractors in the emerging *gig economy*. All the while, the lack of a social safety net—particularly universal health care—keeps many locked in to insecure or dead-end jobs that maintain lives on a razor's edge, effectively constricting the so-called birthright of "freedom" for many Americans. Workers increasingly face the dystopian prospect of millions of jobs being lost to rising automation and artificial intelligence,[49] and people feel rising uncertainty, insecurity, and vulnerability around climate change and the disruptive and unpredictable weather events it churns out. The 2020 COVID-19 pandemic has been an acute shock to the system, showing just how vulnerable millions of Americans are not only to a deadly virus but also its economic fallout, and how deeply unprepared the state is to protect us in an age when austerity has so hollowed out our shared institutions.

The Material Consequences of the Neoliberal Era on Public Health

Such societal conditions exact a toll on our collective well-being. Americans rank among the most anxious people in the world, with a self-reported stress rate 20 percentage points higher than the global average.[50] Indeed, lack of mental health care is a massive problem in the United States, with 129 suicides a day (40,000 annually) and 130 deaths a day from pain-killing opioids.[51] Life expectancy declined in the United States for three consecutive years, from 2015 to 2017—the longest sustained decline since the Spanish flu and World War I decimated the global population from 1915 to 1918—with rising "deaths of despair" linked to suicide, alcoholism, and substance abuse playing a central role.[52] In 2019, the United States ranked a distant 45th in world rankings of life expectancy.[53]

As the early 21st century has been shaped by widespread disparity, austerity, and precarity, it has sown deep emotional pain, frustration, alienation, and powerlessness. People are weary of living with constant insecurity under austerity regimes; of being considered disposable commodities in their jobs and perpetually pitted against one another in market-based competition; of being interminably barraged by advertisements; of not having enough money to meet their needs; of feeling isolated and lonely; of losing trust, solidarity, and a sense of connection to neighbors in our sprawling neoliberal landscape.

As a sense of dislocation has built, so too has anger. It was particularly galling to many people that while the Great Recession wiped out tremendous wealth and retirement savings and led to mass foreclosures for ordinary folks, no systematic prosecution of Wall Street malefactors was ever undertaken. Essentially, the Obama administration, which had accepted nearly $15 million from Wall Street during his 2008 presidential run,[54] handed out no-interest loans to these massive centers of power, while average Americans were made to accept deeper "austerity measures" and essentially suffer for the mistakes of the rich.

Such machinations have made it increasingly impossible for many to ignore the fact that nearly everyone in the "big club" of Congress is a millionaire and that special interests continually dominate our politics and override the popular will. A study by political scientists at Princeton University has famously established that the preferences of wealthy elites, corporations, and trade associations (that is, the 1%) have dramatically more impact on policy change than average citizens, who appear to have only what researchers called "a minuscule, near-zero, statistically non-significant impact."[55] Knowing that both neoliberal parties are almost entirely subservient to big business and the ultra-wealthy donor class (with five lobbyists for each member of Congress[56]) and openly hostile to working-class interests and policy preferences has a poisonous effect on public trust of democratic institutions,[57] with studies showing that 57% of Americans believe there is no point in voting because elections and policy are controlled by the wealthy, corporations, and "dark money"—that is, a functional oligarchy rather than a representative democracy.[58,59,60] In the 2016 presidential election, this disillusionment was manifest in the nation's largest voting bloc being the 100 million registered voters who simply elected to cast no ballot at all.[61,62]

In short, if we were to treat America as if the country were a patient, we would be well justified in diagnosing it with a clinical dementia (see text box 1).

While elements of the American political class—including Donald Trump—responded to our current crisis of capitalism with populist appeals that redirect the pain people feel at the declining political-economic situation to scapegoats (immigrants, refugees, racial minorities, Russia, and so on), while promising a return to national greatness (Make America

THE ONSET OF AMERICAN DEMENTIA

Clinical dementia is a condition that affects individuals, characterized by memory loss and other cognitive difficulties, such as decision making, language, and perceptions that impair activities of living.

Cultural dementia is a condition that affects communities, characterized by collective patterns of dysfunction in thinking, valuing, and acting.

Over the past four decades of hyper-capitalism, society has been progressively afflicted by an American dementia, causing us to suffer from

- lack of executive function and attention deficit (inability to act decisively against major challenges/crises of our time, such as income and wealth inequality, lack of universal healthcare, national lead poisoning, climate change)
- mania (psychotic focus on the market, on individualism, on divisive culture war issues)
- amnesia (forgetting important lessons of the past, like the success of social democracy in the mid-20th century)
- apathy (inability to motivate change from an unhealthy status quo)
- agnosia (failure to recognize or act upon the underlying drivers of popular discontentment)
- alienation (disenchantment from nature, loss of trust/solidarity, political disillusionment)
- lack of imagination and creativity (political, cultural, economic, and scientific stagnation)
- loss of foresight (inability to see connections, think holistically across systems)
- psychological suffering (widespread agitation, depression, despair, precariousness, self-harm, and mental health crisis)
- impaired activities of daily living (inability to change behaviors necessary to alleviating widespread suffering, falling lifespans)
- social disinhibition and self-centered attention to individual needs (inability to be a functional member of the global community and pursue collective goals, political corruption, transactional relationships, viewing people as commodities, commitment to austerity and callousness toward suffering)

Great Again), the public is also mobilizing in life-affirming ways that go beyond xenophobia and tribalism.[63]

As exemplified by Occupy Wall Street and the rising popular mobilizations of our time, regular people are pushing back, defining our *real* enemies and calling for public officials to rein in the zombie economy raised by neoliberalism and bring about a more fair and inclusive political-economic system capable of caring for populations humanely, dealing with rising public health and ecological threats, and achieving a minimum set of guarantees for all citizens (for example, healthcare, education, jobs, housing, and retirement security) that allow for human flourishing. The storming of Zuccotti Park was not just about punishing the big banks; it was a primal scream for a world with better politics, better values, and a sense of solidarity with others—in short, a healthier society.

There has been much cultural turbulence as we seek out a new path forward, and our age has been marked by justified anger and contempt at "establishment" political and media institutions, which are serving extreme wealth and corporate power but no longer working for normal citizens. Across the world, people have increasingly sought solutions outside the political establishment, with the election of Trump in the United States, the Brexit vote in the UK, and the *gilets jaune* movement in France serving as symbols of an era of working-class discontentment, resentment, and anger over the failed neoliberal policies that have reordered the global economy since the seventies and worsened material conditions for the working class.

Yet another major life-affirming expression of this global mood has been a renewed embrace of *social democracy*, the venerable post–World War II economic project that broadly supports government's role in putting the beast of capitalism back on a tight leash and enacting policies that promote fairness, justice, and solidarity within the framework of a sustainable capitalist economy. While the dominance of neoliberalism has led to a collective amnesia about social democracy in the United States, the model is once again ascendant in the Western world. Understanding this countervailing force to free-market capitalism is essential to our vision for healthier brain aging and—while not a panacea—is a necessary step in beginning to correct the collective dementia that has afflicted America and spread elsewhere in the Western world via globalization.

SOCIAL DEMOCRACY: 21ST-CENTURY REVENANT

Rather than wholly embracing the extreme neoliberal ideals of unfettered free markets fueled by competition and profit or the oppositional Marxist vision of workers overthrowing capitalism and "seizing the means of production," proponents of social democracy hold that democratically elected governments ought to act to maintain high levels of wealth distribution and income equality in ways that foster greater shared prosperity. This means using progressive taxation to provide basic services as universal civil rights (health care, housing, child/elder care, education, social security, and so forth) to create the conditions for more humane and egalitarian outcomes for all citizens and to reduce hierarchies. As Albert Einstein observed, "The real purpose of [democratic] socialism is precisely to overcome and advance beyond the predatory phase of human development."[64]

Indeed, the basis of social democracy is that people living in wealthy modern countries should not have to endure lives defined by the unholy trinity of *disparity, austerity,* and *precarity*—that different choices by our political "representatives" aligned with popular will (rather than the will of the 1%) can deliver a healthier and more egalitarian world with less needless suffering and cruelty. Whereas hyper-capitalism prizes independence, self-interest, and free markets, social democracy balances individual and collective interests while valuing empathy, fairness, and inclusive prosperity. Accountable government is regarded as an instrument in bettering the lives of citizens and ensuring that peoples' basic needs are met and that our fates do not psychotically hinge on the vagaries of the market. Senator Bernie Sanders, a leading modern proponent of democratic socialism, has said that, to him, social democracy means "having, in a civilized society, the understanding that we can make sure that all of our people live in security and in dignity."[65] Similarly, representative Alexandria Ocasio-Cortez told an audience on the television show *The View* in 2018 that her definition of social democracy is simply: "In a moral and modern America, no person should be too poor to live."[66]

As mentioned, this governing approach is often associated with the economist John Maynard Keynes and was the economic philosophy adopted by many Western countries in the 1930s and '40s. In *Capital in the Twenty First Century*, economist Thomas Piketty argues that the collapse of the rabidly unrestrained markets of the Gilded Age into the wreckage of the Great Depression and chaos of the two world wars imposed uniquely devastating social conditions in the mid-20th century, creating an unprecedented crisis of capitalism not unfamiliar to our current day.[67] Threat of a full-scale revolution hung over modern industrial countries, and populist political movements demanded widespread reforms from society's elite. Western countries in turn embraced Keynesian social democratic policies to tackle mass unemployment, highly regulate capitalism, and quell restive populations. In doing so, an "armistice" was forged that effectively suppressed class conflict between the 99% and 1%. As acknowledged by Franklin Delano Roosevelt, who ushered forward the New Deal in the United States, social democracy was a necessary antidote *to protect capitalism from itself*: "I want to save our system, the capitalistic system," said FDR. "I want to equalize the distribution of wealth."[68]

To rebalance "demented" societies in disarray, Western nations of the mid-20th century politically reordered their economies around progressive taxation, high public expenditure to support full employment and high wages, business regulation, and robust welfare states and social programs (education, healthcare, social security, and so forth). These aggressive policies—enacted by politicians across the political spectrum—helped heal war-torn populations, producing nearly full (white male) employment, greater income equality, the highest sustained growth period in history, and a robust middle class in the United States and Western Europe that many still look back on with nostalgia.[69] After World War II, the economy grew 4% per year, with the poor and middle classes gaining more than the rich, and disposable income increasing by 15% in real terms.[70]

Through the Eisenhower administration, the United States would maintain the world's most progressive tax code, with the top marginal tax rate at 91%, the corporate tax rate above 50%, and high levels of social spending.[71] Even as late as 1971, before the neoliberal turn, Republican president Richard Nixon would assert: "I am now a Keynesian in economics."[72] The wave of democratic socialism during this decades-long bipartisan consensus also led to major gains in public housing, health care, and work conditions (paid holidays, vacations, pensions, and so forth), as well as improving other social determinants of health that enhanced overall population well-being and materially benefited brain health.[73] Unlike the frothing deranged beast of unfettered capitalism that would belch out an age of record inequality in the late 20th and early 21st centuries, mid-century social democracy ushered in what economists Claudia Goldin and Robert Margo have called "The Great Compression" of inequality,[74] a more egalitarian balancing of social forces contributing to healthier societies. Keynes, for his contributions, was honored in 1965 as *TIME* magazine's "Man of the Year." Still today, many of our most popular public programs remain socialist in nature: Medicaid/Medicare, social security, K–12 public education, police and fire departments, the interstate system, national parks, and so on.

SOCIAL DEMOCRACY TODAY

Neoliberalism has wholly transformed the United States and other Western countries, leading to an era defined by historic levels of wealth and income inequality, surpassing the Gilded Age. Meanwhile, social democracies continue to thrive in Scandinavian countries like Norway, Sweden, Finland, Iceland, and Denmark, which also happen to consistently rank not only among the "happiest" countries in the world (all appeared in the *World Happiness Report's* top 10 in 2019)[75,76] but are also annually recognized by *Forbes* as the "best countries for business."[77] Driven largely by organized workers movements that protect the broader population from exploitation, these nations have found ways to sustain a social contract that supports commerce while harnessing collective wealth to foster better lives for everyone—free universities, free day care, universal health care, low poverty rates and homelessness, greater voter participation, a robust safety net, and so on.[78] The success of diverse social democracies in Scandinavia, which rely on a combination of high taxation, high social spending, and strong unions, is particularly potent because it reveals that capitalism and free markets are neither natural truths nor inevitable, and that there are living, breathing, sound-minded alternatives that are entirely feasible.[79]

Even so, the dominance of hyper-capitalist logic has spun stigma around the very word *socialism*, often inappropriately conflating it with the more totalizing, repressive, and dreary political system of authoritarian communism. Such tactics have long been in the arsenal of market fundamentalists. As Harry Truman observed in 1952: " 'Socialism' is a scare word they've hurled at every advance the people have made. Socialism is what they called public power, social security, deposit insurance, and independent labor organizations. Socialism is their name for anything that helps all people."[80]

As a political-economic formation, social democracy, in existing between the poles of free-market fundamentalism and communism, tolerates some degree of inequality in the market and protects individual liberty while preventing extreme concentrations of wealth and equalizing opportunities for people to lead healthy and dignified lives.[81] In recent years, fear-mongering efforts to conflate a desire for social democratic policies like universal health care with the gulags, purges, and show trials of authoritarian Stalinist Russia have been revealed as folly.

Just as FDR realized in the wake of the Great Depression, people in our era—defined by a similar crisis point of capitalism—are increasingly coming to view a reembrace of social democratic principles as a form of compromise necessary to save the capitalist beast from eating itself. As Nobel Prize–winning economist Joseph Stiglitz has written, "The neoliberal fantasy that unfettered markets will deliver prosperity to everyone should be put to rest."[82] Even more directly, Senator Sanders has written that the legitimation story of market fundamentalism has simply lost its explanatory power: "From an economic perspective, from a moral perspective and from a philosophical perspective, the ideology of Milton Friedman is dead wrong."[83]

Since the Great Recession, there has been a groundswell in the United States to embrace some form of social democratic policies as a counterbalance to the excesses of our current neoliberal economic order and the grave disparities in wealth produced by the zombie economy. For instance, Bernie Sanders' political ascendency last decade was built on a popular agenda offering basic social democratic policies, like progressive taxation, a living wage, free public university tuition, and Medicare for All, that would simply bring America up to par with standards in other Western countries. Minds are changing fast. In 2019, 43% of Americans (and 57% of respondents of color) said socialism would be a good thing for the country.[84] Millennials—whose pay, employment, and home ownership prospects were hit hardest by the Great Recession—increasingly harbor more favorable views of socialism than capitalism.[85,86] The anger and indignation unleashed by Wall Street and channeled by Occupy, as well as politicians like Sanders and other upstart citizen groups are permeating the culture and gradually weakening the pallid but firm death grip the zombie economy has had on our collective imagination. A new political-economic reordering and an era of regeneration and revitalization finally feels possible.

WHAT DOES THIS HAVE TO DO WITH BRAIN HEALTH AND ALZHEIMER'S?

The Innovation Fantasies of Neoliberalism

Diseases are always embedded in particular historical milieus, and thus our understanding of them is forged by the dominant political, economic, social, and technological forces present within a culture at a given time. So too are our bodies and brains materially affected by the dominant political-economic organization that characterizes particular historical junctures. Alzheimer's disease—now regarded as the most common global cause of *dementia* (defined as a syndrome of impaired cognition, usually involving memory as well other thinking abilities)—was "discovered" in the early 1900s but lay mostly dormant as a clinical diagnosis for decades, only to reemerge in a different form as a prominent global "epidemic" in the mid-1970s over the *precise* timespan that neoliberalism has become internationally dominant.

As such, our cultural story of Alzheimer's, now said to affect nearly 50 million people globally, has been powerfully "produced" by the hypercapitalist order and organized around two fundamental beliefs:

1. The "holy trinity" of science, biotechnology, and free markets will yield a "fix" for Alzheimer's.
2. In the absence of a "fix," we can prevent the disease through enlightened rituals of individual consumption, self-help, and self-care.

Despite billions of dollars spent, neither neoliberal "innovation fantasy" has come to fruition, and tens of millions of people and their caregivers still cope with age-related cognitive impairment and the social stigma associated with Alzheimer's. For those of us who have worked in the field for decades, it's clear who *isn't* suffering—namely, big pharma, diagnostic companies, segments of the stock market, researchers, clinicians, consultants, fee-for-service health systems, advocacy organization executives, and sundry hucksters who have benefited from the current neoliberal, market-based approach to Alzheimer's.

While this reductive, consumerist milieu has enriched a multibillion-dollar, fear-driven industry, it has narrowed our imaginative thinking about how to rise to the collective challenge of brain aging. As we have fixated on the molecular "black box" of the disease, anticipating that biotechnology and free markets will deliver us from the crisis of Alzheimer's via a cure and narrowly defining prevention and brain health as a matter of individual consumption in markets (eating blueberries, taking supplements, doing crossword puzzles, playing brain-training apps, and so on), we have lost sight of the many political-economic, social, and environmental inputs that surround cellular processes, materially affecting our bodies and brains across our lives to engineer shared vulnerability to brain aging. Our fixation on cure and on market-based, consumer-level interventions is an indictment of the neoliberal fetish of individualism and "innovation," and a distraction from the deeper societal power structures that are collectively damaging our brains in this troubled era, particularly among our most vulnerable citizens. Those are the structures that this book—in interrogating the "demented" organization of our unhealthy society—aims to change.

Thinking about Brain Health across Lifespans and at the Societal Level

We are not saying that we cannot act as individuals to address our aging brains, only that this perspective is not enough. Our lifespans are embedded within historical circumstances and socioeconomic/geographic environments that materially alter our exposures to risk and protective factors as we age. As humans, we are delicate, adaptable organisms who respond with great physiologic sensitivity to periods of war and peace, starvation or excess nutrition, access to education, working and living conditions, technical innovations, cultural practices, and healthcare, and our risk for dementia is thus entangled with such micro and macro events engineered by cultural circumstance.

The major political-economic shifts in the mid-20th century associated with the decades-long dominance of social democracy may have lowered lifetime exposure to dementia risk factors and increased protective factors for brain health that are now helping current elders postpone the clinical manifestations of dementia. To fully grasp this historical wisdom—which has only emerged in recent years—and apply it to our own lives, we will need to widen our aperture beyond the individual and think across lifespans, historical eras, political-economic regimes, and populations. The charge of *American Dementia* will be to advance beyond our neoliberal amnesia and "recall" the lessons of the past so as to inspire current and future actions around a basic concept: that we as humans are *interdependent beings* with complex, psychological, social, emotional, spiritual, and ecological lives, and the *political-economic organization of a given historical moment* (that is, the "health of our societies") *will always affect the health of our brains.*

The Three Evils of Society

One of the most damaging effects of our market-fundamentalist understanding of Alzheimer's is that crass individualism and faith in science, biotechnology, and markets have caused the field to almost totally lose sight of what Martin Luther King, in a famous speech at Riverside Church in Manhattan on April 4, 1967, defined as the "Three Evils of Society"—poverty, racism, and war[87]—corrosive forces that not only are still lurking in our zombie economy and afflicting us today but are intimately interwoven with society-level risk factors for brain aging. Far from being a molecular riddle to be solved through technical mastery and market forces, Alzheimer's is a heterogeneous, age-related, multifactorial manifestation of a complex neurologic system in disarray that requires broader and more imaginative thinking about root causes, lifespan risk factors, and *social determinants of health*—in essence the socioeconomically patterned differences in the material conditions in which people are born, grow to adulthood, live, work, and grow old.[88,89]

In trying to adapt to the massive public health challenge of Alzheimer's, we must learn to look less to doctors, drug companies, bench scientists, biomedicine, and biotech companies and more at what we can collectively do to redress the damaging social policies and programs, grossly unequal economic arrangements, and political-corporate malfeasance of the neoliberal era that drive the social determinants of health that affect our bodies and brains. The decisions we make at the level of our shared societal systems matter far more than any we make as individual consumers in the task of self-care. Put simply: *the pursuit of a healthier society is the best tool we have for improving brain health.*

This book aspires to jolt the Alzheimer's field just as the Occupy protestors shook the world from Zuccotti Park in 2011. Our vision is to reorganize our societal approach to brain health around a new narrative—one that shifts a sense of hope from the neoliberal innovation mythology of a market-based panacea and salvation through individual rituals of consumption and self-care and back into the domain of social democracy, public health, prevention, community building, civic action, and protection of our most vulnerable citizens. Here in this realm, we can reckon with the material, spiritual, and, importantly, *cognitive* costs of the "evils of society" and the social determinants of health that they influence to affect brain aging. Such a reckoning will require no less than what Dr. King called a "revolution of values."

Indeed, when we view Alzheimer's through a different lens—not merely as an individuated biomedical disease but rather as a phenomena produced in part by the unjust political-economic structures, values, and priorities of our time—it can empower us to see how neoliberalism is not merely fixing our understanding of Alzheimer's in a limiting way, it is *actively driving* society-level risk factors for brain aging. Just like Wallace's proverbial fishes swimming in water, blissfully unaware, this is happening all around us every day, as the hyper-capitalist order

- transfers wealth upward, deepening poverty, and widening inequality to levels surpassing the Gilded Age;
- cuts protective social services under the guise of "austerity measures";
- intensifies precariousness and competition in workplaces that drive stress, anxiety, self-recrimination, depression, record rates of mental illness, and "diseases of despair" from suicide, alcoholism, and accidental poisonings[90];

- attacks the unions that protect workers and demands unsustainable levels of productivity while stagnating wages below a livable standard and making workplaces more dangerous, competitive, and inhospitable;
- limits access to high-cost resources like healthcare and higher education that are highly protective for our brains;
- strips away environmental and economic regulations that have allowed the poisoning of our soil, water, and air with environmental neurotoxins like lead and mercury, especially in low-income neighborhoods;
- promotes unhealthy foods and drives up rates of chronic disease;
- fuels endless wars abroad that put troops at risk for traumatic brain injuries and posttraumatic stress disorder (PTSD);
- weakens the protective ties and social infrastructures that bind our communities, while estranging people from public and political institutions and from one another, driving widespread loneliness; and
- contributes to a warming of our climate and environmental deregulation that puts our most vulnerable (particularly the elderly and the poor) at risk.

In Foster Wallace's words, the "immediate point of the fish story is that the most obvious, ubiquitous, important realities are often the ones that are the hardest to see and talk about."[91] Over the course of this book, we build a new story about Alzheimer's that shows how these and other hard-to-see "evils" of neoliberalism are materially damaging our bodies and brains in insidious ways, placing us at greater collective risk for neurodegenerative syndromes like Alzheimer's as we age. Far from being an idle concept, *neoliberalism is a public health threat* that is making us sicker[92] and must be regarded—alongside age—as one of our *most prominent risk factors for Alzheimer's.*

How's the water? Well, not so great.

ALZHEIMER'S: A RAPIDLY CHANGING PARADIGM

Last century, philosopher Thomas Kuhn developed a framework for understanding how science changes over time, including our concepts

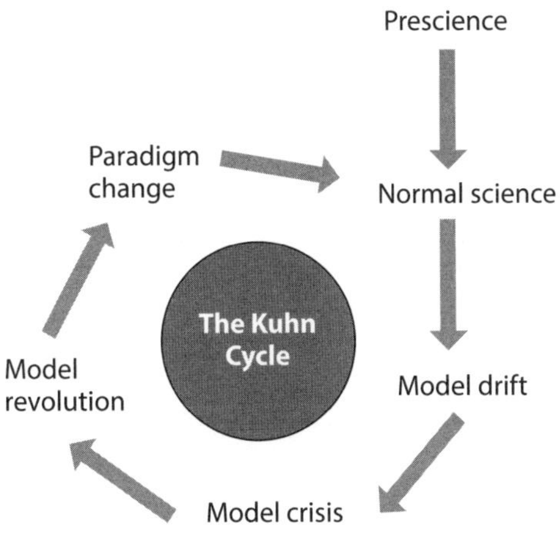

Figure 1.2. Thomas Kuhn's theory of scientific paradigms
Source: Created by Daniel George.

of disease. Kuhn referred to the medical stories that predominate at a particular time as "paradigms."[93] Like everything else, paradigms were subject to change, and Kuhn helped articulate the general social processes through which the organization of scientific-medical knowledge is continually produced. Although Kuhn's model has been oft critiqued for being overly simplistic and in places historically inaccurate, the idea of the importance of dramatic shifts in scientific and cultural understanding has taken hold in the broader culture (figure 1.2).

When we wrote our first book, *The Myth of Alzheimer's*, in 2008, the field was undergoing what Kuhn termed "model drift," when a disease paradigm starts to accumulate anomalies that cannot be solved but which the established order nevertheless tries to defend. A decade later, the field has accumulated such a multitude of anomalies that the concept of Alzheimer's as a singular disease unrelated to aging is no longer tenable. Now, Alzheimer's, not unlike neoliberalism, has entered and is passing through what Kuhn called a period of "model crisis"—a time when the field has drifted so far from its foundational theories that new concepts begin to emerge and compete for legitimacy. We believe we are now beginning to transition into what Kuhn termed "model revolution," a period preceding a full paradigm shift, when people see beyond the cognitive dissonance of their current understanding and begin searching in earnest for new models that better serve the pursuit of truth. This book contributes a new conceptual model for brain health that seeks to drive a field (and society) in crisis away from failed molecular theories promoted by market forces and toward the broader, more life-affirming direction of social democracy, prevention, public health, community support, and greater social equity. Ultimately, improving brain health will require substantial changes in how we are governed, how we care for one another, and the investments we make in one another.

THE JOURNEY AHEAD: FORGING NEW MYTHS, ETHICS, VALUES, AND ACTIONS

Human beings cannot live without stories—they are the universal cognitive vessels that shape our meanings, beliefs, values, and actions, giving our lives shared direction. As the late anthropologist Clifford Geertz wrote, culture is "made up of the stories we tell ourselves about ourselves."[94]

Within a society, then, the emergence of new stories and myths are essential to reorganizing human meanings, inverting existing values and norms, and providing a framework for active resistance.[95] Occupy Wall Street was launched in part by a simple viral story born of material circumstance that interrogated the class antagonism between the 99% and the 1%. In doing so, it helped introduce a new populist mythos into our era, mobilizing people across the world and infusing a moral vernacular of egalitarianism, working-class solidarity, and social and economic justice that remain potent animating ideas. Similarly, a new story connecting brain health to the broader health of our society and structures of power can unleash new meanings, values, and actions that bind us; help us think across generations with greater ethical, intellectual, empathic, and artistic force; and organize actions against shared risk factors in our society that sustain us into the future and bring greater richness, dignity, and compassion into our care for the socially vulnerable, including the cognitively frail. Ultimately, our current reductive story of Alzheimer's is a fiction that exists only because we agree it does. As Kuhn showed us, it can and eventually will be something different.

Why We Must Resist Alzheimer's

In telling a new story about Alzheimer's and brain health, we have carefully chosen to use the word *resisting* throughout the book. Within our current political landscape, the notion of collectively resisting has gained traction by capturing a general mood toward the neoliberal establishment. After decades of mass layoffs, declining living standards, depressed wages, widening income and wealth inequality, endless precarity, destructive wars, rising debt, and environmental degradation at the hands of the hyper-capitalist project, many people are feeling the need to resist and build a political-economic system that works for the people. And while #Resistance emerged in 2017 as a somewhat superficial slogan in opposition to the Trump administration, in a less partisan sense, it can serve as a unifying rallying cry for a more serious and clear-eyed search for ways to address the political, social, and economic causes of human suffering, including dementia, which both political parties have been complicit in. We include a section in many chapters with the heading "How We Can Resist" to guide specific thoughts and actions for healthier brains and societies.

But there is also a scientific rationale for embracing the concept of resistance. As scientists and humanists, we believe the language we use in framing both the scope of our medical problems and our ability to intervene in "fixing" them is critical. For decades, the dominant neoliberal story about the disease has implied that, if given enough time and investment, the trinity of science, biotechnology, and markets will produce a cure that will "end," "halt," "reverse," "conquer," or "arrest" the disease, full stop. Yet, these war-mongering tropes, expertly used by politicians, Alzheimer's advocates, and industry insiders to drive continuous public and private investment in the field, has propagated the dangerously misleading myths about the disease that belie scientific realities of Alzheimer's—a syndrome deeply entangled with normal brain aging that will not likely be amenable to an absolute cure. The late writer Ursula Le Guin once observed:

> A lot of people are getting tired of the huge pool of metaphors that have to do with war and conflict [and] the proliferation of battle metaphors, such as being a warrior, righting, defeating, and so on . . . [O]nce you become conscious of these battle metaphors, you can start "fighting" against them. That's one option. Another is to realize that conflict is not the only human response to a situation and to begin to find other metaphors, such as resisting, outwitting, skipping, or subverting. This kind of consciousness can open the door to all sorts of new behavior.[96]

We believe that by replacing the vernacular of "total war against Alzheimer's" with the notion of *resisting* our most dreaded disease at the level of political-economic organization and public health, we are putting into place the conceptual foundation of a new story that grounds our expectations, behaviors, and hopes in a more honest, accurate, and humane manner while pointing to real solutions. In abandoning current notions that we are at biotechnological "war" against a few molecular antagonists within individuals that "cause" Alzheimer's, we can broaden our focus to more fundamentally understand how brain-aging processes unfold within the context of all our lifespans and learn to see not only the intricate multisystemic, political-economic, social, and environmental interactions that affect cognitive health but also important opportunities to connect with, support, and build solidarity with those most at risk as well as those experiencing progressive cognitive decline. We resonate with our colleague Margaret Lock, author of *The Alzheimer Conundrum,* that focusing on "lifestyle, toxins, poverty, and community support . . . is likely to reduce the prevalence of dementia worldwide to a much greater extent than would an approach confined to expensive micro-medical management."[97]

While not as profitable as drug development, social policies, public health initiatives, and personal- and community-level actions that will, over time, materially succeed in reducing vascular risk factors, oxidative stress, and inflammation; protecting people en masse from traumatic brain injuries; promoting social engagement and lifelong learning; reducing exposure to neurotoxins; and providing care, purpose, and engagement for those with memory loss represent our most powerful resistance to Alzheimer's. Indeed, *resisting* is an appropriately aggressive way of framing the challenge ahead of us, and it also contains a valuable leaven of humility. In contrast to the grandiose innovation fantasies of neoliberalism, it connotes that while we cannot fully "cure" Alzheimer's, we *can* attempt to delay, disrupt, postpone, and become more resilient through our efforts as individuals and, more importantly, as a society.

No less strong is our belief that the severe *stigma* around Alzheimer's must also be resisted. One thrust of our work over the years has involved challenging the dominant language and metaphors borne of the market-oriented shaping of the field since the seventies, which have increasingly pitied people with dementia as "lost selves" and reduced them to little more than an economically unproductive surplus of "zombies" who "burden" the culture with rising costs. In contrast to the military and horror tropes that overwhelmingly guide our understanding of Alzheimer's in the neoliberal era, we are proponents of the person-centered care movement and more humanizing concepts like age- and dementia-friendly communities, which point us toward a more compassionate and solidaristic embrace of people with cognitive challenges. We have ourselves pushed back by creating intergenerational schools, youth reading programs at nursing homes, medical school courses held in dementia care units, farmers' markets, and other community-based initiatives that provide a blueprint for how to resist stigma, age segregation, and "social death" for the cognitively frail. This will be a critical part of the new story we tell about how we can best pursue brain health via building healthier societies.

BOOK LAYOUT

This book is presented in 10 chapters. In chapters 2–7, we look in depth at the onset of our American dementia—in essence, how neoliberalism has deranged and distorted the Alzheimer's field—and share surprising evidence revealing how social democratic policies of the mid-20th century appear to have had a more dramatic material impact on brain health than any market-based biotech intervention. You will learn

- why Alzheimer's, an obscure illness until its rise to international prominence in the 1970s, is the hallmark disease of neoliberalism, shaped by its internal logic and contradictions;
- how the current paradigm of Alzheimer's has been unable to overcome certain "inconvenient truths" that confound a cure, and how a new paradigm focused on prevention, public health, and enlightened collectivism is emerging;
- how the crass individualism fostered by many of our billion-dollar "marketplace of memory" products (that is, brain-training games, supplements, nutraceuticals) has warped our thinking about prevention;

- how soaring inequalities of our era are damaging to our brains;
- why there is a strong evidence-based argument that social democratic policies, including single-payer healthcare, a living wage, and universal access to free higher education and technical training programs, will build collective resilience to dementia, and how we must fight for them;
- why Flint, Michigan, holds some of the most powerful and painful lessons about hyper-capitalism, austerity, and Alzheimer's but also contains a hopeful blueprint for how we can act to resist dementia at the population level and across generations;
- the many ways in which poverty, disadvantage, loneliness, lack of sleep, and stressful life events tied to material inequities of our neoliberal era shape the brain and affect risk for Alzheimer's; and
- ways in which climate change has become a major risk factor for dementia and an existential threat to our most vulnerable citizens.

In chapters 8–10, we take on the ageist tendencies in our culture that disadvantage both vulnerable youth and elders, promoting strategies for resistance that show how local communities can rise above the atomization and alienation of our era and rally around the moral challenge of caring for our struggling neighbors, including the cognitively frail. You will learn

- how nursing homes are being reinvented around an ethos of care and mutual support rather than just profit, and how all of us can "occupy" and reinvigorate these formerly moribund spaces by contributing our talents, passions, and interests;
- how "socialceuticals" and other elder care interventions informed by the arts are proving far more effective than pharmaceuticals in helping persons with dementia and their caregivers;
- why the emerging age- and dementia-friendly community movements are providing a framework for better caring for people old and young; and
- how people with Alzheimer's diagnoses are staying actively engaged by mentoring and learning alongside elementary schoolchildren in inner-city schools.

CONCLUSION

In 1968, with civil rights protests bracing the country, Martin Luther King Jr. observed that such actions represented "the language of the unheard," a phrase that again powerfully resurfaced in the national Black Lives Matter protests in 2020. So too was this dynamic at play when Occupy protestors massed in Wall Street four decades after King's death, calling into question a corrupt government that painstakingly shored up its financial institutions in the midst of crisis while largely ignoring the declining lives of its citizens. While the tents are long gone from Zuccotti Park, the "language of the unheard" that the protests unleashed has not only become part of our shared vernacular ("We are the 99%") but also galvanized a wave of civic energy. As Eric Blanc, a journalist who has covered the aforementioned teachers strike movement has told us, "We are witnessing the biggest strike wave in forty years. We are starting to fight back."

The ideas, energies, and actions unleashed by the movement are transforming our culture and can even serve as tools to help us think about how best to pursue brain health in an era of soaring inequality, austerity, melting icecaps, pandemics, and lead-poisoned water. After all, as George Orwell famously wrote, "all issues are political issues," and that encompasses health as well. Ultimately, the story of brain health is a story about rebalancing political-economic organization and structural power to better serve population health.

This book is based on the simple but powerful premise that a healthier society built on social democratic principles, guaranteeing the basic material and environmental security and dignity of every human being at every age, will also be protective of our brains. While markets are unlikely to produce an absolute cure or prevention for Alzheimer's, you will see how the political-economic choices we make as a society—particularly those that serve all citizens more equitably than markets—affect the material substrate of our brains and thus our resilience to dementia. In this moment of crisis, we can collectively evolve away from neoliberalism and its zombified economy and in the direction of more humane values and actions that lead to greater collective wealth, freedom, and security.

In the chapters to come, we examine how Alzheimer's disease has been constructed within the arc of hyper-capitalism. As we move through the book, it will become increasingly clear that the struggle against Alzheimer's and for brain health is, at its core, a "fight" for one another and for a healthier society.

2

Alzheimer's and the Neoliberal Turn

"Politics of Anguish," Visions of a Cure

As historians of science like Thomas Kuhn have taught us, conceptions of disease are not sacrosanct. What we conceive of as "diseases" are the products of the society in which they emerge—not merely an outgrowth of the science of the day but constructs forged by particular historical and political-economic circumstances and the dominant technologies, institutions, ideologies, and beliefs of an era. Over the last 100 years, Alzheimer's has been reborn several times as a concept due to changing circumstances, and each time these factors have played a key role in the evolution of the paradigm.

In the next two chapters, we explore how the story of Alzheimer's has unfolded and why our current medicalized, individuated, market-based conception—a paradigm forged in the fires of the dramatic political-economic neoliberal reordering of society since the 1970s (that is, the onset of our American dementia)—has been so limited in its scope while driving a billion-dollar drug development enterprise. We delve deeper into why certain "inconvenient truths" make a cure for Alzheimer's an extraordinarily difficult proposition, and explore how the zombie economy of hyper-capitalism has spawned a problematic *marketplace of memory*, which has rapidly expanded beyond the realm of drugs. Putting together a coherent history of Alzheimer's in its many phases of development is critical to envisioning a better future for brain health. Let's start at the very beginning.

THE CONCEPTUAL BIRTH AND REBIRTH OF DEMENTIA AND ALZHEIMER'S

Origins of Dementia

Dementia is today conceived as a syndrome of impaired cognition, usually involving memory as well as other thinking abilities, that develops in previously intellectually intact people, most often later in life. While symptoms of dementia have been noted in the written records of human communities for thousands of years, dating back to the medical papyrus scrolls of the ancient Egyptians circa 1550 BC, the formal diagnostic label (which literally means "out of mind" in Latin) was invented in the mid-1800s, with the prototype being *dementia paralytica* due to the progression of syphilis, an infection that can cause dementia when it reaches the brains of those affected in its tertiary stage.

Diagnostic and treatment approaches for dementia were limited in 19th-century medicine, and techniques to microscopically examine the brain had not yet been developed. Theories of causation varied but included paradigmatically dominant ideas that morally dissolute behaviors, such as excessive drinking or sexual lasciviousness, played a causative role in dementing illness. In the latter part of the 19th century, a major technological advancement in describing clinical conditions and examining brain tissue at the microscopic level allowed scientists to develop more nuanced categorizations of different types of dementia and thereby banish these spurious theories of "moral causation." These changing circumstances laid the foundations for our current paradigms of Alzheimer's.

Alois Alzheimer Meets Auguste D.

During this period, Alois Alzheimer, a psychiatrist from Marktbreit, Germany, received his formative scientific and clinical training in Frankfurt. There, he came under the mentorship of Emil Kraepelin, the foremost psychiatrist in Europe and a man professionally committed to establishing a scientific basis for major psychiatric conditions, including age-related dementias. Alzheimer was later invited to work in Kraepelin's clinic in Munich, where he achieved some renown both as a clinician who developed innovative uses of therapeutic baths for patients and as a talented histologist who pioneered the then-new technique of photomicroscopy.

Beginning in 1901, while in Frankfurt, Alzheimer spent five years closely tracking the case of one particular patient, a German housewife

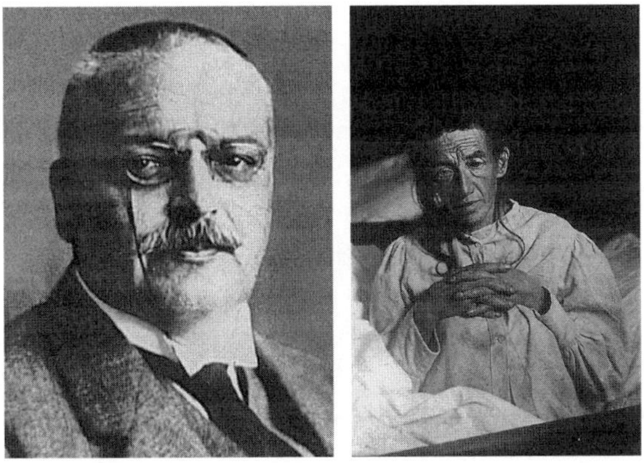

Figure 2.1. Dr. Alzheimer and his patient Auguste D.
Source: Public domain images from "Alois Alzheimer," Wikipedia, last updated May 20, 2020, https://en.wikipedia.org/wiki/Alois_Alzheimer; and "Auguste Deter," Wikipedia, last updated May 9, 2020, https://en.wikipedia.org/wiki/Auguste_Deter.

named Auguste Deter (Auguste D.) who experienced a precipitous decline into dementia in her early fifties. Because of Auguste D.'s relative youth, Alzheimer was captivated by her case and kept meticulous notes of all their interactions, as well as handwriting samples (figure 2.1).

Upon Auguste D.'s passing in 1906 from sepsis associated with a bedsore, Alzheimer, who was a pioneer in using cell stains, microscopes, and photography to study the structure of tissue, used a recently developed staining technique to discover numerous neuritic plaques with a core of *amyloid* along with neurofibrillary tangles inside neurons and a loss of cells in various regions of her brain (figure 2.2).[1] Amyloid, which is derived from the Greek word *amylon*, meaning "starch," was first described and named by Rudolph Virchow, another 19th-century German pioneer of modern medicine and a fascinating figure in the story of Alzheimer's disease in his own right. Because of the technological limitations of his day, Virchow erred in arguing that amyloid was a type of starch, and later discoveries would show it to be composed of various proteins, including the beta-amyloid family.

Despite Virchow's understandable mischaracterization, his contributions to medicine, politics, and public health were formidable. In addition to being a foundational figure in biological medicine who helped develop theories of disease based on cellular approaches, he was also a leader in the advocacy movement for modern water and sewage systems, which

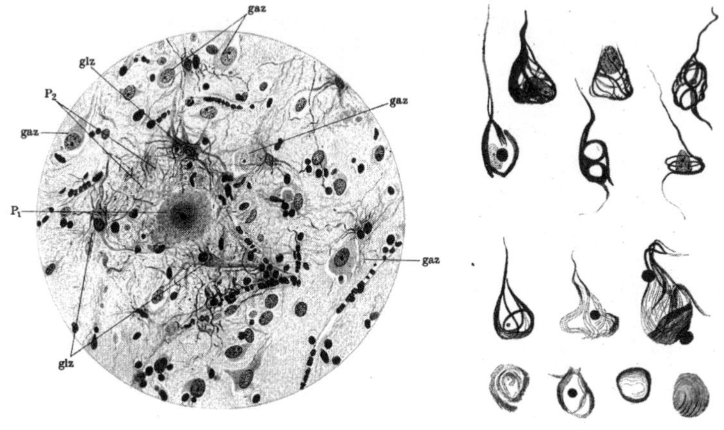

Figure 2.2. Illustrations of the original plaques and tangles from Alzheimer's 1911 article describing the cases of Auguste D. and Johann F.
Source: Alois Alzheimer, "Über eigenartige Krankheitsfälle des späteren Alters," *Zeitschrift für die gesamte Neurologie und Psychiatrie* 4 (December 1911): 356–85.

would substantially reduce the spread of death and disease over the 20th century. Also an anthropologist, Virchow helped found the field of social medicine, which is predicated on the aforementioned understanding that disease is never purely biological but is powerfully influenced by social, cultural, and political-economic factors. Arguing that many diseases resulted from the "unequal distribution of civilization's advantages," Virchow called for public provision of medical care for the poor, promoted universal education, worked to outlaw child labor, developed hygiene standards for schools and public buildings, and improved food inspection. One of his most famous aphorisms—"Do we not always find the diseases of the populace traceable to defects in society?"—remains as true a critique of our current unhealthy society as it was when Virchow and Alzheimer practiced in the late 19th century.[2] After a prolific career, Virchow passed away in Berlin in 1902, just as Alzheimer was first beginning to document the case of Auguste D.

Just a few years later, after Auguste D.'s passing in 1906 and Alzheimer's examination of her brain pathology, he was confounded by the question of whether his patient's "peculiar" case in her early fifties had represented a condition that could be distinguished from "senile dementia," a form of cognitive decline that afflicted people later in their lifespan. Since Auguste D.'s range of behavioral symptoms and pathological features were also observed in a great number of older persons in their seventies and eighties who were diagnosed with senile dementia, Alzheimer was apprehensive about formally classifying her condition as a separate specific disease process outside the spectrum of processes that occurred later in life, including "normal" and pathological changes.[3]

Quite revealingly, the second young-onset case study recorded by Alzheimer involved a 56-year-old laborer from Munich named Johann F., who suffered a similar range of clinical symptoms as Auguste D. but showed only plaque-related pathology and no tangles.[4] So it took just *two cases* for Alzheimer to encounter a significant pathological variation in these young-onset patients, a theme that still complicates drug development efforts today. Alzheimer (and even Kraepelin) retained ambivalence about establishing the nebulous condition he had observed in Auguste D. and others as a medically discrete disease. The rapidity of the progression of young-onset cases, the pattern and severity of cognitive symptoms (for example, language impairment), and the frequent presence of major behavioral features (such as psychosis), suggested some differences in the phenomenology of presenile and senile cases, but was it enough to categorically differentiate the younger manifestation as its own disease? To that question, Alzheimer concluded: "There is no tenable reason to consider these cases as caused by a specific disease process. They are senile psychoses, atypical forms of senile dementia. Nevertheless, they do assume a certain separate position so that one has to know of their existence."[5]

Alzheimer's Becomes a Disease

Despite this ambivalence, the preeminent Kraepelin used the term *Alzheimer's disease* for the first time in the 1910 edition of his influential textbook *Psychiatry*.[6] Medical historians believe Alzheimer might have assented to publishing this concept before some of these issues concerning the relationship to aging were clarified because he and Kraepelin were competing with other schools of brain psychiatry—including Arnold Pick's lab in Prague and Sigmund Freud's school of psychotherapy—to determine who would lead in describing specific types of brain diseases and their causes. Just as in our contemporary scientific landscape, the researchers who struck first in understanding age-related dementias could position themselves to capture scarce scientific resources and dominant professional status. Kraepelin's aggressive medicalization of the phenomena observed by Alzheimer was as much tactical within the political economy and dominant societal institutions of early 20th-century Germany as it was scientific.

Over a century later, we now know that many young-onset cases are due to rare mutations in three genes (amyloid precursor protein, presenilin 1, and presenilin 2) that alter amyloid processing and result in the clinical presentation of dementia usually before age 65. In essence, these are *autosomal dominant* genes, which will *cause* the illness when only one gene is present and inherited from one of two parents, hence creating a 50/50 risk of passing it on. Ironically, modern analysis of the original tissue taken from Auguste D.'s microscopic slides demonstrated that she might have possessed such a mutation,[7] although this finding has recently been disputed.[8]

After the initial description of Alzheimer's disease in 1910, the diagnosis was rarely used by medical professionals. Alzheimer passed away in 1915, and scientific inquiry into the condition linked to his surname tapered off as World War I diverted manpower and resources from basic laboratory work.[9] The presumption of those living and writing during the first half of a 20th century marked by world wars and the Great Depression was that the *Alzheimer's disease* terminology simply referred to cases such as Auguste D.'s and Johann F.'s, which featured younger onset of symptoms, even though these cases were arguably not fundamentally different from senile dementia.[10] The term *presenile dementia* was used in patients under the age of 65, an arbitrary threshold picked in part because that was the age of eligibility for the German version of social security in existence at that time. A new paradigm of Alzheimer's disease had asserted itself but quickly receded into obscurity.

The Longevity Revolution: Extending the Lifespan across the 20th Century

While the diagnosis of Alzheimer's disease was reserved for rare presenile patients like Auguste D. through much of the 20th century in the United States and elsewhere, shifting social and political-economic tides were creating the conditions for the reemergence of the label as more than just an obscure classification of younger onset dementia. Specifically, as the decades unfolded after Alzheimer's death, people living in

Western industrialized nations like the United States began experiencing a *longevity revolution* that dramatically extended the average lifespan. When Alzheimer died in 1915 in his early fifties, this was consistent with the average age of mortality of people during his era. In less than a century, however, Western industrialized countries would push the average life expectancy up by nearly two decades, into the mid- to late seventies.

Scholars who have studied the phenomenon commonly identify several areas of major impact, all of which contributed, in sum, to healthier societies and longer lives:

- One clear contribution was the near universal uptake of *germ theory*—the concept promoted by Virchow and other scientists that microbes caused disease—into the state public health apparatus of industrialized nations. Such transformational knowledge enabled widespread standardized adoption of more sanitary practices (boiling water, sterilization of medical instruments, and so on) that protected people from disease and infection and, in particular, helped increase survival of infants.[11,12]
- Another clear impact was made via *public health infrastructure* (for example, improved sewage, water, sanitation systems, and sanitary reforms), established by modern states (again at the urging of advocates like Virchow), which saved and improved the quality of countless 20th-century lives.[13,14]
- Still others point to the *economic growth linked to social democratic policies* that more evenly distributed wealth and resources throughout societies in crisis after the Great Depression and two world wars, establishing robust welfare states and other collective investments that promoted the lifespan well-being of whole populations, including the most vulnerable.[15,16,17] Programs such as workers' compensation, national health care systems, social security, unemployment protections, universal education, environmental agencies, nutrition programs, housing, and other planks of the Keynesian welfare state that emerged across the Western world as part of the postwar social democratic consensus produced a societal undergirding that supported millions of citizens in industrialized countries in living longer, healthier lives. Further, trade unions helped bring about improved working conditions (for example, five-day work weeks,

eight-hour workdays), better wages, and child labor protections, which also substantially improved peoples' quality of life.

- Other scholars have identified more specific *environmental factors* like the gradual eradication of lead from gasoline, paint, and drinking water as having a major influence on longevity—a crucial argument that we return to in chapter 5, when we visit Flint, Michigan.[18,19,20]
- Of course, *medical technologies* also made a significant contribution to improving 20th-century health. The development and mass production of drugs such as penicillin (used in medical practice) and vaccinations (distributed through populations via public health immunization campaigns) reduced deaths from infections and virtually eliminated illnesses like polio, typhoid, diphtheria, and smallpox in developed countries.[21] Around the mid-20th century, biomedical innovations such as dialysis machines, the mass commercialization of insulin, and advanced surgical procedures such as transplants further extended the lives of those who would have hitherto perished.[22] Epidemiological research also began uncovering some of the causes of major chronic diseases, such as lung cancer (smoking) and heart disease (diet), and allowed resources to be mobilized to act on modifiable risk factors at the population level.

Across the 20th century, the confluence of these social, political-economic, scientific, and technological forces acted on social determinants of health *across whole societies* to dramatically transform population health. As Cambridge researcher Carol Brayne told us, these changes were especially powerful "for the generations experiencing in early life, including early adulthood, the collective actions following the Second World War—i.e., stronger health, welfare and education systems." Such societal adaptations have materially transformed life in the 20th and 21st centuries, ostensibly making a dramatic impact on longevity increases.

When the first formal use of the term *Alzheimer's disease* occurred in 1910 in Kraepelin's textbook, during the early stages of many of these societal changes, only 4.3% of the US population was over the age of 65; however, by 1970, that had grown to almost 10%, and numbers are still increasing.[23] As more Americans survived longer, people in turn accrued more neurodegenerative changes in their brains and acquired increased risk for cognitive decline. In the United States, the changing demographics of a graying society intersected quite profoundly with the rise of neoliberalism in Western governments in the pivotal decade of the seventies, forever altering the Alzheimer's paradigm.

THE NEOLIBERAL TURN

Whereas postwar social democratic policies informed by Keynesian macroeconomics had helped extend lifespans and produce high rates of growth in advanced capitalist countries in the fifties and sixties, the stagflation crisis of the seventies opened the door for market-fundamentalist ideas to be implemented by Western governments. Not only did the unleashed free-market-based economy emerging in the seventies promise to pull lagging domestic and global markets out of the quagmire of stagflation, it was also imagined as a period that would give birth to the type of revolutionary technological innovations presaged by 1969's moon landing.[24] In the United States, the convergence of the neoliberal economy with the societal response to population aging proved a watershed moment, resulting in the Alzheimer's disease (AD) paradigm reemerging from the medical wilderness and into the global spotlight—this time, not as a rare and "peculiar" illness afflicting a small number of people like Auguste D. in middle age, but as a widespread scourge that had now entered the crosshairs of science and the free market as a *medicalized* disease potentially amenable to a cure through technological innovation.

"Politics of Anguish" and Visions of a Cure

In 1974, a US Congress forced to confront the country's aging populace passed the Research and Aging Act, bringing into existence the National Institute on Aging (NIA) to provide leadership on age-related issues. Psychiatrist Robert Butler was named the first director of the NIA, and quickly went to work developing a strategy to make aging-related disorders a national priority. As a leader of this fledgling institution, Butler executed several key organizational decisions that profoundly shifted the cultural trajectory of AD.

The first decision concerned Butler's choice to strategically define Alzheimer's as a specific tragic disease that would essentially replace the vaguer and more fatalistic concept of *senility* that had been common parlance across most of the 20th century when referring to the physical and cognitive decrements associated with advanced age. Butler would famously explain his reasoning for making this push in the seventies by saying, "I decided that we had to make [Alzheimer's] a household word. And the reason I felt that, is that's how the pieces get identified as a national priority. And I call it the health politics of anguish."[25]

No longer would Alzheimer's be an obscure reference to rare, discrete cases of young-onset dementia like those of Auguste D. and Johann F.; instead, Butler and NIA colleagues, such as Zaven Khachaturian, in building the capacity of a national organization within an aging country, argued with great vigor and success that the two-word phrase *Alzheimer's disease* should replace what was previously considered *senile* dementia. Increasingly, academic researchers advocated for the expansion of the AD label to people aged 70 and beyond who experienced what had previously been understood as "being senile." Indeed, in 1976, one of Butler's influential colleagues, scientist and advocate Robert Katzman, published an influential editorial in the journal *Archives of Neurology* that collapsed the former classificatory distinctions of the 20th century. As he argued, "Both Alzheimer disease and senile dementia are progressive dementias . . . that are indistinguishable by careful clinical analyses . . . the pathological findings are identical."[26] As academic and advocacy support mobilized around the resurgent medicalized understanding that rare young-onset cases of dominantly inherited familial AD, such as that genetically possessed by Auguste D., could be categorically merged with the late-life cases of sporadic dementia formerly understood as senility, the size and scope of AD swelled—as Butler had intended—into a major public health issue for an aging society (figure 2.3).

In addition to leading the charge to make *Alzheimer's* a broadly applicable household phrase (and thereby a national priority), Butler's other strategic decision was to leverage the emerging economic zeal for technological innovations characteristic of the post–moon landing era and articulate a vision of a cure that might eventually halt or reverse the cognitive decline of older Americans. In executing the dramatic "politics of anguish" strategy, Butler frequently invoked the triumphant eradication of the polio epidemic earlier in the 20th century, arguing that unless effective treatment or prevention was found for dementia, the health care system would be crippled by the coming demographic wave of baby boomers. In

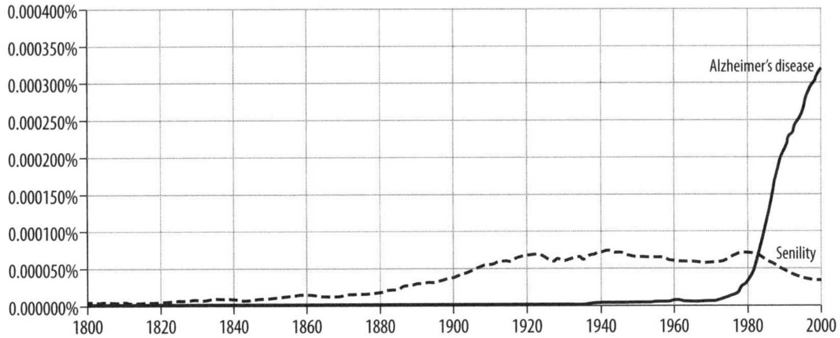

Figure 2.3. A Google Ngram demonstrates the effectiveness of Butler's "politics of anguish" strategy in promoting the nomenclature of *Alzheimer's disease* over *senility*. *Source:* Created by Daniel George and Jesse Ballenger based on Google Ngram data.

congressional testimony in the early eighties, Butler directly conflated the two "disease epidemics" while striking a tone of medical triumphalism: "In 1935, a March of Dimes was started. In 1961, less than 30 years later, the last polio epidemic occurred . . . Senility could fall the way polio did, if we invest now . . . We cannot wait until the first baby boomer turns gray in the year 2011 to declare war on senility."[27]

Whereas Alzheimer had expressed doubt that the cases he observed in the early 1900s were worthy of being considered a specific disease, by the Reagan era, in the eighties, a new cultural narrative was forming. The aging population in the United States could now envision a cure for the condition-formerly-known-as-senility that extrapolated past success against infectious disease into a forward-looking faith in the scientific innovations that would surely arrive with time and market investment in biotechnology. As the famous British psychiatrist Tom Kitwood, a key progenitor of the person-centered care movement in the nineties, argued, the cultural success of Butler's "politics of anguish" strategy—against the backdrop of a society increasingly optimistic about scientific progress—had the gradual effect of creating a new paradigm defined by an "obsessional search for technical fixes."[28]

Indeed, as the upstart Alzheimer's field began reconstituting itself around the search for rational drug targets, a vast national research infrastructure quickly grew. In the eighties, the NIA began establishing multiple Alzheimer's Disease Research Centers (ADRCs) across the country, which allowed public and private resources to flow to the biotechnological study of Alzheimer's. (I, Peter, would train at Johns Hopkins in one of the first ADRCs and years later go on to develop one in Cleveland.) Advocacy organizations arose nationally and internationally to drive funding and attention to the search for a molecular cure. In the United States, the Alzheimer's Association was established in 1979 as the Alzheimer's Disease and Related Disorders Association, composed of a national patchwork of family support groups. From its inception, the organization struggled with a strategic balance between emphasizing care or cure—a quandary that continues to this day and has led to major internal political challenges for the national headquarters and its local chapters.

Nonetheless, its leaders and advocates soon learned that fundraising and lobbying efforts were dramatically more effective when framed around the NIA's articulated vision of a cure, and that's where both the NIA and the Alzheimer's Association began allocating the vast majority of their public and philanthropic money. As one fundraiser was quoted as saying during the early eighties: "The name of the game is 'Alzheimer' . . . you can sell 'Alzheimer.' "[29] In other words, in a society increasingly infatuated with the innovation fantasies of the era, it was easier to drum up funds around the prospect of finding a cure to a specific medicalized disease than to focus on, say, improving care or public health prevention, as someone like Virchow might have advised given the lessons of the 19th century.

Thus, the national Alzheimer's Association became existentially committed to promoting Butler and the NIA's "politics of anguish" and pursuing a roadmap to a cure. In the early eighties, the organization hired a consulting firm to lobby and maximize visibility in Washington, thus increasing its access to representatives and senators. Soon Alzheimer's became a frequent talking point in Congress. So politically effective was this strategy that in 1983, the US House of Representatives proposed a resolution declaring November of that year to be National Alzheimer's Disease Month in the hope that "an increase in the national awareness of the problem of Alzheimer's disease may stimulate the interests and concern of the American people, which may lead, in turn, to increased research and eventually to the discovery of a cure."[30] By 1985, the NIA had established ten ADRCs across the country.

Organizational growth was also occurring globally around this new medicalized story of Alzheimer's. In 1984, Alzheimer's Disease International (ADI), a confederation of national Alzheimer's groups, was founded with encouragement from the World Health Organization to serve the needs of people with dementia and advocate for a research-driven quest for future fixes to the "disease." With a global advocacy infrastructure in place to "fight" Alzheimer's, the pharmaceutical industry was only happy to jump in with capital investment. After all, if AD was, like polio, a discrete medical "disease" that could be defeated, there existed the prospect of profitable cures in a largely untapped and burgeoning drug market, which would only grow as societies around the world aged. Throughout the eighties, AD quickly became a new business frontier, organized around the emerging neoliberal faith in the holy trinity of science, biotechnology, and free markets to eventually produce solutions to medical problems. Such a coupling reflects an age-old dance in capitalism—that science requires investment, and investment requires motivation. As James Watson, the father of DNA, famously observed, "Nothing attracts money like the quest for a cure for a terrible disease."[31]

Of course, paradigmatically framing Alzheimer's as a disease-to-be-cured began a decades-long process of diverting precious societal resources—many billions of public (taxpayers) and private donor dollars—not only away from *prevention* but also from patient and family caregiver education, as well as from psychosocial research and resources aimed at improving the safety, quality of care, support, and quality of life of people living with dementia. So too did important issues like prevention of abuse and neglect of these individuals in the community and long-term care homes, evidence-based person-directed care, and timely support and education for underserved individuals and carers take a back seat to a potential cure.[32] As member of various advisory and fiduciary boards of Alzheimer's organizations, I (Peter) witnessed this imbalance in priorities firsthand. From the eighties onward, psychosocial research was always made handmaiden to clinical inquiry, which, in turn, often gave way to the seductions of molecular, market-based, individual-oriented approaches to cure. While advocacy groups like the Alzheimer's Association have consistently provided resources—(for example, 1:1 care consultations with professionals, 24/7 helpline, online forum, online resources, classes, support groups, in-person support, education, forums, events)—the organization has, over the decades, come under increased scrutiny by disproportionately privileging the search for a cure over these other socially valuable areas.

A Thriving Market Comes of Age: The Political-Economic Milieu of the 1980s

Ronald Reagan's two-term presidency from 1980 to 1988 accelerated the hyper-capitalist reordering of the United States. In opposing Jimmy Carter, who had presided over grinding years of stagflation and early neoliberal reforms, Reagan, under the direct advisement of leading neoliberal economist and White House courtier Milton Friedman (figure 2.4), had campaigned on attacking so-called big government and accelerating market fundamentalism. His victory launched in full a new era committed to dismantling the Keynesian social democratic state, which had put a leash on the free market, and shifting public resources away from welfare programs, including those whose funding was targeted to help the disabled and elderly.[33] Whereas the top tax rate during the massive burgeoning of America's middle class after World War II fluctuated between 74% and 92%, Reagan's Tax Reform Act dropped it to 28%.[34] In the context of an ever-aging culture, this redistribution of resources from state institutions into private hands further shifted the onus of producing a solution to the growing but ostensibly "curable" problem of Alzheimer's disease to the free market, academic research, and the motivated pharmaceutical industry.

During the Reagan years, the proposition that these entities would yield a cure for Alzheimer's ossified into a sort of cultural orthodoxy. As our colleague Jesse Ballenger has written in his brilliant history *Self, Senility, and Alzheimer's Disease*, "I have not found a single instance in congressional hearings during the 1980s and [into] the early 1990s in which a witness or member of Congress questioned the assumption that biomedical science would eventually find a solution to the problem of Alzheimer's disease if it was given enough resources to do so."[35] The political-advocacy infrastructure and emergent forces of neoliberalism had not just pulled AD back from the brink of medical obscurity, they had also set up a new social contract with the American people that the

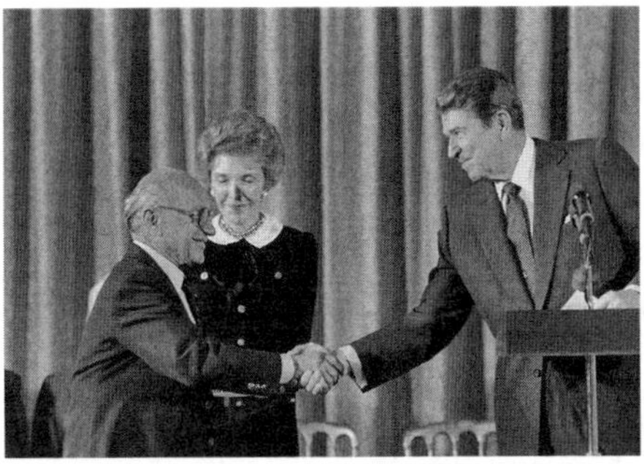

Figure 2.4. Ronald and Nancy Reagan with neoliberal economist Milton Friedman, October 17, 1988.
Source: Reagan Library Archives via Wikimedia Commons, CC BY-SA 4.0.

emerging political-economic order (that is, the unleashed beast of the market economy) would eventually produce a panacea to one of the country's most dreaded diseases.

Bursting Open Markets with Bayh-Dole

Scientific research of the eighties, especially in universities and other public institutions, began refitting itself to meet the needs of industry and global competitiveness in the reordered neoliberal landscape. The Supreme Court decision of *Diamond v. Chakrabarty* in 1980 had enabled the patenting of life and a new understanding of science as *intellectual property*, while in the same year universities were permitted through the 1980 Bayh-Dole Act to become owners of NIH-funded research results. Reflecting the ascendancy of the hyper-capitalist economic order, Bayh-Dole unleashed forces of markets, competition, and profit motive into academic research.[36] Whereas innovations in academia had long been regarded as existing in the public domain,[37] universities sought to gain monetarily from the products of research by creating technology transfer offices and encouraging faculty entrepreneurial behavior in the private sector. Partnerships were formed with biotechnology and large pharmaceutical companies, and some universities made significant financial gains in selling their intellectual property as market commodities. These university-industry collaborations often distorted the scientific enterprise. Secrecy rather than free communication of scientific results emerged, as did mission conflicts between educating students and making money.

Under the spell of the market, conflicts of interest became more problematic for clinicians and scientists. Academics increasingly consulted for industry and even created their own companies, distorting their objective assessments about the likelihood of success for products. The pharmaceutical industry developed the concept of key opinion leaders (KOLs)—experts paid handsomely to provide opinions to guide the search for new medications. After the industry succeeded in developing only minimally effective products for dementia, however, KOLs were used to spread the opinions of the industry, often hyping the value of medications to the advantage of the experts and their client companies but perhaps not to the advantage of patients or payers of health care. And after the initial drugs for Alzheimer's were viewed by most as only marginally successful, experts and companies learned they could nevertheless hype the promise of more powerful future drugs to keep capital flowing—a deception that still goes on today.

Dawn of the Neurotransmitter Drugs (and Madison Avenue's Lukewarm Lasagna)

So what were the underwhelming drugs for dementia that industry began paying KOLs to promote in the landscape created by Bayh-Dole? In the seventies, a drug called l-dopa had been used as a therapy to compensate for dopaminergic cell loss in Parkinson's disease by increasing production of dopamine—a phenomenon depicted in a subgroup of persons who developed Parkinson's disease after a viral epidemic in the major-motion film *Awakenings*. Building on the success of dopaminergic therapies, the Alzheimer's research community wished to find a single neurotransmitter like dopamine that could lead to similar treatment approaches for the emerging Alzheimer's "epidemic."

Early clinical signs suggested that the neurotransmitter acetylcholine might be important since drugs that blocked acetylcholine in animals and humans had been found to cause memory and attention problems. In the early eighties, I (Peter) was the first author on several papers produced by teams of investigators at Johns Hopkins University demonstrating that, in cases of Alzheimer's, the specific cell populations responsible for this loss of acetylcholine were located in an obscure part of the brain located deep under the front parts of the organ called the *nucleus basalis of Meynert*. Various scientists demonstrated that these cells sent their long processes (*axons*) into areas of the brain like the cortex and hippocampus that people had long focused on as being responsible for some of the cognitive impairment in dementia. Yet, it was the loss of the neurons, or cell bodies, deep underneath the cortex that led to the loss of cholinergic markers. This finding motivated the quest to develop drugs that, like l-dopa, might enhance cholinergic functions even in the face of dying neurons.

That quest proved at least partially successful when a type of cholinesterase inhibitor, which could prevent the breakdown of acetylcholine that normally occurs as a part of brain metabolism, was observed to reverse some of the cognitive symptoms of dementia in animals and human beings. While not a cure, these drugs held some promise of treating symptoms in patients with age-related memory loss.

The public and private funds devoted to the early market-based search for treatments since the seventies ultimately yielded five drugs for use in the United States and Europe. Four of the compounds (tacrine, rivastigmine, donepezil, and galantamine) were cholinesterase inhibitors (ChEIs), and the other compound (memantine) acted on a different neurotransmitter system involving glutamate. This first wave of drugs had limitations in their clinical use. Primarily, they did not modify the disease, and although they had been found to be somewhat efficacious (albeit with small statistically significant differences vis-à-vis placebos) in some people in well-controlled studies, they were less effective when brought into clinical practice with a wider range of patients than the populations who normally participate in clinical drug trials. These drugs also cause significant side effects, such as gastrointestinal upset, nausea, diarrhea, muscle cramps, insomnia, vivid dreams, and occasionally nightmares. Even though several drugs are now on the market (including generics), the over-the-counter price for cholinesterase inhibitors has remained steep, at a little less than $5 a day. Although KOL experts do use the drugs in their patients, when advocating for new monies to support novel approaches, they will often reverse course and say that the current medications are largely ineffective.

Despite the failure of this wave of initial neurotransmitter-based drugs to demonstrate major benefits, they have been heavily marketed and commercially successful. This curious legerdemain of neoliberalism is reflected in a now-infamous commercial for Pfizer's cholinesterase inhibitor (Aricept), which has come to be infamously known as the "Lasagna ad."[38] In the spot, a doting Italian grandmother inexplicably forgets to prepare the traditional Sunday lasagna for her family, causing great consternation for her adult daughter. Upon making a clinical visit to address this unsettling domestic peccadillo, a bespectacled doctor straight out of central casting strokes a prescription for Aricept, and in no time at all, the now-medicated grandmother is back to her old self, effortlessly dishing out lasagna to her daughter's family on a future Sunday visit.

The seductive but grossly misleading image of a non-disease-modifying drug inducing a total metamorphosis in someone with memory loss—a message received by millions of aging people and concerned family members in the United States since the commercial aired in the first decade of this century—is perhaps direct proof of English author H. G. Wells's observation that "Advertising is legalized lying."[39] Such widespread airing of pharmaceutical commercials like the Lasagna ad are unique to the United States and New Zealand, the only countries to allow direct-to-consumer pharmaceutical advertising.[40] The billions of dollars spent by the industry on these kinds of Madison Avenue–concocted advertisements are often targeted at primetime television audiences, demonstrating that they *do* affect sales largely by having consumers ask their physicians to prescribe things they've seen on television or in magazines.

As it stands, the last FDA-approved drug (memantine) for use in Alzheimer's came out in 2003. Even then there was considerable pressure to approve this marginally effective compound because of the absence of new drugs coming down the pipeline at a rapid enough rate. Multinational drug companies have also tried to maximize the profit of these drugs by changing formulations, such as dose. One company (Pfizer) has attempted to convince people that a 23 mg dose of Aricept was more effective than the already approved 10 mg maximum dose. Studies showed that the new dose could increase side effects but not benefit the patient; however, the advantage to the company was to extend their intellectual property over this odd and arbitrary new dosage, making it difficult for generics to follow and pilfer market share. Over the past 15 years, shortcomings of neurotransmitter-based drugs like Aricept—while generating billions of dollars in global profits—have nevertheless created dismay and tension in the "normal science" of the Alzheimer's paradigm, driving an influx of new ideas about how to modify underlying neuronal death and produce more effective treatments.

Ascendancy of the Amyloid Cascade Hypothesis

As the turn of the century neared, scientists began gravitating away from obviously limited neurotransmitter therapies and toward a theory about Alzheimer's that had first been ventured in the eighties. Called the *amyloid cascade hypothesis*,[41] this theory had roots in Alois Alzheimer's original early 20th-century observations and held that improper processing of amyloid precursor protein in the brains of people like Auguste D., who carried rare genetic mutations, caused overexpression of an aberrant 42-amino-acid peptide (Aβ42) that was "toxic." The increasing presence of this abnormal toxic peptide in turn triggered a *cascade* of extracellular amyloid accumulation. This accumulation formed plaques that then somehow caused *tau proteins*—the structures providing stability within neurons—to *hyper-phosphorylate* and twist into intracellular tangles. Ultimately, the theory went, this beta-amyloid-driven cascade produced widespread neuronal death in various parts of the brain, which led to dysfunction in synapses and neurotransmitters, a domino effect of cell death and thus progressive dementia. Given the overall thrust of the "politics of anguish" strategy, the idea that beta-amyloid was the first step in the chain of disease progression was extended from rare young-onset cases like Auguste D.'s to all forms of sporadic AD.

Amyloid thus became conventionally understood as a pathogen-like entity, referred to in the scientific literature as "abnormal," a "burden," and a hallmark of a "pathological state" in the brain. Rather than altering levels of acetylcholine in the brain, as cholinesterase inhibitors do, drugs developed in accordance with the amyloid cascade hypothesis were intended to prevent neuronal death in various ways: by directly removing beta-amyloid (the peptide that forms into the plaques noted by Alzheimer in Auguste D.) or some subunits called *oligomers*; by inhibiting and modifying the enzymes involved in the initial generation of these peptides (that is, γ-secretase and β-secretase); or by attacking amyloid aggregation and plaque formation and enhancing clearance.

Initially, two competing camps formed around this theory: baptists believed that *inter*cellular beta-amyloid protein was the causative factor in AD, and tauists argued for the causative significance of the *intra*cellular tau protein. Nonetheless, the former became dominant in shaping a new paradigm of drug development built on the belief that antiamyloid drugs could intercede earlier in the cascade of neuronal dysfunction, before the formation of tangles. Once the field became reorganized around the amyloid hypothesis, baptists dominated the scholarly literature, becoming gatekeepers of "acceptable paradigmatic discourse" around AD. So too did amyloid proponents find disproportionate representation as KOLs on drug company boards who guided market investment, and on NIH study sections that dictated grant funding. Today, the NIH budget for Alzheimer's and dementia, which reached nearly $2.3 billion in 2019,[42] continues to prioritize funding to amyloid-centric research, but this now appears to be changing. As longtime advocate Zaven Khachaturian has observed of the baptist phenomenon, when the field and market coalesced around amyloid with a certain mania, "Things shifted from a scientific inquiry into an almost religious belief system, where people stopped being skeptical or even questioning."[43]

Indeed, while those who zealously championed the dominant amyloid paradigm have, for decades, more frequently attracted accolades, awards, lucrative consulting deals, and well-paid academic appointments, dissenting voices who have opposed the centering of amyloid have often been stifled—their research relegated to lesser journals, their perspectives marginalized at conferences, and their professional status reduced in the research community.[44] Such a dynamic underscores Thomas Kuhn's observation that paradigms establish themselves as a result of the "abandonment of critical discourse" that brings about the lack of debate about certain basic concepts.

Guided by dominant baptist theories since the nineties, scientists have developed hundreds of elegant drugs that act on amyloid through the above-mentioned pathways. Yet, since the early 2000s, more than 400 clinical trials of therapeutics for AD—the majority targeting amyloid—have been registered with a fail rate of nearly 100% in reported trials.[45,46,47] As of spring 2021, no antiamyloid or other disease-modifying drugs for AD have been approved by the FDA. The occasionally claimed successes of early small studies often melt away when larger, more carefully designed studies are conducted. Frequent trumped-up claims that a subgroup of patients may have responded to treatment tend to disappear when replications are attempted.

The Great Zombie Revival

While it has now become clear to us and others that the baptist approach of attacking amyloid late in the disease process when people are already symptomatic is inefficacious, recent drug development has not abandoned the amyloid cascade hypothesis. Instead, in the past decade, the dominant paradigmatic theory has been adjusted around the belief that drugs have been administered *too late* in the disease process, once neurons and synapses are already past the point of rescue. Current hope (and billions of dollars in investment) are now flowing into presymptomatic treatments. Scientists are aiming to (1) use biomarkers in spinal fluid and brain scans to detect levels of amyloid and tau and identify those experiencing Alzheimer's-type changes in the brain without symptoms, and (2) administer antiamyloid drugs to such high-risk people in "predisease" stages.

The main drugs under investigation are forms of immunotherapy against amyloid protein that effectively condition the brain to clear it. Early data are not altogether encouraging (at least to noninvested academic and pharmaceutical researchers like us), and even if vaccines were to somehow prove effective, questions will remain about the safety, expense, and feasibility of administering a drug across decades. So too is it important to factor in the opportunity costs of wasting money on drug development and not applying population health interventions to improve brain health and prevent dementia over the life course.

A case in point is the so-called A4 research study of Lilly's drug solanezumab, an antiamyloid antibody, launched with combined industry and NIA money in 2014. Participants in the study had no symptoms or signs of dementia but were found through PET scans to have amyloid in their brains and were given prophylactic doses of the antiamyloid drug. As the studies began to show signs of failure, doses of solanezumab were raised, and the duration of the study was extended. Unfortunately, these efforts also failed, and Lilly decided not to pursue its own drug, although some studies are still ongoing.

With the dawn of the 2020s, the drug attracting the most attention has been Biogen's aducanumab. While it is another monoclonal antibody like solanezumab, aducanumab has different properties based on where it acts on amyloid molecules. Emblematic of the zombie economy that has defined the American dementia era, aducanumab is a drug that has quite literally been raised from the dead. In March 2019, it failed a so-called futility analysis—a process through which data are analyzed before a study is finished for the drug's likelihood to achieve predesignated clinical outcomes—and Biogen announced that it had halted development. When this occurred, it shook the field, and many pronounced the aducanumab failure as heralding the final death of the amyloid hypothesis. Just months later, however, in November 2019, the company made a shocking and triumphant reversal, announcing that aducanumab was actually alive and that an application for approval would be submitted to the FDA.

What happened to cause this miraculous revival? On one hand, new data not available in the initial futility analysis were received from patients who continued being administered higher doses of the drug after the March announcement. And on the other hand, in the intervening months, the company had also restructured, with a new vice president, new statisticians, different consultants, and ostensibly an organizational imperative to dig deeper in the data during a critical juncture when many industry analysts were arguing that the company's fate hinged on the success or failure of aducanumab.[48]

In Biogen's fall announcements, it teased a major press conference that would be held later and drummed up much fanfare in the media. When the data were presented in a highly choreographed setting, however, they were far from convincing. There appeared to be possible positive results on cognitive and functional loss, but the drug was also observed to have caused microscopic hemorrhages and swelling in the brain, especially in participants who carried particular genetic risk factors (namely, the ApoE4 gene) for Alzheimer's.[49] As a new decade began, the Alzheimer's research community was left pondering the implications of a potentially costly and risky drug with possible minor benefits for people with milder cognitive impairment. Questions raised by the carefully stage-managed press conference went unresolved: Why were the results of the futility analysis and later evaluation so different? How did the reanalysis affect the results in the placebo group? Was the higher dose responsible for the better results in the repeat analysis? Did patient characteristics vary in other ways than dose? Why did people in the second analysis on lower doses seem to do better as well? How did amyloid-imaging results relate to any clinical effects? What about the full spectrum of side effects? What role was the placebo effect playing in the results? Underlying all these questions was whether the bar for approval set in the discussions between the FDA and Biogen had been set too low.

The company claimed that a biologics license application (antibodies are formally called *biologics* rather than *drugs*) would be submitted in March 2020. The submission was delayed until fall 2020, however, perhaps because a major internal Biogen meeting held in Boston in March 2020 was an early COVID-19 *superspreader* event, which had transmitted the virus to some of the company's key leadership.[50] Thus, during the entire six-month period between November 2019 and the time of this writing, Biogen presented essentially the same data on several occasions at international drug development meetings, shedding no new light on any of the pressing questions about their analyses. Ramping up the political process to drive approval was ostensibly more of a priority than transparency, as the company employed a media strategy of hyper-capitalist brinksmanship in practically daring the FDA not to approve its product. In turn, lay organizations and other advocates began talking excitedly about possible approval of not only the first new drug in decades but one that promised to slow the disease. In my (Peter's) many emails phone calls, and Zoom meetings with CEOs, advocacy organizations, and "key opinion leaders," I have attempted to stem the tide, warning that inadequate skepticism would create potentially false expectations that would help drive the momentum for approval.

Ultimately, at this stage (spring 2020), we share the opinion of many experts that the results are too confusing to warrant approval and that other studies that could incorporate higher doses and other experimental features based on what was learned in the futility analysis should be done. We and others are concerned that political pressure from advocacy groups, people with the condition, and the experts who have been promising success for years could lead to an FDA approval of this zombie drug out of desperation. But if the first approved "disease-modifying drug" has such marginal effects that they would be largely unnoticeable to patients and clinicians (as even the best interpretation of the drug data suggests), what would that do to research in other approaches as drug companies developed equivalent therapies? The stakes are too high for letting one company make lots of money while the field loses more credibility and squanders more hope. If Biogen is asked by the FDA to conduct more studies, as it should be, it will be interesting to see if the company's own beliefs are sufficient to motivate it to do more expensive clinical trials to bolster the case for approval or not. In the meantime, Biogen's stock will continue fluctuating wildly, with billions of dollars in value lost or gained in days, depending on the latest presentation or security analyst report—a Wall Street–driven dynamic we explore in greater detail in the next chapter.

Meanwhile, the tension among Alzheimer's experts is palpable. Some proponents of the amyloid approach are aggressively promoting approval of aducanumab (and still seeking the fame and perhaps fortune that would redound to them personally). Other amyloid proponents are more balanced. Most experts are not impressed by the aducanumab results, but some say they would still use the drug if it is approved. Some, however, irresponsibly promote anecdotes of success plucked selectively from the stories of participants in the trials and exclaim their enthusiasm for drug approval. In general, the field is frustrated by not being able to have a new therapeutic emerge from their efforts and the billions of dollars spent trying to find better drugs. Rarely do they ask whether their life's work has been in vain or consider that there are other obvious ways this money could be better spent that would actually affect individual and population brain health. Indeed, no one knows exactly what aducanumab would cost individuals and society financially, but it would likely be in the tens of billions of dollars over the first few years of approval.

Beyond aducanumab, enthusiasm for not just beating but *reviving* the dead horse of amyloid cascade continues. In fact, other studies combining an amyloid antibody with other drugs is being designed, and researchers are shifting to other biological approaches, such as targeting tau proteins that form into tangles. Increasingly, the rallying cry is for *therapeutic cocktails* (that is, combining multiple drugs with different mechanisms into one treatment regimen). Such cocktails would likely be more expensive and lead to more possible side effects from drug interactions, but they remain the latest neoliberal innovation fantasy.

And that fantasy extends to not paying adequate attention to what the goals of therapy might be. In actuality, what would a cure for Alzheimer's look like to the patient and family? Would the brain revert back to "normal," and—if so—what age of normalcy? Moreover, the costs of such therapies are ignored (literally) in conversations, a fact that does not prevent companies and their Alzheimer's Association allies from claiming that billions and trillions would be saved by the "priceless" drugs.[51] Those claims are often based on reducing medical costs, like preventing hospital or nursing home admissions. But seldom is it ever asked whether a truly effective drug that had those outcomes and might keep people alive longer would ultimately incur even greater societal costs associated with longer lives.

Scanning for Profits

In our free-market landscape, which has medicalized, monetized, and individualized brain aging during the last four decades of American dementia, there is also significant money to be made in pushing Alzheimer's diagnostics. Companies such as Lilly, which are trying to patent antiamyloid drugs, are also developing sophisticated amyloid diagnostics. After all, if patients need an amyloid scan (which currently costs around $4,000) to be given an amyloid drug, a company can make money twice over (and if they need genetic counseling to determine risk and benefit, as appears to be the case with aducanumab, that's another cost that must be factored in). Yet, we face an uncomfortable situation where diagnostics for Alzheimer's have been pushed in advance of any existing therapy—the proverbial "cart before the horse." Some people ask whether it is worthwhile (or ethical) even trying to make a clinical diagnosis when a cure, much less a precise therapy, is not available.

Amyloid imaging was FDA approved last decade as a device-based technology and was not required to demonstrate clinical value (tau imaging was approved in 2020). The labeling associated with amyloid imaging is that it can be used to *detect amyloid*, not to *make a diagnosis* of Alzheimer's, yet the concept of detecting amyloid in the brain and diagnosing AD are frequently conflated. In fact, getting the fuzzy images produced by the amyloid scans approved required considerable work because even with experts reading the PET scans, there has been major disagreement about whether the scans show increased amounts of amyloid or not. So when the FDA approved the use of the amyloid-imaging device, the experts apparently agreed that the scans would be labeled as either "positive" or "negative." Of course, an unavoidable reality is that the amount of amyloid in aging brains exists on a continuum of different values, and there is considerable difference between having no amyloid detected and having an amount just below the amount required to make a determination of a positive scan.

In fact, in clinical practice and in research studies, the formal language often used is that the person has either an elevated amyloid level or a nonelevated level. Screened patients inevitably ask, "*How* elevated was my score?" or "*How* close was it to being 'officially' elevated?" But in research studies, specific amyloid levels or associated risks are not given; thus, people who have a slightly elevated amyloid level may very well have an inappropriate sense of gloom about their prognosis. Or, on the other hand, people with levels that are not significantly elevated may believe inaccurately that they have escaped the looming threat of a progressive dementia. Despite this uncertainty, in 2013 the Alzheimer's Association convinced the Centers for Medicare and Medicaid Services (CMS; the government funders of health care for the elderly) to pay $100 million to use amyloid-imaging in a study of clinical practice,[52] based on the belief that deploying amyloid imaging would improve diagnostic accuracy and presumably help patients (see the IDEAS study).[53] At present, this innovation fantasy appears to be not only a waste of money but part of an effort to get expensive so-called diagnostic tests of unclear value into clinical practice in ways that potentially further medicalize Alzheimer's for asymptomatic patients. Initial reports for the IDEAS study claim that such imaging can change practice, but there is a bit of a tautological, self-serving behavior on the part of the dementia "KOL experts" who feel the tests they developed *should* be valuable. Certainly, the tests are valuable to the experts and their client companies, but whether to patients and the public—that is less clear. Again, as we propose throughout the book, there are likely better ways to invest scarce resources at the level of population health and psychosocial care in ways that more likely prevent dementia, support brain health, and improve quality of life on a large-scale.

CONCLUSION

Alzheimer's has existed as a "disease" for just over a century, waxing and waning over the decades in response to shifting political-economic, technological, and cultural forces. Within the last several decades of American dementia, the influence of neoliberalism and the influx of market forces has profoundly shaped our paradigmatic concepts of the disease and our strategies for resisting Alzheimer's. Pursuit of a market bonanza has, in essence, warped decision making and diverted funds away from psychosocial and preventive approaches. We know that pharmacological efforts have largely failed to produce effective therapies, diagnostics, and cures—*but why*? In the next chapter, we examine the inconvenient truths around the illness as it is presently constructed. Further, as drugs have failed, the innovation fantasies and profit-seeking obsession of the neoliberal era have spawned an emerging "marketplace of memory" aimed at finding new and creative ways of extracting revenue from aging citizens increasingly anxious about memory loss and Alzheimer's "disease." Let us now fast-forward to the present moment and examine this more recent zombie market phenomenon that increasingly has many of us in its grips.

3

Alzheimer's Today

Inconvenient Truths in the Marketplace of Memory

There is a good chance you and those you love are being "followed." In the last decade, big tech marketing mavens have created stealthy online software that attaches itself to your internet browser like a digital barnacle, tracking the websites you visit and harvesting this data to better understand the intimate details of your life. Based on your patterns of online behavior, this algorithmic tracking technology will then market targeted products to you via digital advertisements that, quite literally, "trail" you around the internet, popping up in the nooks and crannies of future websites you visit until it wears you down to the point of purchase. Fittingly for our American dementia era, this unrelenting tactic of personalized, profit-seeking marketeering is often referred to as "zombie advertising."

Several years ago, after researching and writing an academic paper[1] about the emerging phenomenon of "brain fitness" products being aggressively marketed to baby boomers, Peter and I were separately pursued for weeks by persistent zombie ads from Lumosity, a leading company in that industry, that kept materializing on websites we would visit. While these ads, which still trail people around the internet today, certainly say much about the zombie economy wrought by hyper-capitalist forces since the seventies, which seeks constant, insatiable short-term profit, they also bespeak the failures of an Alzheimer's marketplace that has yet to produce a pharmaceutical cure and thus has turned its hungry eyes to other products and strategies for revenue.

So how did we get here, and why haven't drugs succeeded in fulfilling the innovation fantasies of neoliberalism that, since the political-economic reordering of the last several decades, have devoutly predicted that the confluence of science, biotechnology, and free markets would yield a cure for Alzheimer's disease? And beyond the brain fitness industry and its fleet of zombie ads tracking anxious online baby boomers and others around the global interwebs, where else has industry turned for profits, and how have the innovation fantasies evolved in the wake of failed pharmaceutical drugs? This chapter answers these questions, beginning by taking stock of what we've learned from the ongoing failures of Alzheimer's drug trials.

THE INCONVENIENT TRUTHS OF ALZHEIMER'S

Amyloid Is Complicated and Pathology Is Not Destiny

The neoliberal turn of the seventies coincided with a rapidly aging population. Out of this changing historical circumstance arose a "politics of anguish" that shaped the paradigmatic contours of the field across decades and helped entrench a dominant public narrative that brain aging is a "battle" to be won by "attacking" beta-amyloid—one of the two hallmarks documented in neuritic plaques by Alois Alzheimer—as if it were a polio-like pathogen. But a funny thing happened on the way to the panacea. Turns out amyloid is a complicated biological entity and that some of its constituent proteins appear to have complex roles in normal brain function. To wit, amyloid-related components have been shown to have antioxidant properties,[2] to be crucial to the growth of cells, synapses, and learning, and to even be involved in stress and immune responses.[3] In fact, the final beta-pleated structure of amyloid found in plaques is a low-energy state that may actually represent inactivity and harmlessness. While amyloid's appearance may be indicative of something "not being quite right" in the brain, reducing it to the level of a pathogen via the analogy to an infectious disease like polio seems to have been an increasingly misguided rhetorical flourish of the "politics of anguish" strategy that has hitherto guided failed drug development in the neoliberal era.

Moreover, population research—including the famous Nun Study, in which researchers examined the aging brains of 678 American members of the School of Sisters of Notre Dame—has repeatedly shown that the amount of amyloid deposition in peoples' brains does not correlate strongly with cognitive performance.[4,5,6] In fact, amyloid deposition frequently occurs in cognitively intact elderly persons without causing symptoms, with up to 40% of nondemented elderly reaching some level of neuropathologic criteria for AD.[7] Similarly confounding is that around 25-30% of people clinically diagnosed with Alzheimer's are, upon postmortem analysis, observed to *lack* neuropathological criteria for AD.[8] One recent antiamyloid drug study even showed that 40% of people enrolled (who had been clinically diagnosed with AD) were actually *amyloid-negative* when researchers used imaging to look at biomarkers in the brain.[9]

When it comes to amyloid and Alzheimer's, pathology is not destiny, and there is an uncomfortable disconnect between its appearance and the symptoms of illness. Whereas many markers of advancing age and AD pathogenesis (such as synaptic loss, tangles, and microglial activation) increase with the course of dementia, the amount of amyloid deposited in the brain has been observed to plateau even as cognition continues to decline. Cognitive symptoms are actually better correlated with the presence of tau tangles than amyloid, and tangles can occur in the absence of plaques. If, as the baptist's hypothesis holds, amyloid is *driving* the cascade of the "disease," why is this the case?

Such findings raise three fundamental questions:

- Have we mistakenly regarded disease-associated proteins like amyloid as "toxic"?
- Is the appearance of amyloid merely an *effect* of earlier damage rather than a *cause*?
- If so, are we "attacking" a process associated with normal brain aging that might be part of the brain's protective response?

That the field has not yet abandoned its amyloid-centric focus but rather doubled down in the baptist holy war to now "attack" it in presymptomatic stages is discouraging. In chapter 2, we discuss at length the still-unfolding story of Biogen's aducanumab, the drug that was "killed" in early 2019 and then raised from the dead months later to possibly haunt us for some time to come. For those of us who have watched the field "evolve" since the seventies, tracking the billion-dollar enterprise of drug development and the litany of aducanumab-like pratfalls has felt a bit like being in the middle of Van Gogh's painting *Prisoners Exercising*—with

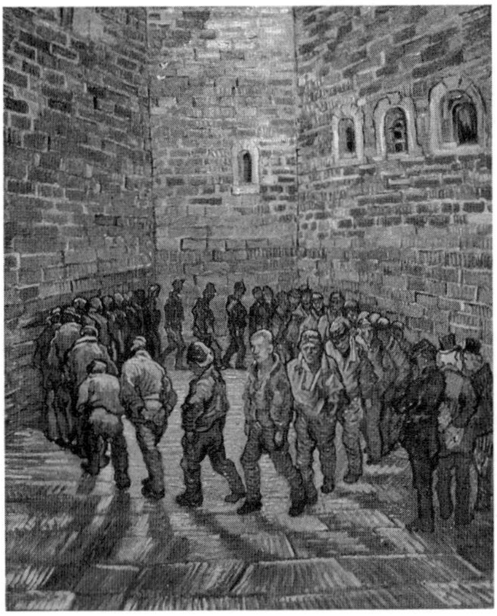

Figure 3.1. The Alzheimer's field, with its fixation on curing the "disease" by removing amyloid, has felt increasingly like Vincent Van Gogh's painting *Prisoners Exercising*.
Source: Wikimedia Commons.

industry and researchers going around and around in circles, pursuing different tactics contra amyloid with little forward progress (figure 3.1).[10] Brought into its modern existence over the same timeframe during which the hyper-capitalist era was unleashing the zombie economy across the globe, the Alzheimer's field seems now to be similarly walled in by circular thinking, obsessively organized around short-term profit and instrumental solutions, and challenged to truly think creatively.

Lessons about the Heterogeneity of Alzheimer's Disease(s)

Another emergent finding is that even while we have, since Butler and the NIA's push for the aggressive medicalization of senility in the seventies, come to conventionally refer to Alzheimer's as a singular "disease," it is in reality a highly *heterogeneous* condition.[11] This heterogeneity applies at the level of genetics, risk factors, age of onset, clinical presentation, progression, response to drugs, and—perhaps most importantly—brain pathology. When scientists examine Alzheimer's at the molecular and cellular levels, "it" appears to be not the result of a single protein or process, but rather the outcome of multiple overlapping pathological abnormalities. In fact, a majority of so-called AD cases show signs of *mixed dementia*. This means that they encompass not only the classic hallmarks of plaques and tangles first documented by Alzheimer, but also other overlapping pathologies like vascular lesions (large infarcts, microinfarcts, lacunas, and hemorrhages associated with atherosclerosis; arteriolosclerosis; hypertension; and other unknown factors and cerebral amyloid angiopathy), accumulation of alpha-synuclein (the abnormal protein that makes up Lewy bodies), abnormal proteins called TDP-43, hippocampal sclerosis, white matter disease, and other variably identified and even more poorly understood inclusions such as argentophilic grains.[12,13,14,15,16,17,18,19,20,21,22,23]

What this well-established phenomenon means is that there are multiple pathways to neurodegeneration in persons clinically diagnosed with AD (a finding harkening back to Alzheimer's divergent first two cases with Auguste D. and Johann F.), and that these pathways frequently "mix" and overlap. *Alzheimer's disease* is thus not explicitly definable as a singular entity but is rather a catch-all term for various pathologies and clinical manifestations occurring on several different trajectories, which we used to refer to as *senility*. Put otherwise, Alzheimer's is perhaps best thought of as a multifaceted protective response of the brain to numerous insults that occur across the lifespan.

As such, we and others continue to argue that it would be much more appropriate to speak of *Alzheimer's diseases* (plural) or *Alzheimer's syndrome* than to continue the "politics of anguish" conceit that we are dealing with a singular disease that can be instrumentally fixed.

Given the reality of the underlying heterogeneity of Alzheimer's, it is perhaps unsurprising that our current generation of drugs targeting *single aspects* of this apparent diffuse syndrome—predominantly beta-amyloid—have almost universally failed to provide clinical benefit. While current amyloid-based therapies are organized around the theory that *all* clinical Alzheimer's can be effectively treated pharmacologically by focusing on pathways that converge on beta-amyloid, this has left untreated a significant proportion of the associated conditions in the AD phenotype that are not related to plaque and tangle pathology (for example, vascular damage, Lewy bodies, white matter disease).[24] Instead of treating multiple *disease processes* in brains affected by Alzheimer's syndrome, the field continues to operate as if patching one hole in a roof riddled with openings is enough to stop a major leak.[25]

As John Hardy, an Alzheimer's researcher at University College London, has said about heterogeneity: "I wouldn't say it's a dirty little secret. Everybody knows about it. But we don't know what to do about it."[26] Of course, the question lurking behind this "dirty little secret" is this: If you can't properly define what a condition is, how can you realistically posit a cure?

Lessons about Entanglements of Alzheimer's and Aging

The strategic decision to establish Alzheimer's as a disease wholly separate from aging went hand in hand with the neoliberal turn in the seventies. Despite billions of public and private dollars flowing into the pursuit of diagnostics and cure, there remains no definitive way to distinguish someone with so-called Alzheimer's disease from someone with severe brain aging. Increasingly, the field is moving from what our colleague Margaret Lock has termed theories of "localization" (that Alzheimer's is a specific disease—the result of *local* molecular mechanisms amenable to treatment) to theories of "entanglement" (the belief that Alzheimer's is a syndrome intimately associated, or *entangled*, with numerous brain-aging processes).[27] Most scientists (at least in private) would concede that the notion of brain aging and Alzheimer's arising from clearly distinct physiological processes—that is, the premise of localization—is simply not proven. Our British colleague Carol Brayne and colleagues have referred to this "dis-entangling" of Alzheimer's and aging as the "great Alzheimer's mistake," as age is far and away the strongest associated risk factor for dementia.[28,29]

In retrospect, the narrative recasting of senility as a curable disease called Alzheimer's in the seventies was far more defensible as a logical *political* and *business* stratagem of the era than as a *scientific* thesis. In 2013, Lock wrote a landmark book, *The Alzheimer Conundrum*, in which she shared an interview with the aforementioned neurogeneticist John Hardy, one of the most famous and well-funded researchers in the field since the hyper-capitalist turn and someone in competition for the much sought-after Nobel Prize. Lock captured a moment of truth in which Hardy, reflecting on the medicalization of Alzheimer's as a singular condition separate from aging in the political-economic transition of the seventies and eighties, acknowledged that this "was just a political maneuver to get funding, and some people then actually came to believe that this is the case."[30] Such admissions shake the foundations of the dominant scientific paradigm. So too do they demonstrate quite profoundly how Alzheimer's has functioned much more effectively as a political shibboleth than a precise scientific concept, and why this dominant narrative helped manufacture consent for free-market forces to transform the field in pursuit of innovation fantasies. Many of the best minds in AD research and advocacy acknowledge the uncomfortable reality of the entanglement of Alzheimer's and aging, mostly privately, and these controversies remain largely out of public view.

As a result, the paradigmatic understanding of Alzheimer's as a singular curable "disease" is in crisis even while modern advocacy continues to publicly present the syndrome as a singular disease, caused by beta-amyloid, that is wholly separate from aging. The polio analogies launched by Butler still proliferate in modern discourse, serving as justification for maintaining the search for an absolute cure. For instance (emphasis added):

- In 2009, US politician and Alzheimer's advocate Newt Gingrich implored the American public to "imagine ... if we discovered a cure—a breakthrough for the disease like the *vaccine for polio.* The financial and social impact on this country and the lives of millions would be immense."[31]
- In 2010, former Supreme Court justice Sandra Day O'Connor cowrote an editorial in the *New York Times* that argued: "If we could eliminate [AD], *as Jonas Salk wiped out polio with his vaccine*, we would greatly expand the potential of all Americans to live long, healthy and productive lives—and save trillions of dollars doing it."[32]
- In 2017, Lisa Genova, a neuroscientist and author of the novel-turned-film *Still Alice*, wrote of her belief that "we will soon have a prevention, treatments or even a cure for Alzheimer's, much as we've seen with tuberculosis, typhoid, diphtheria, *polio*, certain cancers, HIV and heart disease."[33]

The public health campaign against polio was certainly a remarkable success and a key part of the longevity revolution we discussed in chapter 2, but the syndromal, heterogeneous, age-related entity that is *Alzheimer's disease(s)* categorically does not appear to be an illness resembling polio. Moreover, success in one medical area does not imply that success will occur in another, and the analogy undergirding our search for a cure over the last four decades has helped usher the field into what increasingly appears a stagnant and untenable situation.

There is growing acknowledgment that the age-related aspects of Alzheimer's syndrome need to be embraced and accepted for any progress to occur. As John Morris, a professor of neurology at Washington University in St. Louis, has said: "We can't avoid the fact the number one risk factor for Alzheimer's disease is age, and many of these other pathologies are age-associated. We don't see them in younger people."[34]

The Way Forward: Moving Beyond the Elephant in the Room

When we talk about the state of the Alzheimer's field, we often reference the parable of three blind men and an elephant. In most retellings, three men who are visually challenged happen upon an elephant and lay their hands on different regions of the creature's body—the tail, tusk, and leg. Because they become fixated on single components of the creature, the men vehemently disagree about its very nature.

Similarly, the paradigm of Alzheimer's formulated during the neoliberal turn has promoted the belief that we are dealing with a singular condition, and those involved in drug development have laid their hands on amyloid and built a theory around the reductive concept of "one protein, one disease, one drug."[35] Like the elephant in the parable, however, Alzheimer's is not just *one thing* but rather *various processes* that are intimately related to severe brain aging that we will all experience to one degree or another as we age. Myriad studies have claimed that these processes include overlapping factors, such as:

- inflammation
- vascular deterioration
- oxygen deprivation
- changes in glucose metabolism
- oxidative stress and mitochondrial dysfunction
- alterations in balances of ions such as calcium
- loss of synapses
- alterations in neurotransmitters and growth factors
- the misfolding of neural proteins such as beta-amyloid and tau

In essence, given what we know about the heterogeneity of Alzheimer's, a more apt parable might place the blind men in a petting zoo, where they unknowingly encounter different animals while trying to come to a singular understanding of what "it" is. Such a predicament produces an even more fragmented view of scientific reality than the proverbial elephant.

The age-related, heterogeneous nature of Alzheimer's carries profound implications. As mentioned above, we would perhaps be best served to think of the illness as a syndrome entangled with aging processes that is multifactorial across the lifespan and starts decades before symptoms appear. We ought to increasingly entertain the possibility that (1) amyloid is not *just* toxic but rather an adaptive response to upstream damage, and (2) paradigmatic theories that have organized the field for decades are no longer useful. Furthermore, given the challenge presented by Alzheimer's disease(s) we must set our sights on treating other forms of dementia that co-occur with traditional Alzheimer's pathology, and not merely fixate on amyloid like blind men huddled around an elephant. The age-related nature of Alzheimer's means drugs should increasingly target the biologies of aging listed above; this does, of course, necessitate that we realize our challenge is tantamount to "curing or treating aspects of aging."[36]

Such paradigmatic shifts in the drug and advocacy marketplace are already in motion. Interestingly, in 2017, when Bill Gates donated more than $50 million from his unfathomable personal fortune to Alzheimer's research, he expressed his desire to focus less on "mainstream" approaches involving amyloid and tau and more on backing "scientists with different, less mainstream ideas [since] a more diverse drug pipeline increases our odds of discovering a breakthrough."[37] It is worth noting that, even while correctly identifying the "elephant problem," Gates also invoked the neoliberal doctrine "that science and innovation are going to solve most of the tough problems over time."[38] As we discuss further in subsequent chapters, it is necessary to question whether the allocation of such massive wealth and resources to public health might be a more sure-fire investment. For instance, as we explore in chapter 5, cities across our country, such as Flint, Michigan, have no clean drinking water because of the contamination of lead, a known neurotoxin, in the public water supply. Fixing Flint's service lines is estimated to cost around $60 million—just a billionaire's hair over the amount of Gates's donation to biomedical science. Would such a straightforward and effective *brain health intervention* not be a better investment of resources than throwing more money into a pharmacologic lottery?

As we see the "whole elephant" and recalibrate our understanding around the notion of Alzheimer's as a heterogeneous, age-related, multifactorial condition, we must bear in mind that multiple pathways for developing the syndrome mean that there are also multiple ways for resisting it, and that risk factors for the various aging processes we see in Alzheimer's disease(s) are quite similar and overlapping. We believe that the nature of the multifactorial, age-related illness means we ought to act on *collective* risk factors (vascular disease, oxidative stress, diabetes, exposure to neurotoxins, and so forth) at the level of *society*. Moving away from our reductive, profit-oriented, individual-based neoliberal model demands the perspective of public health and a broader return to principles of social democracy that have been "forgotten" in the era of American dementia—a critical theme that we fully crystallize in the next chapter.

Regarding drug development, it is fair to ask where things go from here. In 2018, the pharmaceutical giant Pfizer folded its research and development operation for Alzheimer's and Parkinson's. Since the turn of the century, Pfizer has sponsored or cosponsored 99 clinical trials of 24 Alzheimer's drugs with only one approval (Aricept, which was initially developed by a different company, Eisai). The clinical pipelines of the other nine largest pharmaceutical companies are also drying up and list only eight Alzheimer's drugs in development. Four of the companies—Johnson & Johnson, Bayer, GlaxoSmithKline, and Gilead Sciences—list none.[39] The search for a solution to Alzheimer's has, quite frankly, been both a financial and a PR disaster for the industry. In addition to the cascade of failures, several antiamyloid trials have had to shut down because of patient deaths (from inflammation and meningoencephalitis) and increased skin cancer incidence. After all, inhibiting things on the molecular level can have all kinds of unwanted biological consequences.

Despite this rash of failures, the Alzheimer's Association and its aligned expert KOLs in the United States and elsewhere continue to state that the ultimate goal of research is "finding a cure." Since the "politics of anguish" was launched in the seventies amid neoliberal reordering, it has been promised that we will possess something like a cure in just a few years; conventionally, predictions are projected to arrive at the starting or midpoint of decades (for instance, 2020, 2025). These arbitrary promises continue to drive fundraising efforts even in the face of scientific evidence that problematizes the very notion of a cure.

We appear to have crossed a threshold wherein the great neoliberal innovation fantasy of Alzheimer's—that the trinity of science, biotechnology, and free markets would yield a "fix"—is beginning to crumble. Such findings bring to mind a pithy observation by surgeon-writer Atul Gawande: "There are, in human affairs, two kinds of problems: those that are amenable to a technical solution, and those which are not."[40] Alzheimer's syndrome, it seems, may well be the latter.

THE MARKETPLACE OF MEMORY: MODERN MANIFESTATIONS OF NEOLIBERALISM AND THE ZOMBIE ECONOMY

A Thriving Market for Failed Drugs

Even with the bevy of pharmaceutical failures since the eighties, a striking paradox of the American dementia era is that Alzheimer's research continues to be an engine for revenue in private markets *regardless of whether drug development yields any actual benefit for patients.* Wall Street traders have generated enormous sums of money by betting against (that is, *shorting*) the future stock prospects of companies that have unsuccessfully invested in antidementia drugs.

Perhaps predictably, this market force dynamic has led to historic financial crimes in the Alzheimer's field. Take the case of Sid Gilman, a neurologist and respected department chair at the University of Michigan, who last decade was involved in the largest insider trading case ever brought by the federal government. A prolific researcher and established expert in the Alzheimer's world, Gilman became a KOL and a consultant to big drug companies, research/tech firms, and Wall Street, where he enjoyed a lucrative role as a go-to expert for hedge fund companies looking to invest in the pharmaceutical market. This side gig earned Gilman hundreds of thousands of dollars a year along with the fringe benefits of travel in limos, luxury hotels, and private jets.[41]

In 2003, Gilman had been invited to join a "safety and monitoring committee" for a Phase II trial of an antiamyloid antibody (bapineuzumab) being developed by companies Wyeth and Elan. This compound had arrived just as the amyloid cascade hypothesis was cresting, and the

Alzheimer's field and financial markets were awash with excitement and optimism about its therapeutic potential. Hopes continued to rise over the next several years as the drug showed vague signs of promise in initial experiments. In turn, hedge funds sunk major investments into the partner pharmaceutical companies as the Phase II trials were carried out. One company, CR Intrinsic, an affiliate of the hedge fund SAC Capital Advisors, went in bullishly, amassing $700 million in Wyeth/Elan securities in June 2008. A month later, however, before the public release of unsuccessful Phase II trial results for bapineuzumab, the company spontaneously unloaded all its stock investments in the companies.

This abrupt volte-face drew the suspicion of the Securities and Exchange Committee and launched a massive federal inquiry. What investigators would eventually find was that, in 2006, Gilman had been set up with a consulting gig in partnership with a portfolio manager named Matthew Martoma, who oversaw the CR Intrinsic fund for SAC Capital. Martoma had carefully cultivated the relationship with Gilman, becoming a close colleague while paying him more than $100,000 as a consultant. Two years later, and against his better judgment, Gilman had used his insider status on the bapineuzumab safety and monitoring committee to pass along detailed information about the impending negative Phase II results and adverse side effects associated with the drug. So too had Gilman illegally shared with Martoma an encrypted PowerPoint summary of the upcoming results along with the password to open it. Secretly—and illegally—in possession of the knowledge that their investment was toxic, SAC capital shorted the drug by selling its shares to bet on failure. In doing so, the hedge fund generated profit and avoided losses totaling $275 million. Shortly after, Martoma received a $9.38 million bonus.[42]

While this historic case of insider trading is a rather dramatic example of the neoliberal zombie economy's grasp on the Alzheimer's world, it nevertheless reflects the surreal predicament we find ourselves in when drug failures are nevertheless monetized as part of a larger profit-seeking game of casino capitalism on Wall Street.

Diagnostic Creep and Mild Cognitive Impairment

Additionally, the forces of hyper-capitalism that helped animate both the Alzheimer's field and the broader zombie economy in the seventies have driven monetization of other aspects of brain aging via the creation of new, untapped markets. One approach has involved the literal creation of new disease categories that extend the diagnosis of Alzheimer's to milder and milder forms of the syndrome, chiefly to widen the potential consumer base for the current minimally effective FDA-approved drugs.

Sometimes called *diagnostic creep*, this process has occurred most obviously through the recent "discovery"—or, perhaps more accurately, "social construction"—of a condition called mild cognitive impairment (MCI). A supposed precursor to progressive dementias, like Alzheimer's, MCI has been defined as existing in a liminal state between the boundaries of normal aging and disease. While MCI first appeared as a concept in the fifties, its resurgence as a clinical label in the last decade (it was formally added to the *DSM-V* in 2013, coded as "Mild Neurocognitive Disorder," just as "Dementia" was changed to "Major Neurocognitive Disorder") reflects the field's paradigmatic acknowledgment that changes in the brain begin well before the manifestation of major cognitive-clinical symptoms of Alzheimer's syndrome.

Traditionally, the MCI label has been given to patients who present with a memory complaint and some changes in intellectual function as determined by neuropsychological testing, but who have relatively little impairment in activities of daily living. A range of subclassifications, however, has recently emerged that implies different "stages" of MCI: pre-MCI, early MCI, and late MCI. Reflecting the field's more recent focus on using the imaging biomarkers we reviewed last chapter to identify early stage or even asymptomatic individuals, an even more upstream classification of preclinical Alzheimer's has been embraced, this being a situation further in advance of early MCI, in which beta-amyloid and tau are identified in a person's brain or spinal fluid absent any clinical symptoms.[43] Not to be left out, clinicians have extended an even newer label, subjective cognitive impairment (SCI), also called subjective cognitive decline (SCD), for people without impairments detected by objective neuropsychological testing but who simply complain of their memory challenges (figure 3.2). Who, one might ask, does *not* have some form of SCI?

These predisease classifications were originally proposed as research categories, but their clinical use is actively being pushed by the Alzheimer's Association, as well as academic and commercial interests that desire to profit from diagnostic testing using amyloid imaging and eventually sell powerful drugs by effectively "medicalizing" individuals who

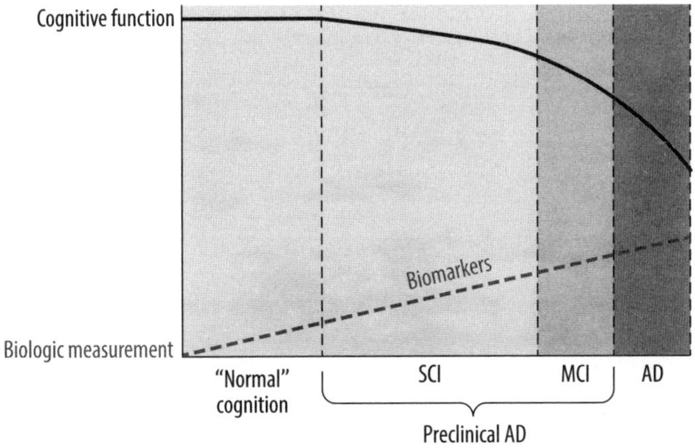

Figure 3.2. In the face of pharmacologic failures, industry-supported *predisease* categories like mild cognitive impairment (MCI), preclinical Alzheimer's disease (AD), and subjective cognitive impairment (SCI) have created lucrative new markets for existing drugs and diagnostics. *Source:* Created by Daniel George.

have no symptoms. This outcome would perhaps represent the ultimate market expansion in the zombie economy of Alzheimer's.

Indeed, the social construction of MCI and its variants has been largely supported by industry because of the potential to widen market share for existing drugs by many millions of consumers. Big pharma has funded some of the expert panels in establishing the diagnostic parameters for MCI and preclinical Alzheimer's as well as publishing papers in the academic literature. As the diagnostic predisease categories have become reified as scientifically acceptable classifications, the armamentarium of potential drugs in the pipeline to treat MCI has ramped up. According to clinicaltrials.gov, in 2019 just under 900 pharmacological and nonpharmacological trials were registered related to "mild cognitive impairment,"[44] demonstrating a sizable industry and academic investment in MCI—a condition that did not formally exist until last decade. Already, cholinesterase inhibitors and memantine—very limited neurotransmitter-based drugs—are being prescribed for MCI, even though studies have not shown significant benefit.

As one might expect, the diagnostic creep of MCI within the larger neoliberal economy has generated profound scientific, clinical, and ethical questions. The greatest controversy surrounds the heterogeneity observed in cases of MCI, the vagueness of its diagnostic criteria, and a lack of specific ability to predict the "disease" trajectory. Conversion rates of MCI to dementia vary significantly, and some studies observe that well over a quarter of people labeled with MCI do not progress to AD,[45] and between 14% and 41% of individuals with MCI have reverted back to "normal" cognitive functioning.[46]

Naturally, this raises questions about the accuracy, usefulness, and ethical soundness of a label that is supposed to represent a clinical precursor to AD. For instance, imagine that a loved one has some memory loss, but their activities of daily living are not affected—would you want them to be clinically labeled with MCI? When does the forgetfulness we may all be touched by as our brains age cross the line to "disease"? And should a clinical diagnosis be freely given by the physician or should it also require a subjective complaint from the patient or his or her family? Materially speaking, how much power should doctors (and the pharmaceutical industry) have to define and dictate the terms of how individuals experience disease, which can have such devastating effects in the lives of their loved ones? Does this trend push toward the danger of overmedicalization and overtreatment of asymptomatic people? With respect to the last question, as our colleague Ken Langa, a physician-researcher from the University of Michigan, has said: "If we start treating everyone with preclinical Alzheimer's, we'll treat a lot of people who would never have gone on to have dementia at all."[47]

Indeed, it's important to remember that while markets and shareholder profits may be enlarged by such diagnostic schemes, ultimately sentient human beings with fragile, finite lives and bonds must bear the biopsychosocial consequences of disease labels.

MCI is particularly confounding to patients since it portends a threat that our colleague Stephen Katz of Trent University in Canada has rightly called "ambiguous, variable, and uncertain."[48] Social scientists who have studied the effects of an MCI diagnosis, such as our aforementioned colleague Margaret Lock, as well as John Bond and Tiago Moreira in the UK, concur that the label is experienced as liminalizing, stigmatizing, and distressing since the diagnosed person becomes neither "normal" nor "demented" yet is warned their MCI *may progress* to dementia.[49] Scholar Renee Beard has found that while receiving the label can be a relief for some ("whew, it's not full-blown dementia!"), it more often produces "troublesome identities" for people with mild problems and low risk who must reconcile a frightening and uncertain future with their families.[50]

There is justifiable concern that the psychological harm that may arise from this fraught and uncertain diagnosis, which puts people on the brink of a highly stigmatized full-blown disease label—especially in the absence of effective treatments—may itself negatively affect the underlying brain-aging process.[51] In 2014, the satirical newspaper the *Onion* deftly captured this Kafka-esque modern dynamic in an article darkly titled "Aging Mother Knows Any Wrong Move Could Be Taken for Telltale Sign of Dementia."[52] People live in their diagnoses, and current behaviors and future expectations are colored by these potentially damaging diagnostic categories.

Ultimately, in the last decade of the "construction" of MCI, we see the paradigmatic goalposts of Alzheimer's disease shifting, in part, as a result of political-economic forces within the culture voraciously seeking new markets for diagnostics and drugs. To frame this process as being played on the moral high ground of addressing the suffering of others often avoids the more hidden game in which privileged and powerful economic actors (big pharma, diagnostic companies, the stock market, industry-cozy researchers and KOLs, fee-for-service health systems, and so on) benefit from hastening diagnostic creep and moving people into new consumer markets. These actors frequently argue that patients want to know "the truth" about their condition and that we shouldn't be paternalistic by *not* sharing test data. But data are not knowledge, and they are certainly not tantamount to wisdom. Giving people labels and information about which the experts are themselves confused while pretending that such knowledge is scientifically valid and useful borders on the unethical. And what about the common argument that we need this clinically obtained information to attract and enroll people into clinical trials? Fundamentally, it is an ethical error to conflate research with clinical care, and advocates too often dangerously blur the two when using research diagnoses and tests in their regular clinics. Do we want Medicare to pay part of the process for enrolling people in trials of unproven therapies? These are all questions demanding answers in the near future.

Of course, as you know from the "zombie ads" that may tail you around the internet should you use search terms related to aging, MCI, and dementia, one other zombie neoliberal force of our time that is fueled by societal anxiety around early memory loss is the massive industry that churns out consumer products targeting individuals who worry they may be in the early stages of MCI. Let's examine that space.

The Brain Health Marketplace

Into the therapeutic void created by hundreds of failed Alzheimer's drugs during the past several decades has emerged a vast marketplace of supposed memory-enhancing "brain health" products. This massive industry has traditionally been targeted at anxiety-addled baby boomers with money to burn, offering everything from "smart drugs" to enhance brain function (biological products, herbs, vitamins, nutraceuticals, and so forth) to legions of digital gadgets, including video games and computer software, phone apps, and other products proclaiming to maintain or enhance the memory, concentration, visual and spatial skills, verbal recall, and executive functions of individual users. More recently, however, the industry has begun marketing its wares to young professionals and college students, who are trying to survive in the highly competitive and mentally taxing knowledge economy workplaces and universities of the neoliberal era, which place a premium on optimizing cognitive performance.

This shift in marketing focus reflects the dominance of a hyper-capitalist order that has succeeded in creating an obsession with individual productivity, self-improvement, and meritocratic achievement—values that, as David Foster Wallace might have noted, have become the "water" of modern society in our era of American dementia. In expanding into billion-dollar global markets, the brain health industry has deployed aggressive, manipulative, dishonest, and, at times, unlawful advertising campaigns. Let's take a closer look at the products pushed by this industry, all of which are sociocultural objects deeply imbued with the contemporary values and ideologies of neoliberalism.[53]

NOOTROPICS (SMART DRUGS)

The concept of a *nootropic*—a drug or supplement intended to improve memory and learning—was coined in 1972 by Romanian scientist Corneliu E. Giurgea. Today, there is a booming market for edible nootropic supplements in the form of pills, chewable tablets, and drinks, and these "smart drugs" represent over $3 billion of the $49-billion-a-year supplement industry in the United States, which is dominated by familiar names like Pfizer, Johnson and Johnson, Novartis, and those of other multinationals.[54]

There's a reason the market has experienced such rapid growth in the 21st century. In 1994, the Clinton administration passed industry-friendly federal laws that imposed minimal reporting and labeling requirements on the makers of vitamins, minerals, and herbs. The law dictates that unless the FDA can prove a particular product is unsafe, they cannot prevent companies from selling that product. Businesses must inform the FDA that they have created a dietary supplement, but the law does not require any information about what ingredients are in the product. Companies are further prohibited from claiming that their products treat specific diseases like Alzheimer's, but the lines are often blurred when claims of "memory enhancement" are made.

Over the past several decades, this deregulated landscape has unleashed a rapidly expanding market flooded with products of dubious value that promise "brain-boosting" benefits—usually focus, attention, clarity, mood, and memory.[55] For instance, a popular nutritional drink from the San Francisco–based company BrainGear—a concoction of 13 allegedly "neuron-friendly" supplements, vitamins, and amino acids—is marketed as a "brain booster shot" that is "clinically proven to optimize brain function."[56] The company positions its product, which it brands as "One Small Bottle, One Big Meal For Your Brain," as an elixir that is—somewhat incongruously—capable of both speeding up and slowing down the brain, on demand. As one advertisement says, "If you struggle with brain fog, BrainGear will help you feel clearer. Or, if you're a person who struggles with your mind racing before bed, you may notice that BrainGear helps you relax and become more balanced."[57] Of course, it's impossible not to wonder whether an actual "big meal" (perhaps a plant-based dinner shared in good company) would be exponentially better for your cognition and quality of life than a processed nutritional shot.

Another high-profile supplement has been pushed by actress Gwyneth Paltrow's controversial company Goop. Unlike the BrainGear concoction, however, Goop has developed and branded a café au lait–flavored chewable anti-"brain fog" supplement called Nerd Alert. This "synergistic blend" of caffeine and L-theanine (a compound found in green tea) is said to give consumers a "bite-size mental boost" that will make them "more effective at improving scores on tests of memory, accuracy, and attention."[58] The top-selling nootropic on Amazon, a soluble formula called Genius Consciousness, dangles an even more lofty promise, suggesting that its product both facilitates "the creation of new brain cells" and, perhaps more cosmically, "opens the mind to limitless possibilities."[59]

Yet another herbal supplement product, Alpha Brain, is endorsed by famous actor-comedian and podcast host Joe Rogan and marketed as "another gear for the brain." Most notable about this capsule product is how the company (Onnit) explicitly embraces neoliberal doctrines of individualism, self-improvement, and meritocracy. Its website conjures a societal landscape transformed by hyper-capitalist logic as it positions the supplement and customer within a ruthless marketplace of winners and losers, alphas and betas: "Competition is unavoidable. No matter how altruistic your intentions, you are competing. If you are in the corporate structure, you are competing for a promotion. If you are in the stock market, you are competing against other investors. If you run a small business, you are competing against other companies. If you are dating, you are competing against other suitors. If you are a parent, you are competing to create more time to do what you love."[60]

Of course, despite the soaring claims of nootropic marketing departments, there is insufficient evidence to recommend their use. In 2019, an evidence-based review examined current efficacy data of brain health supplements and concluded that no ingredient, product, or supplement formulation designed for brain health could be endorsed. The authors' main practical tip for consumers was that "Buying supplements to benefit your brain health is likely a waste of your money."[61] Rather than turning to supplements to boost brain health, the authors wrote, consumers would be wiser to choose dietary patterns known to support a healthy brain. Somewhat humorously, other research conducted by a San Francisco–based startup called HVMN, backed by former Yahoo CEO Marissa Mayer, found that in a clinical trial comparison, one of its best-selling nootropic supplements was less effective than a simple cup of coffee.[62]

Given the surging sales, dubious evidence, and potential for unwanted side effects, the government has begun to regulate the veritable wild west market of oral, injectable, and topical nootropics. In 2019, the FDA sent warning letters or advisories to 17 companies selling about 60 supplements with names like Cogni-Flex and Mind Ignite.[63] The warnings pointed out that the companies had touted these products as working like anti-

Alzheimer's drugs, "but naturally and without side effect," or as "clinically shown to help diseases of the brain, such as Alzheimer's." Moving forward, those companies implicated in the crackdown are required to submit applications for approval or cease making such marketing claims,[64] but their products remain on the market.[65] The stark lesson: buyer beware.

BRAIN FITNESS DIGITAL GADGETS

Adjacent to the nootropic marketplace is a booming industry of digital devices aimed at improving brain fitness. Ranging from video games and computer software to mobile phone apps and handheld devices, these commercial products make similar promises about instrumentally enhancing memory, concentration, visual and spatial skills, verbal recall, and executive function in individual users. Presently, revenue in the digital brain fitness marketplace alone is estimated at $1.98 billion and projected to grow to $8.06 billion by 2021, as global populations age.[66]

In the advertising language used in this marketplace, the word *neuro* frequently appears as a prefix for terms, such as *neuro-enhancing* or *neuro-boosting*, that focus consumer attention on how products tangibly benefit the function of a single organ—the brain.[67] Concepts such as *neuroplasticity* (the brain's capacity to rewire itself throughout life by creating neural connections in response to mental activity or some brain potion) and *cognitive*, or *neural*, *reserve* (the brain's built-up resilience to age-related pathological changes) give the impression of scientific certitude that consumer products are not only capable of improving cognitive function but are also physically reordering the brain at the molecular level, encouraging the growth of synapses and dendrites, and enhancing cognitive health, just as aerobic workouts improve pulmonary health and increase cardiovascular health (for example, *neurobics*). As with nootropic supplements, such products are often inappropriately said to be "clinically proven" to improve cognitive performance in users of all ages, while other marketing campaigns boast that their products are "designed by neuroscientists" or endorsed by medical professionals (such as the Japanese physician Ryuta Kawashima, who has given his imprimatur to the best-selling Nintendo Brain Age games, a series of puzzles and logic tests). Occasionally, more far-reaching claims will surface, such as the promise that brain fitness technology can affect the brain to the point of preventing, slowing, or reversing dementia.

This manipulative marketing language contributes to a *fetishization* of the brain that renders the three-pound organ in our heads an atomized object in itself. Rather than being understood as one of many vulnerable organs within an intricate biological system that exists within layered and overlapping environments and societal structures (households, neighborhoods, communities, political-economic systems, built environments, and natural ecosystems), the brain is perceived as a decontextualized, privileged entity that healthy monadic individuals in competitive jobs and elite universities or in the latter stages of life must constantly stimulate, rewire, rebuild, nurture, and attend to via enlightened consumerism if they are to maintain normative soundness of mind and selfhood. Mass marketing slogans, such as "Give your brain the workout it needs!"[68] (Nintendo Brain Age) and "Flex your brain the fun way!"[69] (Big Brain Academy) allude to the rather demanding relationship these technological products instantiate between users and their brains. Posit Science, a leading software company, has even suggested to potential consumers in its advertisements that, in return for playing brain fitness games, "Your brain will thank you"—a slogan that personifies the brain as a separate entity from the user altogether! Mirroring the neoliberalism-inflected marketing pitches of herbal supplements, a highly downloaded app called Elevate promises users that it will "boost productivity, earning power and self-confidence."[70]

In placing a preponderance of focus on atomized *individuals* optimizing their brains and its many functions to better position themselves on a trajectory of successful aging and cognitive performance (within a ruthlessly competitive marketplace and meritocracy), the objects of the brain fitness industry clearly embody the neoliberal faith in the capacity of science, technology, and markets to deliver fantastical innovations that contribute to human well-being, as well as a deep belief in the ethos of self-help, self-improvement, self-care, and lifestyle change. Being expressly designed around the neoliberal doctrine of self-actualization through individual consumption, this generation of products tends to ignore the importance of collective community needs, shared risk factors, and the interdependence and shared destiny of our species.

Indeed, the very nature of modern brain fitness products has been *physically shaped* by the ideologies of the modern zombified marketplace. While some products may feature and encourage multiperson functionality, many are sold in single units and marketed for individual consumption on personal computers, individual video-game consoles, PDA-like devices, or mobile phones. Although some long-term care facilities and other organizations such as hospitals and schools have purchased multiple copies of programs and are beginning to foster interaction through peer collaboration, and some emerging web-based products are designed to encourage social networking, brain fitness products themselves have dictated that brain healthy activities generally occur during private, sedentary moments in the seclusion of one's home rather than in the context of interpersonal interaction. The prevailing meaning conveyed by marketing departments is that when consumers use products in a disciplined manner, they can enhance their neural pathways, thereby perfecting themselves from the molecular level outward and, in doing so, slowing or preventing the encroachment of neurodegeneration. The Nintendo Brain Age slogan has promised that users will be "getting the most out of [their] prefrontal cortex,"[71] even though, ironically, users might ultimately get the best out of this brain area responsible for executive functions (such as decision making) by more carefully evaluating their purchasing habits and outsmarting the marketing machinations of Madison Avenue!

Beneath the glossy sheen of modern marketing, what is most concerning is that, like nootropics, empirical support for the efficacy of brain fitness devices in meaningfully improving cognition is generally insufficient. Relatively few products have been rigorously evaluated or reported in peer-reviewed journals, and existing studies have failed to establish clinical or practical benefit for prevention of cognitive decline and dementia.[72,73,74] Consumers of digital brain fitness games and training programs may marginally improve at the games or tasks themselves, but—despite some small positive signals[75]—such benefits have not yet definitively shown that they can extend to global cognition, everyday tasks, or quality of life.[76] The technologies may offer more profound benefits for acute recovery from conditions like stroke and brain injury, and video games like flight simulators do transfer practical knowledge and skills into capabilities and real work.

Experts have felt growing concern about the excesses of marketing departments. In 2014, nearly 70 scientists cosigned a consensus statement through the Stanford Center on Longevity, concluding, "We object to the claim that brain games offer consumers a scientifically grounded avenue to reduce or reverse cognitive decline when there is no compelling scientific evidence to date that they do. The promise of a magic bullet detracts from the best evidence to date, which is that cognitive health in old age reflects the long-term effects of healthy, engaged lifestyles. In [our] judgment . . . exaggerated and misleading claims exploit the anxieties of older adults about impending cognitive decline. We encourage continued careful research and validation in this field."[77]

Given this absence of evidence, companies have been called to task for misleading marketing. For instance, in 2016, Lumosity, the company that unleashed the online zombie ads on us several years ago and that has accumulated 100 million users since 2007, reached a $2 million settlement (allegedly reduced from a larger $50 million fine originally suggested) with the US Federal Trade Commission (FTC) for making unsupported claims that its products helped users perform better at work and in school and reduce or delay cognitive impairment.[78] "Lumosity preyed on consumers' fears about age-related cognitive decline, suggesting their games could stave off memory loss, dementia, and even Alzheimer's disease," wrote Jessica Rich, director of the FTC's Bureau of Consumer Protection. "But Lumosity simply did not have the science to back up its ads."[79] As long as evidence remains lacking, the industry's claims should be viewed as the unwarranted hype of marketing departments rather than genuine hope earned through robust scientific inquiry.

In general, a good antidote to industry marketing is asking about the deeper and broader aspects of brain health. For instance, how should brain health activities relate to one's life purpose? How can brain-friendly activities be made social, undertaken with other purposeful people? How might such activities even support our legacy after we pass on? As others have suggested, it is also useful to conceive of digital products as *games* rather than *medical interventions*.[80] For those looking to stay apprised of the industry, the independent market research team Sharp Brains has generally done a comprehensive job consolidating information on emerging digital brain fitness products and retaining a critical edge, although they are not always adequately skeptical about their potential.[81]

PERSONALIZED PLANS TO "END ALZHEIMER'S"

There has been another recent phenomenon of researcher-entrepreneurs hawking "personalized plans" to prevent or reverse cognitive decline. Dale

Bredesen, a doctor at UCLA, has conducted very preliminary (though widely publicized) research claiming to find that multifaceted prevention strategies may produce functional improvement for people with memory loss (Alzheimer's, MCI, and SCI). Bredesen's embrace of the multifactorial, heterogeneous, age-entangled nature of Alzheimer's disease(s) and recommendation of multifaceted prevention strategies is perhaps a positive direction for him, particularly because early in his career he was predicting a rapid cure. But ultimately, he has parlayed his preliminary research demonstrating some positive signals into yet another commodified, revenue-generating product in the marketplace of memory.

In addition to his best-selling book (*The End of Alzheimer's*), Bredesen developed a trademarked functional medicine-type "protocol" that retails at $75 a month and entails getting regular blood tests to track markers such as insulin resistance and inflammation, as well as following a low-carb, high-fat diet, intermittent fasting, and supplement regimen. It is suggested that this protocol be preceded by a so-called ReCODE report (retailing at $1,399), which covers assessments, blood labs, and genome tests prepared by a certified ReCODE practitioner.[82] With "data" in hand, Bredesen's company uses a computer-based algorithm to provide granular analysis of an individual's problem and recommend a personalized, targeted approach to reverse cognitive decline. Much of the advice that Bredesen sells about diet and exercise has support from science, and the information is available for free, but the specific money-making aspects of his and other such efforts are not.

Like the panoply of products in the marketplace of memory, Bredesen's personalized treatment approach is fundamentally limited by its focus on the individual consumer, catering to the rarefied few with the disposable income to aggressively treat themselves with what are, ultimately, mostly common-sense interventions that people should be doing anyway (for example, healthy diet, exercise, and mental stimulation). Like supplements, nootropics, digital technologies, and the like, Bredesen's product is inspired by a hyper-capitalist calculus: one must establish an intellectual property position (own a patent, copyright, or trademark) to make money. It is more difficult to lay claim and potentially profit from something entangled with the common good, and interventions to improve population health and the circumstances in which we all live and age are distinctly noncommodifiable. Again, to move beyond the confines of the American dementia era, we urge a higher moral charge: for you to think about not only personalized prevention strategies and rituals of consumer-based self-care within markets but also about what must be done at the level of population and local community health to support healthy brain aging for the many, not the few.[83]

GOING BEYOND THE BRAIN HEALTH MARKETPLACE

Ultimately, the reductive mentality that consumption of commercial goods can forestall the heterogeneous, multifactorial, age-entangled processes of brain aging that occur across the life course—a mentality that has hitherto driven the development of failed pharmaceuticals—is now increasingly being projected onto new breeds of technological products heavily advertised to aging members of society in the hope of cultivating new markets. The consequence of reductive innovation fantasies, however, is that they disregard the myriad overlapping factors that influence brain health across the lifespan for all of us (such as diet, exercise, exposure to neurotoxins, psychosocial stress, formal education opportunities, access to healthcare, head injuries, and so on), to which we necessarily turn our attention in coming chapters.

Humans are not merely brains devoid of context; in fact, our brains are embedded among many other vital organs in the bodies of individual selves who are interdependent members of families, neighborhoods, local communities, national constituencies, and natural ecosystems. Manifold forces at each of these levels affect neurodegenerative processes from womb to tomb, with *cognitive health* being the emergent property resulting from the interaction of these inputs across our lives. To ignore the complex etiology of neurodegeneration, and thus to fail to frame brain aging as a public health and broader social issue, is a misapprehension fostered by a hyper-capitalist, market-focused approach to brain fitness that we aim to course correct in this book.

Advancing a broader understanding of brain health requires us to go beyond the reductive individualism and abdication of collective responsibility of the current brain health marketplace and ask how our political-economic organization can play a role in cognitive and psychosocial wellness. After all, once we accept that humans are not just discrete brains but rather intricate, interconnected beings with psychological, social, emotional, spiritual, and ecological dimensions, whose very tissue, sinew, and cells are affected by a multitude of insults over the course of our lives, it follows that our brain health activities should mirror the complexity of our nature rather than be dictated by the short-term profit-seeking organization of the marketplace.

A DIMINISHED ROLE FOR PUBLIC HEALTH

As the individualizing, market-oriented logic of neoliberalism has pervaded our public discourse around not just Alzheimer's but improving human well-being writ large, it has also stunted our thinking about public health. As the marketplace of memory embodies, when we think about strategies to improve public health, we usually seek to increase the well-being of *individuals*. If we do that millions of times over, it is believed that the health of "the public" will have become better by default. This logic is reminiscent of the old proverb: "Look after the pennies, and the dollars will follow." Indeed, former UK prime minister Tony Blair, an avowed neoliberal, gave voice to this belief while in office, when he expressed that many public health problems were "not, strictly speaking, public health problems at all. They are questions of individual lifestyle—obesity, smoking, alcohol abuse, diabetes, sexually transmitted disease . . . These are not epidemics . . . they are the result of millions of individual decisions, at millions of points in time."[84]

The consequence of this sort of thinking is that we no longer perceive the health of the public to be different from the health of many individuals multiplied. As strongly reflected in products of the marketplace of memory, the emphasis is on making as many *individual consumers* as we can healthier via personal actions within markets rather than thinking on a wider, more structural scale to make *entire populations* healthier via collective policies and actions. The practical effects of the neoliberal turn can be seen in the largely stagnant federal expenditures on public health since the seventies (figure 3.3), a dynamic that reared its ugly head in 2020 when the COVID-19 pandemic exposed America's lack of systemic institutional preparedness.

Over the last several decades, prevention of diseases like Alzheimer's has largely come to be viewed as a personal project, best pursued through particular rituals of enlightened self-care and market-based consumption that help one accrue a sort of "individual health capital" that may, over time, provide a cognitive "return on investment." Today's *neoliberal subject*

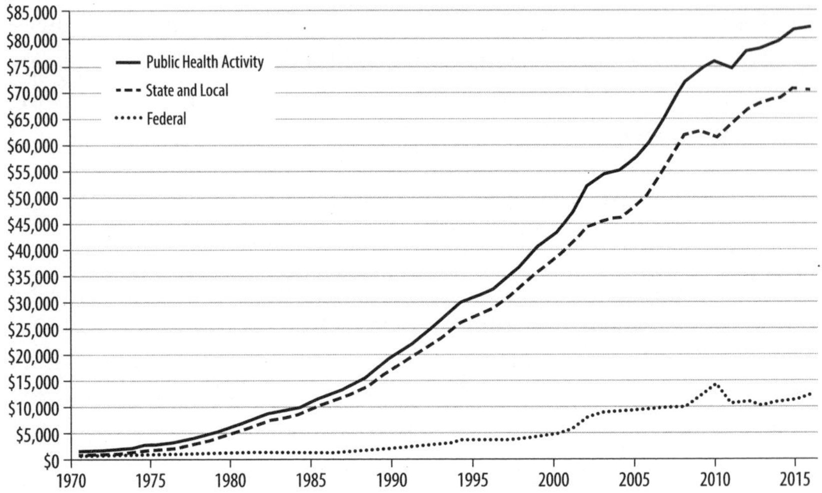

Figure 3.3. Federal expenditures on public health—represented by the lowest line on the graph—have largely plateaued over the last several decades.
Source: Adapted from "Local and Federal Expenditures on Public Health, 1970-2016," Peterson-Kaiser Health System Tracker.

is surrounded by certain manias of individualist approaches to healthy living—obsessing over diets, joining trendy gyms, riding Peloton bicycles at home, or attending CrossFit classes (and creating montages of self-care rituals on social media); counting steps on wearable devices or cellphones; learning mindfulness techniques to quell stress; choosing from an endless deluge of self-help books; and "training" our brains on expensive devices. Political leaders like Blair implore us to eat healthier and exercise more; employers link salary incentives to performance on corporate personal wellness programs;[85] even doctors are inclined to frame our health exclusively as a matter of making better decisions. We, as neoliberal subjects in the American dementia era, are empowered as the problem solvers of our own lives—the monadic maximizers of our own utility. Effectively, by setting up a proposition whereby *prevention* of Alzheimer's is a function of individual consumption habits or lifestyle choices, we *decontextualize* and *depoliticize* our health and avoid confrontation with the power structures causing harm across populations. Private Band-Aids (yoga, mindfulness meditation, step counting, and so on) are recommended as a solution for collective political-economic failures.

One of the starkest illustrations of the neoliberal imprint on our thinking about public health was a series of nearly 20 best-selling books written over the past decade by Oprah-endorsed media darlings Mehmet Oz and Michael Roizen, all with the title *You*: *You: On a Diet*, *You: Staying Young*, *You: Stress Less*, and *You: Breathing Easy*. On each book cover, a cartoon index finger juts out, Uncle Sam–like, at the reader from within the *O* in the word *YOU*, an aggressive in-your-face reminder that staying healthy was a task for *you* and *you alone*. The fetishization of individual health and self-care embodied by these books is a living monument to our era's totalizing market-fundamentalist logic—one that collapses large-scale health issues like chronic disease, stress, and aging, which are intimately interwoven with aspects of our culture and political economy, into an individualized quest for a good life through enlightened consumption. In this paradigm, poor health is a personal failing—the result of *your* maladaptive thoughts, behaviors, rituals of self-care, and insufficient participation in markets.

This cultural conditioning has over time politically neutered us and forestalled thinking about how to improve community and public health. As Margaret Lock has written with specific reference to brain health and political economy, "In the haste to find cures, less often marked is another problem, namely a shift of attention away from social, political, and environmental factors, including poverty, inequality, discrimination, and racism—factors deeply implicated in disease causation. These are the variables that thus far have received the least attention in the Alzheimer's disease world . . . [a] public health approach to aging and Alzheimer's will have a much greater effect in reducing the incidence of Alzheimer's disease worldwide than will the technologically oriented molecular approach."[86]

In correspondence with us, our colleague Carol Brayne has similarly lamented: "Although there is excellent public health research to demonstrate that, in fact, individualized health promotion is far less effective than collective action such as legislation or improved environment this approach has come to be the dominant paradigm in western societies, also exported to other parts of the world." Yet, as the world responds to the growing crisis of capitalism (and thus the global spread of American dementia) in the 2020s, a new understanding is within our grasp, and it is possible to think of public health as something more than simply the collective noun of individual health, and to treat *whole populations* as recipients of medical care via structural changes to the political economy. Elsewhere in the world, people and organizations (such as the World Health Organization, Alzheimer's Disease International,[87] and even the

Alzheimer's Association[88]) are coming around to the notion that "Alzheimer's" is *not* a single curable disease, and that our most effective means of driving down risk is by changing the political-economic structures, institutions, and policies that materially influence society-level risk factors for millions across the life course (access to basic material necessities, guaranteed healthcare and education, lead abatement, and so on).

Even in gently abandoning the notion of an absolute cure for Alzheimer's, there is hope for human beings' cognitive vitality as we age. We can create communities with more inclusive prosperity, where we support one another in humane ways, moving from an ethic of self-care to one of *other*-care. Again, social democracies provide the blueprint for such a shift. As Anu Partanen, the author of *The Nordic Theory of Everything*, has written in response to the finding mentioned in chapter 1 that Scandinavian countries are consistently rated among the "happiest" in the world: "In the U.S., there's a lot of focus on achieving happiness, but often the solution is to do more yoga or to meditate—happiness is what you make of it. For governments, happiness shouldn't be some sort of internal thing that a person has or doesn't have, or that they have to figure out for themselves. It's about helping citizens gain better quality of life."[89]

An ethic of other-care is at the heart of another possible paradigm for brain health and where we'll head in the next chapter as we examine how the most powerful "interventions" for "Alzheimer's" are to be found, not within the marketplace of memory, but rather in noncommodifiable actions we take to help everyone and thereby "treat" whole populations. Such public health–oriented approaches (providing access to physical and mental health care, ensuring housing and safe working conditions, and so forth) have dramatically improved material conditions for people for the last hundred years, and a disciplined attention to enhancing these structures and systems is where our focus must be as we pursue healthier brains in healthier societies. Fixating on the marketplace of memory and its limitless individual consumption while failing to address the broader political-economic forces that affect everyone's brains is akin to treating malaria cases without combating the mosquito population.

THE SHOCK POLITICS OF ALZHEIMER'S AND OUR ENDLESS WAR

In the face of the monumental pharmaceutical failures we've covered in the last two chapters, it is fair to ask with no small wonderment how the

Alzheimer's industry and advocacy establishment have continued driving public and private funds into drug development. The simple answer is that Robert Butler's original "politics of anguish" has proved an effective and durable long-term strategy. And yet the tactic of using a *shock politics* approach—one defined by provocative language, imagery, and rhetoric—to guide the public in thinking and acting with respect to dementia has exacted a serious human toll. Over time, it has contributed to what some term an overwhelming "tragedy discourse of dementia,"[90] which keeps us fixed on the fear and crisis of the biological scourge of Alzheimer's and has too often precluded broader and more imaginative thinking about how to adapt to the human challenges of brain aging.

Since the seventies, Alzheimer's shock politics rhetoric has been principally centered on the well-accepted crisis proposition that we are perpetually at "war" against the disease, with funding largely marshaled to "attack" amyloid. When Butler and the NIA made their intentional effort to blend the domains of an infectious (polio) and a chronic (brain-aging-related) disease through a provocative war metaphor, they launched a powerful meme that has over time crystallized into a cultural truth—that cognitive frailty was the result of a single disease process called Alzheimer's that existed outside the spectrum of normal age-related changes and could be specifically attacked and defeated. The dominant framing of a perpetual "war," amplified in the popular media, has been a major factor in driving untold billions of public and private dollars into research for decades, even in the face of continual pharmacologic failures.

Of course, the overarching "war on Alzheimer's" and the emotionally overwrought rhetoric that sustain it have also caused other forms of collateral damage. Those who bear the Alzheimer's label have shouldered the greatest cost of shock politics. All too frequently, their day-to-day existence has been depicted as that of passive victims to a disease that causes a complete and total "loss of self." Besides being factually incorrect—there are rich, life-affirming ways to preserve and support the personhood and quality of life of even those with severe cognitive loss—this rhetorical strategy has too often stigmatized and caricatured those so labeled and stripped them of their humanity. At times, it has led to deeply insulting depictions. For instance, during a NIH conference on Alzheimer's in 2010, one high-powered representative of the Alzheimer's Association went so far as to evoke zombie imagery in describing the plight of people with dementia: "We are going to see in most of the cities in the world demented people wandering the streets because there is simply no place to put them, no way to prevent their dementia from occurring, and that's going to be a public health disaster that we just can't face up to."[91]

These sorts of eldritch guiding images of people with dementia as an oncoming zombified horde threatening economic growth proliferate not just in the United States but across cultures.[92] In 2009, the French Alzheimer's Association produced a series of vignettes about Alzheimer's for national television. The film grimly depicts several "Alzheimer's victims" in varying states of haunted disorientation. One woman wanders through the streets of a sketchy neighborhood alone in her nightgown; a man unwittingly scoops spoonfuls of canned dog food into his mouth; another woman stares numbly at the wall with no recognition that her head bears a gruesome wound from a recent fall; elsewhere, an addled pensioner fulminates at his aggrieved grandchildren. Last, but not least, a doddering woman squats to urinate in a grocery store aisle.[93]

Such "shocking" tropes may be rhetorically useful in sustaining the war on Alzheimer's and the influx of funds in the modern marketplace of memory, but their iterative use across cultures has advanced a persistent stereotype that is deeply alienating, dehumanizing, and damaging. In accentuating and thereby leveraging the most extreme abhorrent aspects of the dementia experience to "sell Alzheimer's," such imagery propagates the reductive narrative that dementia is a dread condition that uniformly ravages selfhood and reduces individuals to undignified shells of themselves. Through such depictions, we are made to observe poor, deteriorating souls with horror and shame rather than with empathy and common humanity, and we can scarce imagine such "victims"—much less their families, caregivers, and support systems—continuing to grow, develop, or have any meaningful role in society.

Christine Bryden, an author and advocate who has been writing about living with an atypically slow dementia for over a decade, has captured this tension: "The stereotype tugs at the heartstrings and loosens the purse strings, so it is used in seeking funds for research, support, and services. It's a Catch-22, because [organizations] promote our image as nonpersons and make the stigma worse."[94] Advocates in France were even more forceful in their opposition to the aforementioned vignettes and sent a letter to the president of their Alzheimer's Association in protest of the commercial, which resulted in its removal. They wrote:

> You probably hope to help increase the resources allocated to research, but in reality, you have aroused fear, you further isolate these people and can thus hinder any attempt to integrate them (including an intergenerational perspective) to develop them and ultimately to help them. Instead of presenting a simplistic vision of apocalyptic Alzheimer's disease . . . your association should rather encourage the public to think otherwise [about] Alzheimer's disease, to consider that brain aging may be expressed in many forms, more or less problematic, and depend on many factors, understand that in addition to drugs, there are many other means of prevention and intervention (psychological and social) and finally to realize that, even in the most problematic expressions of aging, people retain their humanity. It is high time to tell another story of Alzheimer's disease and your organization should contribute.[95]

Yet another technique of Alzheimer's shock politics has been to emphasize the enormous "burden" caused by the disease, both for caregivers and for society at large. Here, the apocalyptic tropes tend to shift from shambling zombie-like elders who are a drag on the economy to imagery of demographic tidal waves, silver tsunamis, and other natural disasters that visit great suffering on human societies. For instance, Newt Gingrich wrote in his book *Winning the Future*, "The cost of treating Alzheimer's will make Katrina look like a bargain . . . We have to act now while the storm clouds are still on the horizon."[96] Again, such "shocking" rhetoric further builds fear of the disease and antagonism toward those who are affected by cognitive challenges. Aging populations come to be analogized to one of the most catastrophic natural disasters to make landfall on our soil. Such depictions have a human toll. Indeed, Alzheimer's is consistently rated by the public as one of society's most feared illnesses, without any cure or effective treatment on the horizon. Due to this fear, it is not uncommon to see stories of people diagnosed with Alzheimer's preemptively embracing suicide.[97]

Such a cultural narrative also fixes us in perpetual war against a disease that, as we know, may not be amenable to a cure. Since the seventies, military metaphors have seeped into our understanding of the syndrome of Alzheimer's, where in the absence of specific pathogens, they are perhaps even more deleterious than in the realm of infectious disease.[98] Metaphor is such a pervasive tendency in human thought and speech that researchers have established that we utter one metaphor for every 10 to 25 words, or about six metaphors a minute.[99] This holds true in medicine and public health, wherein our prevalent, ever-evolving metaphors of disease have the social power to position people and resources within a culture and affect us biopsychosocially. Achieving moral transformation around Alzheimer's and brain health will require many changes, and key among them is being more mindful of the moral failings interred in the strategic metaphors, speech, and thought-patterns that have predominated since the neoliberal turn and the unfolding of the "politics of anguish" strategy in the seventies, which are in our power to challenge and correct. A major form of resistance must be the tendencies we have to dehumanize people with dementia and reduce them to "diseased bodies"—a theme to which we return in future chapters.

CONCLUSION

The last two chapters have shown how we've gone from one case of Alzheimer's (Auguste D.) to a "global crisis," with hundreds of millions or more affected by something that is impairing cognition. This is a critical time to reflect honestly on what we have learned in the last several decades of research—even if those truths are inconvenient. The primary lesson is that Alzheimer's disease(s) encompasses many illnesses that combine to cause many forms of dementia—ultimately, the label is an umbrella term for many age-related processes that has fundamentally been miscast to the public as a singular disease separate from aging.

While we would obviously like to see a cure to ameliorate suffering for many millions of people affected by memory loss and the families who support and care for them, the market has failed to deliver even a modest treatment, and there remain fundamental challenges with the very possibility of a cure or effective preventive commodity. We continue to be uncomfortable with the unrealistic expectations and hype, and the many ways our cultural understanding of dementia has been warped by neoliberalism and its zombie economy, with market forces shifting focus to the individual and to biotechnology rather than to the collective good, and sowing fear and dehumanization in our public understanding of brain aging for material gain rather than solidarity and compassion.

As we discuss in the next chapter, *we can choose a better path*, one that embraces social democratic reordering, public health initiatives, and other humane, generationally minded actions that can act on social determinants of health, reducing vascular risk factors, modulating oxidative stress and inflammation, protecting against traumatic brain injuries, promoting social engagement and lifelong learning, reducing exposure to neurotoxins, and encouraging generative social relationships. These postmarket approaches will shift the conversation away from the dominance of the neoliberal paradigm of Alzheimer's and have larger repercussions than any drug, supplement, or device in the marketplace of memory.

4

Treating Populations

Collectively Strengthening the Brain Health of the Many, Not the Few

In mid-November 2016, as the world was calibrating to the reality of celebrity mogul Donald J. Trump becoming president-elect, the Alzheimer's field was rocked by two landmark studies. First, the antiamyloid drug solanezumab, which had, for years, been hyped by the pharmaceutical company Eli Lilly and its baptist proponents as the long-awaited pharmaceutical innovation to reverse memory loss, was announced to have failed in its latest trial. Later that week, as the dust was settling from the solanezumab disappointment, a major study in the prominent medical journal *JAMA Internal Medicine* published findings showing that the rate of dementia for people over age 65 had actually been *dropping* in the United States over the past decade—from 11.6 percent in 2000 to 8.8 percent in 2012.[1] While such a trend had been detected before,[2,3,4] this study was robust, drawing data from a nationally representative sample.

As Trump spent the rest of November traversing the American heartland on his victory tour, having won on a populist platform critical of unfettered global capitalism and heralding a return to greatness for hard-luck citizens, the paradoxical story conveyed by these two studies— "Drug fails . . . *but* dementia rates drop!"—also percolated in front-page headlines. Such a narrative powerfully countered the usual shock politics warning of the coming "tsunami" of dementia destined to drown us in societal expense in the absence of a pharmacologic fix for Alzheimer's. In this chapter, we explore what might be going on with this surprising twist in the (literal and figurative) story of American dementia, and what critical wisdom the research offers us as we pursue healthier brains in healthier societies.

A POPULATION REVELATION

In fact, dementia rates have been falling not just in the United States, but also in a host of developed Western countries: Sweden,[5] the Netherlands,[6] the United Kingdom,[7] Canada,[8] and France.[9] While *overall* numbers of people affected by dementia continue to rise in these nations—as we would expect, given the growing population of aging individuals who are living longer—there has been a general *decline* in both dementia incidence (the number of people diagnosed per year) and prevalence (the number of people diagnosed relative to the total number of people in the population) over the past four decades.[10,11]

In other words, this unexpected "population revelation" in the United States and western Europe appears to be showing us that in a growing number of countries, the real risk of elder citizens developing dementia in their lifetimes is *decreasing*. Just how much? A 2020 study[12] that aggregated all available data from those regions between 1988 and 2015 calculated that the incidence rate of dementia has been consistently declining by 13% per calendar decade (with risk for developing clinical Alzheimer's also falling by 16% per decade). In practical terms, this means that the risk of someone developing dementia in 2021 is 13% lower than it was in 2011. As our colleague Ken Langa, a researcher at the University of Michigan and lead author of the 2016 *JAMA Internal Medicine* study, told us: "The idea that there's been a decrease in dementia risk in high-income countries is well accepted now. This is a real trend—it's impossible not to at least acknowledge the consistency in these studies."

While this unforeseen phenomenon has hugely exciting public health ramifications, the findings have gone underreported and underdiscussed because they simply don't fit our normal "politics of anguish" scripts about what should be *expected* to drive dementia rates down. After all, the drug, supplement, and biotech companies competing in the marketplace of memory haven't yet produced a pill, potion, or product—how could we possibly be scoring such remarkable victories against dementia?

To properly wrap our minds around what might be going on in the population revelation studies in the United States and elsewhere, it is necessary to depart from the 21st century, put on our anthropologist hats, and take a broad evolutionary perspective on human health that will ultimately lead us back to the 2020s.

TREATING POPULATIONS: THE LIMITS OF TECHNOLOGY AND THE POWER OF REDUCING SOCIETAL INEQUALITIES

Biomedical technologies (surgeries, drugs, vaccines, and so forth) have made an important contribution to health in contemporary civilization. In the long sweep of human history, however, medical technological advancement has had relatively little influence on our collective health—a tragic irony given just how dominant the market-based search for new biomedical technologies has become in the modern quest for better health and cures to medicalized illnesses like Alzheimer's.

When we extricate ourselves from the innovation fantasies of neoliberalism and take a deeper evolutionary perspective, it becomes apparent that the most fundamental factors influencing health outcomes across human history—and especially in the last hundred years—have been changes in political-economic organization that have profoundly reduced inequality and universalized access to health-promoting services, programs, resources, and infrastructure. Stepping back and considering the longer evolutionary view will help us understand the population revelation studies from the United States and western Europe in proper context, and perhaps also appreciate why aforementioned movements like Occupy Wall Street, which have interrogated deep societal inequality, were responding to something much more fundamental to our nature. Let's explore that very nature.

The Complexities of Human Nature

For two million years—essentially 99% of our species history—our human forebears, including anatomically modern humans who emerged between 200,000 and 300,000 years ago—evolved in tightly knit hunter-gatherer societies that anthropologists refer to as *egalitarian*. In such societies, which have existed on every continent and across nearly all ecological niches, inhabitants forage, hunt, and gather foods, sharing resources without formal notions of private property. Given the frequent movement of hunter-gatherer groups, it is logistically difficult to store food, wealth, or accumulated possessions. Thus, the very nature of egalitarian societies has tended to preclude major hierarchies of disparate wealth, social status, and power, and hunter-gatherer bands have generally (if imperfectly[13]) been organized around norms of mutual fairness, reciprocity, empathy, social intelligence, ad-hoc decision-making, and cooperation. For thousands of generations, this form of social organization created long-term political conditions that were favorable to the natural selection of altruistic traits in human beings.[14,15] In fact, social scientists still identify egalitarian and altruistic norms as being strongly reflected in the foundational stories and myths of the few modern hunter-gatherer societies that remain today.[16]

That said, it is easy to fall into a trap of romanticizing hunter-gatherers and exaggerating what we can know with certainty about their social organization. As anthropologists have argued, however, hunting-and-gathering egalitarian societies are believed to have evolved as a response to a deeper, more primal tendency toward hierarchy and social dominance, which we see powerfully reflected in our closest primate ancestors (chimpanzees and gorillas). Given this natural inclination to form social dominance hierarchies,[17] our hunter-gatherer forebears developed complex sanctioning strategies deliberately intended to prevent abuses of power and excessive inequity in resource distribution. Upstarts who sought undue power over others, failed to share resources (for instance, distribution of meat from a hunt), or otherwise transgressed against egalitarian values would be subject to unified forms of resistance from subordinates, which spanned shaming, humiliation, ridicule, ostracism, and, even in rare cases, executions. Such governance strategies were an early form of "checks and balances" that limited the political power of would-be alphas and ensured equitable distribution of resources within small human bands living in ever-tenuous circumstances. Throughout the long arc of human evolution, a unified, politically vigilant moral community acting in defense of altruistic values has been our most formidable check on abuse of power and inequity.

While a full accounting of human nature is beyond the scope of this book, an honest assessment *must* acknowledge that we have within us the contradictory impulses of (1) hierarchy, born of our ancient mammalian and primate past; and (2) egalitarian social governance, a more recent and cognitively complex development of leveling mechanisms to curtail or counterbalance our hierarchical tendencies.[18] Put otherwise, both hierarchy and egalitarianism are arguably conditions of humanity that inhere in all of us, just as they did our Paleolithic ancestors who assiduously sought to organize their social lives around the latter.[19]

The Dawn of Civilization: Tilting toward Hierarchy

Egalitarian hunting and gathering was the dominant form of social organization for human beings until quite recently—roughly 12,000 years ago, when humans in the Neolithic era gradually began transitioning to agricultural communities.[20] Embracing an agrarian way of life—cultivating food in situ rather than locating it via foraging and hunting—fundamentally disrupted the long-standing egalitarian governance structure of hunting-and-gathering communities—most substantially by creating the possibility for disproportionate accumulation of private property (farmed and stored foods, established territories, and so on) as well as objects of symbolic wealth (such as jewelry and textiles). This tectonic shift in human relations began allowing individuals within emerging agrarian groups to acquire proportionally greater resources and status than others, for the first time imposing differing economic "ranks" on members of settlements. Eventually, the trend toward social stratification, class, and hierarchy in early agrarian civilizations produced the phenomenon of centralized leadership (chiefs, for example).

Around 5,000 years ago, early settlements began expanding from agrarian outposts into more powerful centralized "states" in different world regions—the Middle East, Egypt, China, India, Sub-Saharan Africa, Peru, and Mexico. These civilizations offered a basic proposition straight out of *Game of Thrones*: the elite with excess wealth, resources, and power would provide walls, basic security, and services to inhabitants in exchange for tithes, taxes, and consented sovereignty. Over time, these powerful hierarchical civilizations grew into empires, absorbing and reducing remaining egalitarian societies—only a small number of which have persisted until the 21st century. In the last 300 years, industrialization and globalization have further centralized hierarchical state bureaucracies and led to the formation of modern nation-states. Now, 195 nations exist, and some, like the United States, stretch across whole continents and over vast oceans, integrating diverse peoples into the same political-economic "communities," which are highly stratified.

Civilization's Three Public Health Disasters

Civilization has no doubt been a remarkable achievement for our species. Yet, increasingly, scholars like Yuval Noah Harari and Jared Diamond have taken to referring to the agriculture-based societies that emerged around 12,000 years ago, at the dawn of the Neolithic age, not as a great leap forward for humanity but rather as "history's biggest fraud"[21] and "the worst mistake in the history of the human race."[22] This is because the relatively recent manner of human reorganization in agrarian societies has, by contravening several million years of human evolution exclusively defined by egalitarian social arrangements, imposed several public health disasters on human beings in civil societies that are still affecting us today. Here, the term *disaster* takes on somewhat different connotations than normal—less a sudden catastrophic event than gradual changes in the practices of our species that have produced long-term unforeseen health consequences.

The first disaster has been *agriculture itself*. While agrarian methods and technologies have enlarged sums of food available to humans and contributed to a global population explosion into the billions, this hasn't necessarily translated to better diets or quality of life. Instead, the forced reliance on a few staple crops (relative to the smaller-scaled but highly diverse diets of hunter-gatherers) has, over the last 12,000 years, made humans more susceptible to micronutrient deficiencies, famine due to drought and crop disease, sedentary lifestyles as a result of harvest seasonality, warfare and violence stemming from competition over scarce resources, injuries due to the physical toil of farming, epidemics emerging from close contact with domesticated animals, and disparities in access to resources. Even in today's age of commercial abundance, we suffer from diets lacking in diversity as well as sedentary modes of living that make us less healthy than our ancestors, who foraged daily for their sustenance and largely shared the fruits of their collective labor.

The second disaster imposed by civilization has been *urbanization*. As cities have grown from agricultural outposts into crowded urban spaces, our species has no doubt benefited from the mass concentration of resources and rich opportunities for cultural creativity, innovation, and exchange. But so too has urbanization imposed severe ecological and social consequences, with humans in the agricultural era experiencing an explosion in the spread of deadly infectious disease, increased virulence of deadly epidemics (particularly those that cross over from animals to humans, as has been made all too real during the COVID-19 pandemic), and susceptibility to illnesses born of poor hygiene and sanitation and exacerbated by inadequate nutrition. Accordingly, archaeological evidence consistently demonstrates the physical cost of these cooccurring disasters: not only do skeletons of our agricultural ancestors show more markers of malnutrition, biologic stress, and epidemic disease than hunter-gatherer specimens, they are, on the whole, smaller in stature.[23]

But perhaps the most damaging public health disaster imposed on human communities by agriculture-based civilization—and the one most relevant to our consideration of Alzheimer's disease(s) and the population revelation studies—has been *class-based inequalities*. The reality that a lower socioeconomic position within a hierarchical society is linked with poorer health outcomes and shorter lifespans is as true now as it was when our ancestors began building walls and canals around early settlements. This historical rule governing 12,000 years of human civilization, however, was remarkably disrupted in the mid-20th century, when people in industrialized countries began experiencing gains in human health, stature, and longevity.

Such benefits were not the product of technology alone but rather the outgrowth of uniquely reorganized political-economic circumstances that emerged in the wake of the crisis of the Great Depression and two world wars. Those collective traumas gave rise to the dominance of more egalitarian governance strategies (such as Keynesian social democracy), which traced a philosophical through line back to our hunter-gatherer societies and potentiated major state investments in public health, economic growth, and a more inclusive prosperity through managed capitalism. By gradually providing national public health infrastructure (sanitation, nutrition, and medicine) that protected people from disease and infection; using progressive taxation to more evenly distribute wealth and resources throughout society, including through social welfare states that provide universal services (healthcare, education, access to nutritious foods, and so forth) to people regardless of social position; setting up programs like guaranteed minimum wages, national pension systems (social security), jobs programs, and labor protections for all citizens; and reducing overall environmental exposures, industrialized nations of the 20th century effectively mobilized resources to *treat whole populations* across the lifespan. Such initiatives included—albeit imperfectly—members of vulnerable low-status groups who had been excluded from economic and social benefits.[24]

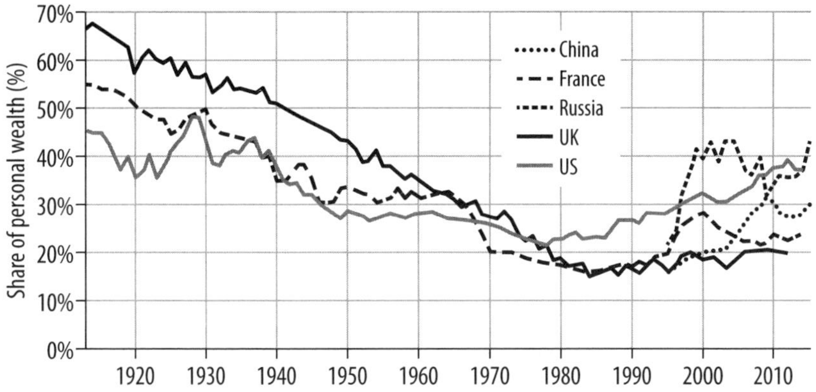

Figure 4.1. Post–Great Depression efforts to reduce wealth inequality through more egalitarian governance strategies produced greater equality in the industrialized world in the mid-20th century, but neoliberal policies have reversed the trend, shifting resources back to the 1%.
Source: Facundo Alvaredo, Lucas Chancel, Thomas Piketty, Emmanuel Saez, and Gabriel Zucman, eds., *World Inequality Report 2018* (Cambridge, MA: Belknap Press, 2018), https://wir2018.wid.world/.

Reverse engineering governance to be more egalitarian and to embrace direct responsibility for collective well-being during this "age of (relative) equality" not only resulted in 20th-century citizens living longer, but also reduced poverty and compressed class-based wealth inequalities born of unfettered capitalism (figure 4.1). These shifts in political-economic organization produced twentyfold increases in real incomes, creating a burgeoning middle class in Western countries[25] and providing a basic standard of living for many citizens, including Americans, that effectively reversed the trends toward diminished human health observed since the advent of agricultural civilization. The lesson: while it is perhaps true that humans cannot help but live with some form of hierarchy, we *can* structure our hierarchies—today in the form of the postwar nation-state—in more egalitarian ways that limit the disproportionate power and resources of the elite, while setting up institutions that reinforce our altruistic impulses and innate tendency to help one another and ensure that the *whole group* does well.[26]

The Festering Disaster of Inequality in Our Neoliberal Era

Despite the clear gains of last century, in the hyper-capitalist era, we have again begun drifting away from the historical wisdom that *pervasive*

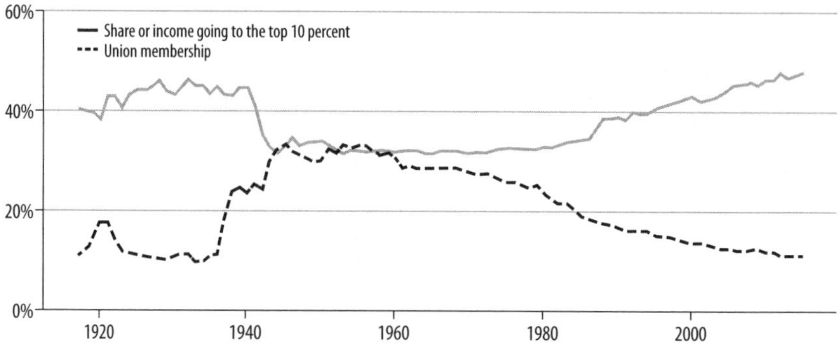

Figure 4.2. As union membership declined from 1917 to 2015, a greater share of income went to the top 10% in the United States. Simply put: when workers have more organizational leverage, there is less income inequality.
Source: Adapted from Economic Policy Institute, "Top Charts of 2017," December 21, 2017.

inequality is itself a public health disaster. In the United States and elsewhere the safety net of the modern social democratic welfare state began to be stripped away in the seventies and has continued apace in the decades to follow. Labor regulations, wage policies, and union membership that protected workers have been rolled back (figure 4.2); progressive taxation has been reversed; and funding for public education and other social welfare programs severely reduced.

Neoliberal political-economic reordering from the Carter administration forward succeeded in gradually privatizing public goods, eliminating and neutering regulations, and creating unencumbered markets to replace the state's role in addressing social problems (for example, vouchers and charter schools, carbon trade exchanges). As public capital—funds traditionally devoted by the state to "treat populations" with programs and infrastructure, which so effectively delivered profound societal gains in health in the 20th century—has fallen in rich countries like the United States during the market-fundamentalist era,[27] private capital hoarded in the hands of a wealthy few has grown (figure 4.3).

So unleashed by the implementation of the policy framework of the four D's, the "beast" of the global free market has done massive systemic damage, tilting us back to pernicious levels of hierarchy and inequality surpassing the Gilded Age. Since the eighties, annual income has expanded by 205% for the richest 1% of the population and by 636% for the top 0.001%, while the average annual wage of the bottom 50% has

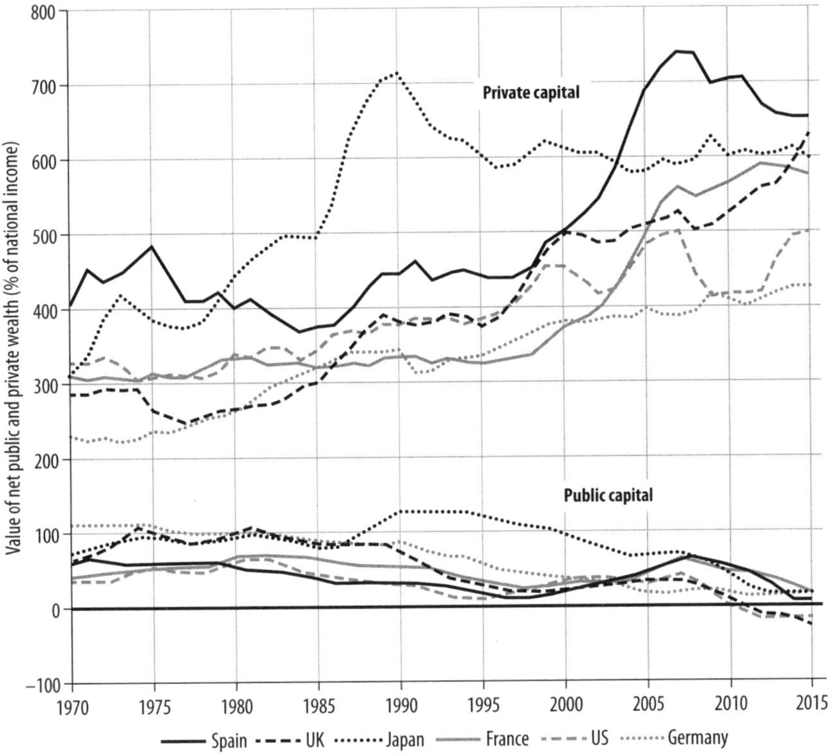

Figure 4.3. The rise of private capital and the fall of public capital in rich countries, 1970-2016.

Source: Adapted from Facundo Alvaredo, Lucas Chancel, Thomas Piketty, Emmanuel Saez, and Gabriel Zucman, eds., *World Inequality Report 2018* (Cambridge, MA: Belknap Press, 2018), https://wir2018.wid.world/.

stagnated, rendering income growth nonexistent for a generation.[28] Consequently, we live in an age of historic income and wealth inequality, when the billionaire class grows while the middle class shrinks, and when the top one-tenth of 1% of the population owns more wealth than the bottom 90%[29] (figure 4.4) and pockets over 80% of the wealth generated annually around the globe,[30] on track to own two-thirds of all wealth by 2030.

This new hyper–Gilded Age has ushered in an era when CEOs of American companies receive well over 500 times the pay of average employees, and three billionaires own more wealth than the 160 million poorest Americans combined.[31] As of 2020, the wealthiest of those billionaires, Amazon CEO Jeff Bezos, had more than $165 billion in personal wealth, on track to become the world's first trillionaire while 32% of

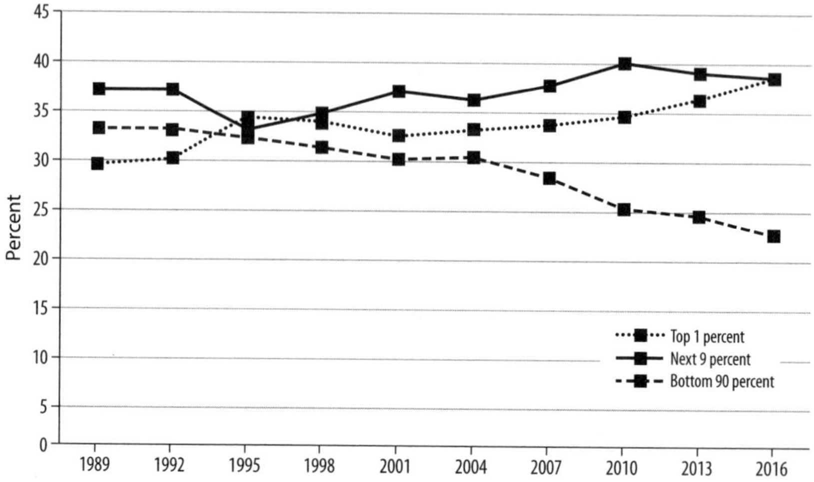

Figure 4.4. Wealth shares by wealth percentile from 1989 to 2016 show how the top 10% have come to own greater wealth than the bottom 90%.
Source: Adapted with permission from the US Federal Reserve.

children[32] (38% of black children) in his home country were living below the poverty line. In a grotesque arrangement that would have likely shocked and horrified our hunter-gatherer forebears, Bezos makes more money every 60 seconds than normal American households earn in a year.[33] Indeed, ours is an age when modern neoliberal governments have allowed rising ranks of millionaires, billionaires, and multinational corporations to brazenly evade taxes and horde unimaginable wealth—perhaps as much as $32 trillion—in tax avoidance schemes, while 1.5 million Americans are living in *extreme* poverty;[34,35] an age when even the International Monetary Fund, echoing the egalitarian, antihierarchical rallying cry of Occupy Wall Street protestors from Zuccotti Park, suggests that market fundamentalism has been "oversold" and that Western governments should force the top 1% of earners to pay more tax to reduce increasingly dangerous levels of inequality.

There is little wonder that aforementioned stories like *Game of Thrones* so captivated viewers in the early 21st century. While set in an imagined medieval world, the show held a mirror up to a society similarly defined by hierarchy, festering inequality, and unjust rule by a privileged, self-serving, and venal elite.

Inequality's Toxic Toll on Our Health

While thinking anthropologically about inequality in deep evolutionary terms is helpful, we also need to understand the health-related devastation that such deep-seated disparities sow in modern societies. In epidemiologists Richard G. Wilkinson and Kate Pickett's book *The Spirit Level*, they used data from the United Nations to show that life expectancy and infant mortality rates are consistently worse in countries with high levels of income inequality. Drilling deep into the data, they evaluated eleven different health and social problems—physical health, mental health, drug abuse, education, imprisonment, obesity, social mobility, trust and community life, violence, teenage pregnancies, and child well-being—finding that overall population outcomes were significantly worse in more unequal countries in *every category*, regardless of the overall economic well-being of those countries (such as their GDP). Looking just at the United States, they found that the same patterns held true: social and health problems were significantly overrepresented in states riven by greater inequality. Given the larger evolutionary context described above, such contemporary findings born of the unfortunate petri dish of historically unequal modern societies should hardly be surprising.

In recent years, researchers have also observed a deeply troubling decline in life expectancy in the United States driven by a surge in "deaths of despair" from suicide, accidental poisonings, addiction, and alcoholism (figure 4.5). This increase in mortality has disproportionately affected poor, uneducated, working-class white citizens who entered the labor market in the eighties, and whose lives have been degraded by aspects of the neoliberal turn (global trade deals, loss of stable manufacturing and mining jobs, low union density, stagnant wages, a stripping away of social services, and so on).[36] As untrammeled globalization has sown disparity, austerity, and precarity, hollowing out small towns across the heartland, into the void has come despondency, opioids, and death. We are losing an estimated 150,000 Americans a year to despair-related deaths.[37] Perhaps unsurprisingly, emerging research[38,39,40,41,42] is showing that rising midlife death rates, among people aged 25 to 64, actually extend across racial, ethnic, and gender lines, as well as into cities and suburbs, although a higher burden remains in the industrial Midwest and Appalachia, where

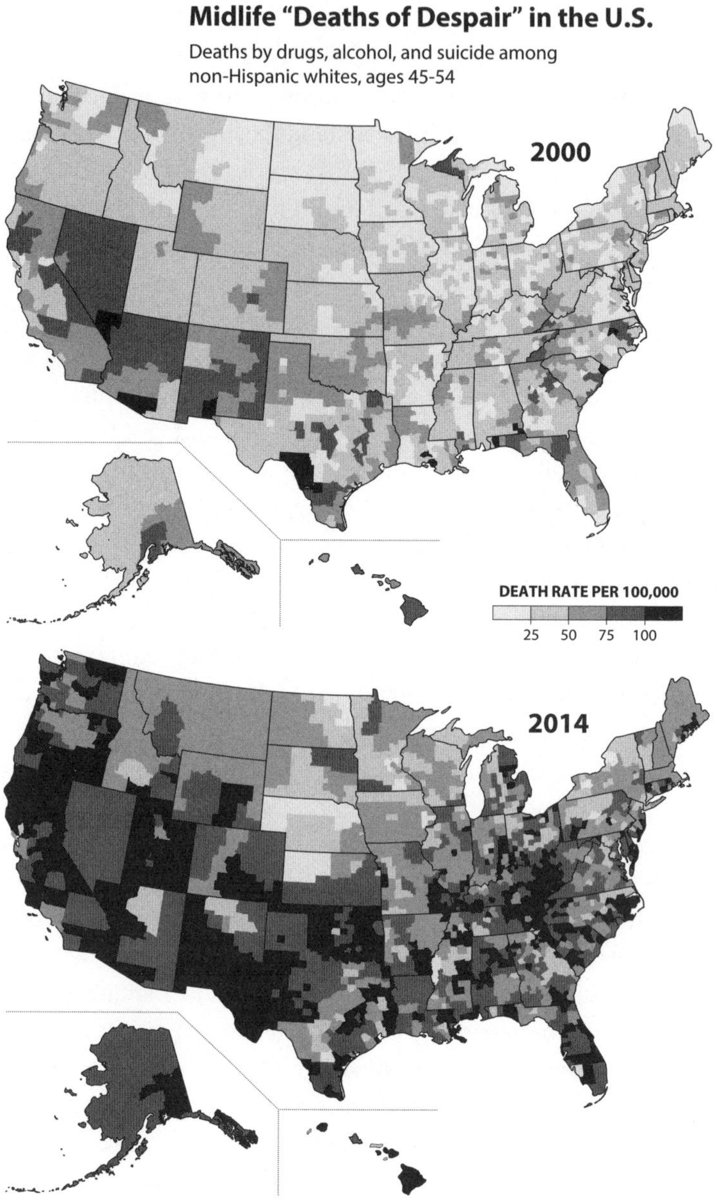

Figure 4.5. The rise of deaths of despair in the United States.
Source: Anne Case and Angus Deaton, "Mortality and Morbidity in the 21st Century," *Brookings Papers on Economic Activity* 1 (2017): 397-476, https://www.brookings.edu/bpea-articles/mortality-and-morbidity-in-the-21st-century/.

during the neoliberal turn deindustrialization, unemployment, austerity, and market fundamentalism have been most damaging.

The underlying lesson is quite simple and harkens back to our egalitarian roots as a species—people *at all levels of the social hierarchy* simply *fare better* when the political-economic organization produces *less inequality*. When political-economic systems fail and become unbalanced, inequality spreads, and people *feel* a rupture of the promise that the next generation can expect to do better than the present. While the election of Trump, the pro-Brexit referendum in the UK, and the Yellow Vest movement in France have all been expressions of discontentment with the hyper-capitalist order, working-class Americans, who are much more atomized, spread out by urbanization, fragmented by corporate media and culture war, and unaccustomed to thinking in terms of class antagonism are disproportionately affected by diseases related to despair than cohorts in other countries. When such deep-seated suffering and alienation does not find public expression, it appears to fester into a sometimes-lethal loneliness and resignation, as people seek escape through drugs, drink, and suicide. That said, researchers have also begun observing the deaths of despair phenomenon in countries like the UK,[43] Canada,[44] and Australia,[45] which have likewise undergone aggressive neoliberal restructuring over the last several decades.

Yet, there is hope. Recent history shows that when we tackle the disaster of grossly inequitable distribution of power, money, and resources, and improve the material circumstances in which people are born, grow, live, work, interact, and age over time, we can expect to move the needle at almost every level of biopsychosocial health for whole populations. This is significant because, unlike the other two public health disasters of agriculture and urbanism, which are inextricably woven into the fabric of civilization, *societal inequality is very much within our power to change*. Indeed, social democracy—a political system designed to reduce hierarchical inequality, poverty, and marginalization—provides a clear and proven pathway to restoring a more egalitarian commitment to treating populations. And that brings us back to the present-day population revelation studies that reflect falling rates of dementia and improved brain health in six Western countries. Let's take a closer look.

WHY DEMENTIA IS ON THE DECLINE

Given the evolutionary and historical context we've established, let's start with the obvious question: What is most likely to have caused the decrease in dementia rates in multiple countries?

When we lift up the hood of the population revelation studies, we see some clear societal patterns for current elders in the United States and other nations who came of age in the postwar Keynesian social democratic consensus of the mid-20th century in ways that appear to have played a key role in protecting their brains and driving down risk for dementia over time. In particular, the data show that elders in these countries have cognitively benefited from two distinct societal changes linked to overall health improvements in the 20th century:

1. improved prevention and treatment of vascular disease
2. increased access to formal and informal education

What might help explain the first pattern? Let's start with the material basis of the brain and work our way outward to material culture.

Getting to the Heart of the Matter

Although we don't tend to think of them as such, our brains are highly vascularized organs deeply intertwined with the health of the heart and blood vessels in the rest of our bodies. Nearly 20% of our cardiac output is committed to delivering oxygen and glucose to the brain, a remarkable percentage considering human bodies are estimated to contain some *60,000–100,000 miles* of blood vessels, which would wrap twice around the globe.[46,47] Across the course of our lives, conditions that affect our vascular system—high blood pressure, high cholesterol, diabetes, obesity and metabolic syndrome, heart disease, sleep apnea, and so on—can impair the heart and its extensive vascular transportation system to, from, and within the brain. Progressive damage to this system, even starting in midlife,[48] makes it increasingly more difficult to oxygenate brain tissue, distribute nutrients, flush out metabolic waste products and toxins, and generally sustain normal organ function over time; such damage can also lead to chronic inflammation and immune response.[49]

All these factors put people at risk for large strokes, associated with big blood vessels, which can damage or kill millions of neurons in one quick moment (through infarction or bleeding), as well as other more chronic forms of brain damage from death of brain tissue (microinfarcts) and sometimes silent bleeds (for example, subdural hematomas).[50] Recall the important "inconvenient truths" from last chapter that vascular brain changes are part of the heterogeneity of Alzheimer's and frequently co-occur with plaques and tangles in the brains of people with the syndrome, implying that vascular pathology and cerebral small vessel disease (thickening of the vessel wall, the presence of inflammatory infiltrates, and so on) may lower the threshold for exhibiting cognitive impairment.[51,52,53,54,55] Vascular disease plays an *intimate* role in Alzheimer's syndrome (and so-called MCI) that is only now beginning to get its due attention.[56,57,58,59,60,61,62,63,64,65,66,67,68,69,70]

While chronic diseases like obesity that burden our vascular system have been a rising concern in Western countries over the past four decades of neoliberal reordering,[71] modern medicine has also, over that same timespan, gotten better at using clinical (such as acute interventions like emergency stroke care), behavioral (rehab programs), and drug-based approaches to manage conditions like high blood pressure (antihypertensives), high cholesterol (statins), and diabetes (insulin).[72,73,74] As Langa frequently points out, the number of people treated for these cardiovascular risk factors has increased significantly just in the last decades alone. In 1990, 58% of people with hypertension received treatment, and by 2008, that had grown to 75%. For diabetes, 74% of people received treatment in 1990, which climbed to 87% by 2011. For high cholesterol, the improvement is even more profound, with the 20% receiving treatment in 1999 more than doubling to 43% in 2010. Worldwide, systolic blood pressure has fallen 1 mmHg per decade since 1980.

Such systemic improvements in healthcare practice, coverage, and delivery have, in turn, driven down risk for heart attacks, strokes, and amputations, in the process benefiting millions of aging brains, including those now being studied en masse by Langa and researchers in other countries. The crucial link between vascular health and the brain cannot be understated. As our colleague Kristine Yaffe has commented, "The same things we recommend for heart health turn out to be important for cognition."[75]

In other words, aggressively treating and preventing cardiovascular risk factors at the population level over the 20th century may be playing a key role in current brain health.

These vascular changes don't exist in a vacuum but are the result of decisions that have affected the political economy over the course of the last half century. Since the mass devastation of the Depression and world wars, every other developed country but the United States has "treated" its population by legally obligating the state to extend universal health care coverage to all citizens. Current elders in those countries have enjoyed full lifespan access to clinical care, which has been instrumental in not only *managing* vascular disease but also *preventing* it. When we consider the intimately vascular nature of the brain within the body—foregrounded against historical lessons about how reduced inequality improves public health—it is logical that extending access to high-quality healthcare for large cohorts of citizens would, in lowering upstream vascular risk factors, push the needle down on downstream dementia rates, as we are now seeing.

It is, however, unavoidably the case that the improvements in vascular health generally observed in the United States have not been enjoyed equally across the socioeconomic spectrum.[76] It might be reasonable for one to assume that where we've been less successful in managing and preventing vascular disease and its risk factors, there will also be higher rates of dementia. And sure enough, if we look at the country writ large, we see the highest current prevalence of dementia across a swath of southern states like Louisiana, Mississippi, Alabama, and Georgia, which are often referred to as the Stroke Belt because of that region's high incidence of vascular disease (figure 4.6). While concerning, the vascular union of stroke and dementia—reflected in the nearly identical appearance of the two figures—is largely unsurprising.[77] And when we compare those images with the state-by-state maps showing disparities in access to healthcare and overall poverty, we see a rather bleak story emerging that returns us to the age-old wisdom: *inequality is a public health disaster* (figure 4.7).

But thinking *just* in terms of modern health care's imprint on larger patterns of vascular disease and dementia is limiting, as it is only one social variable affecting the brain health of people in the population revelation studies. It is equally important to recognize how 20th-century public health initiatives aimed at treating whole populations also made a

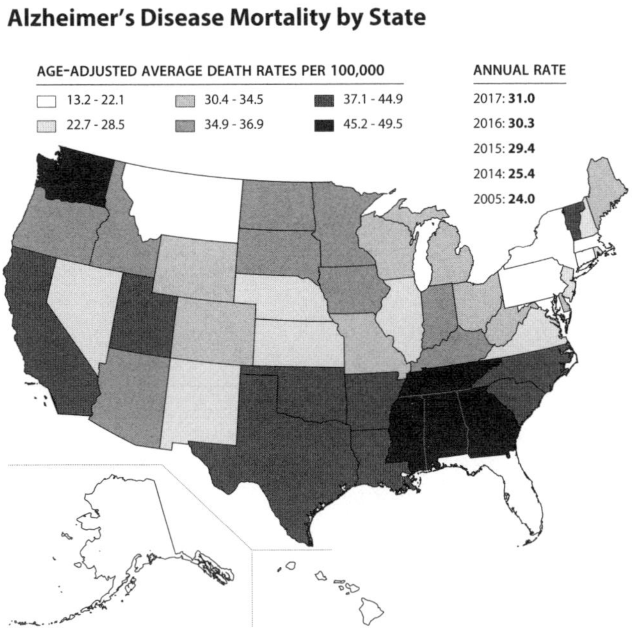

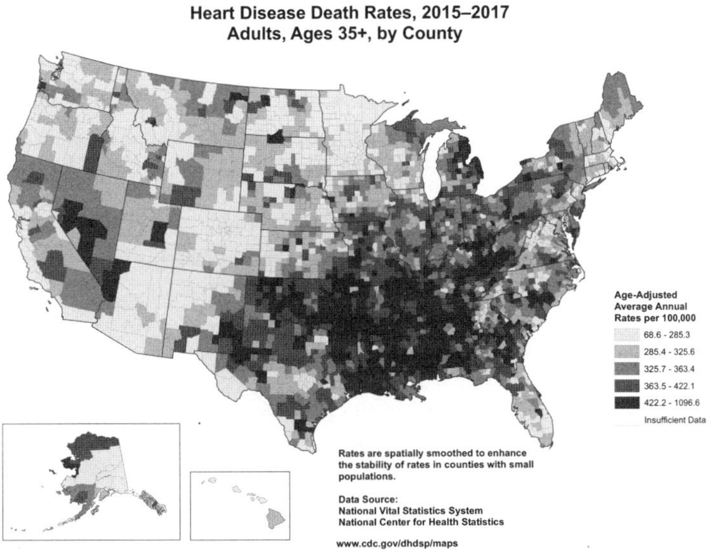

Figure 4.6. CDC data showing prevalence of Alzheimer's death rates (2017) (*top*) versus prevalence of heart disease death rates (2015-2017) by state (*bottom*).

Note: Use of this image does not imply or constitute an endorsement by CDC of any particular organization, product, or service. The views expressed in this book do not necessarily represent the views of CDC.

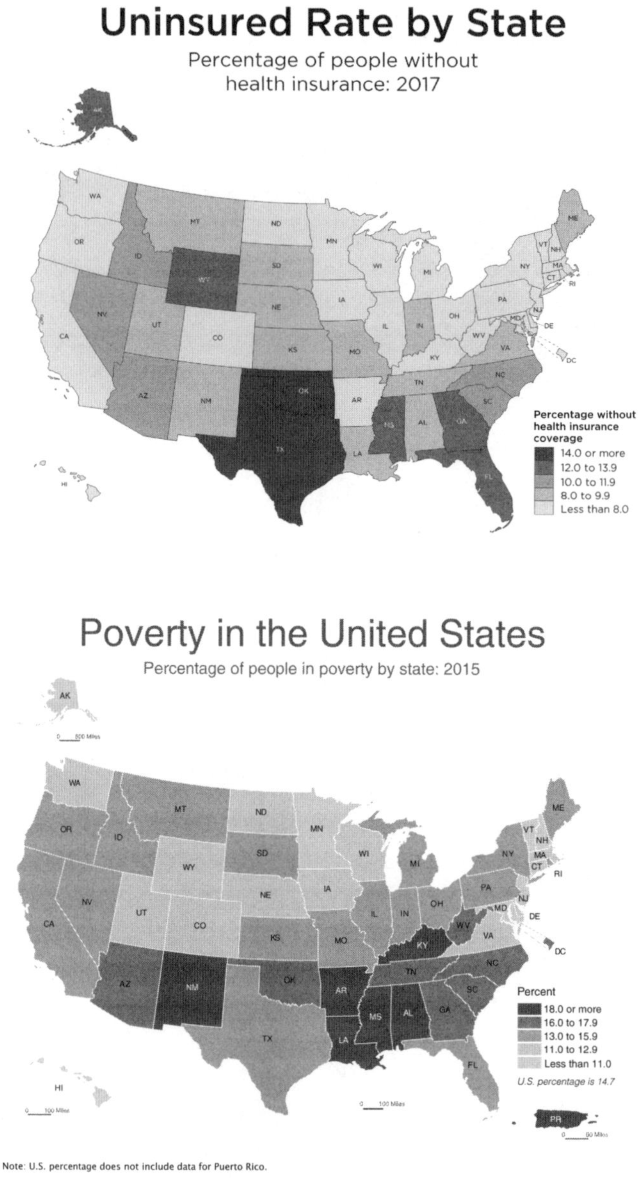

Figure 4.7. Disparities in access to health care (*top*) and overall poverty by state (*bottom*) mirror rates of heart disease and dementia.

Note: Use of this image does not imply or constitute an endorsement by CDC of any particular organization, product, or service. The views expressed in this book do not necessarily represent the views of CDC.

major, if unheralded, contribution to reducing risk for vascular disease for current generations of elders. For instance, in the sixties, the US Congress adopted the Federal Cigarette Labeling and Advertising Act (1965) and the Public Health Cigarette Smoking Act (1969). These laws required a warning label on cigarette packages, banned cigarette advertising in the broadcast media, and called for an annual report on the health consequences of smoking.[78] On top of this, federal, state, county, and local taxes on cigarettes have served as disincentives for developing the habit. Consequently, since 1965, the United States has experienced a dramatic decrease from 42% of adults who smoke to only 14% in 2017.[79] Globally, smoking prevalence in developed countries have mirrored this trajectory, with rates peaking in most nations from the mid to latter half of the 20th century before entering into a steep decline in the following decades, that has largely persisted to today.[80]

Quitting smoking means less-damaged blood vessels, and the steady decline in smoking rates in the United States and elsewhere has corresponded with decreased risk of the vascular diseases mentioned above (cardiovascular disease, heart attack, and stroke[81]) that can precipitate risk for dementia. As our colleague Carol Brayne of Cambridge University argues, the effects of smoking on population health are even more subtle, especially when we consider secondhand benefits of smoking cessation: "Societal actions to reduce smoking have not only improved vascular health in the population with dramatic reductions in stroke and heart disease deaths, they have also manifested in healthier pregnancies, childhoods with less exposure to malnutrition (i.e., brain growth stunting) and infections, and more exposure to education in these periods."[82]

Thus, the synergy of midcentury social democratic and public health policies, which across the Western world pulled multiple societal levers to increase healthcare access and significantly reduce smoking, represent a formidable contribution to vascular health at the population level, and ought to appropriately be considered a key part of the causal matrix of dementia reduction we are now witnessing.

The equation is relatively straightforward: Universal public health programs and societal infrastructure = brain health. As we think about what this means for the future of brain aging, however, an unavoidable reality is that the gains we've made on vascular disease through most of 20th century have started leveling off.[83]

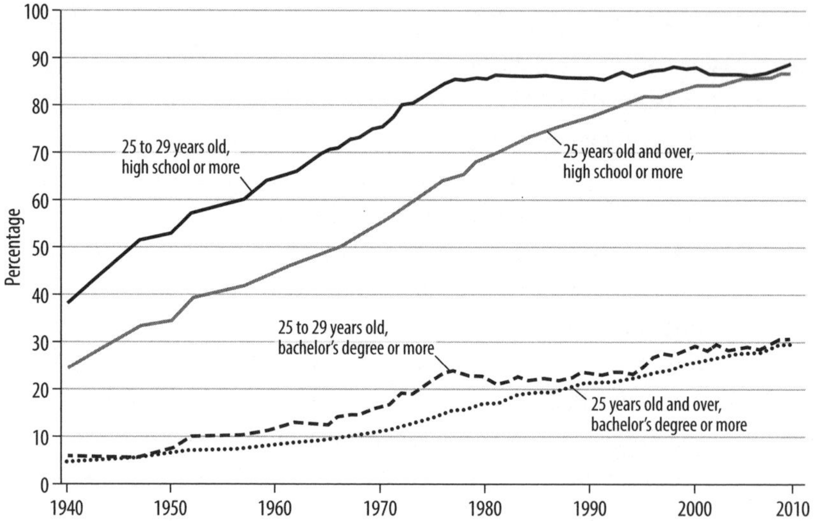

Figure 4.8. Rising percentages of the population completing high school (*top*) or college (*bottom*), 1940-2009.
Source: Courtesy of the US Census Bureau.

Learning to Resist Dementia

The second major societal pattern linking lower dementia rates to more equitable access to formal education is perhaps even more intriguing. Across nearly all the studies, including those looking specifically at aging cohorts in the United States,[84,85] it appears that the total years of education for elders has been rising within national populations over recent decades, tracking with a worldwide trend that has been observed for the last 40 years in developed and developing countries.[86,87,88,89] In Langa's study alone, older Americans age 65 and older who were assessed in 2012 had a whole extra year of schooling relative to their counterparts in 2000.

What this encouraging trend has meant is that, over the last several decades, we are seeing increasingly greater percentages of elders in Western countries who enjoyed access to formal education in their youth. In the United States alone, the proportion of adults age 65 and older with a high school diploma increased from 55% in 1990 to 80% in 2010, and the percentage with college degrees went from 12% to 23% over that same period (figure 4.8). These cumulative years of education appear to now be conferring a strong protective effect on dementia risk, independent of income, race, and other confounding factors. While it can be challenging to suss out the chicken-and-egg question of whether people who are born with more robust and resilient brains end up getting more education or vice versa, the findings from the studies nevertheless confirm a phenomenon that has been observed across multiple countries for decades—that more years of formal education can protect the brain, to some degree, from dementia and other age-related cognitive challenges.[90]

Before we get deep into the protective mechanisms of formal learning on the brain, it is critical to ask *why* education has become more prevalent for current generations of elders. As with improvements in vascular health, the answer leads us invariably back to the political-economic accomplishments of the 20th-century postwar social democratic consensus in engineering more equitable access to cultural resources that demonstrably benefit the body and brain. In the United States, the rise in years of formal education for elders now in their seventies and eighties is *directly linked* to policies implemented during the postwar consensus, which led to a marked increase in access to higher education. In fact, historians refer to the stretch of time between 1945 and 1970—an interval when the cohort of elders who are now 65 and older were in their formative learning years—as education's golden age.

While far from perfect, the "golden age" is said to be "gilded" because it was a time during the Keynesian / New Deal consensus when states were acting decisively to tax the wealthy, invest in educational infrastructure (39,000 new schools),[91] and democratize access to quality learning environments for its younger citizens. In the United States, as World War II grinded to an end, there was a rising moral imperative to integrate returning military personnel into the domestic economy, and Congress passed the Servicemen's Readjustment Act in 1944—better known to us today as the GI Bill[92]—providing subsidies for returning veterans to attend colleges and universities. Over 10 million vets took advantage of this opportunity, significantly increasing the number of people in that generation who gained access to the resource of higher education.[93] Of course, these benefits were not equitably distributed, as black veterans were barred from attending many public universities in the segregationist forties and fifties. Among white veterans who turned 18 from 1941 to 1946, 28% enrolled in college, while among their black peers, the rate was only 12%.[94]

By the mid-20th century, the brutality of the war in Europe had been replaced by a more insidious Cold War with the Soviet Union.

Nevertheless, an era of geopolitical brinksmanship between the United States and the USSR continued intensifying nation-state investments in the brains (and minds) of young Americans through higher education. After the Soviets released Sputnik, the first satellite to orbit the earth, the US government began allocating millions of dollars for educational reform, especially in math and science, but also in advanced studies in "national defense" subjects—foreign languages, anthropology, and political science as well as physics and chemistry.[95] State legislatures were likewise active in appropriating funds to expand colleges, build multicampus systems, and keep tuition rates low. The midsixties would also see the introduction of Pell Grants from the federal government, which were earmarked for students demonstrating financial need, further extending access to higher education across the racial and socioeconomic spectrum.

These Cold War policies combined to increase college access and affordability for entire generations of Americans—namely the silent generation and baby boomers—and gradually expanded the ranks of the formally educated. Consequently, from 1945 to 1975, the number of undergrads increased fivefold and graduate students ninefold. During the sixties alone, the number of students enrolled in college more than doubled from 3.6 to 7.4 million by 1970, and enrollment at public colleges and universities rose from 2.3 million to 5.7 million over that time.[96] By 1970, a public university like Ohio State, which in 1945 had a student body of 8,918, had swelled over five times in size to 46,074.[97]

Of course, the neoliberal turn plays a spoiler role in this story, as the ascendancy of market fundamentalism and the unleashing of the zombie economy in the seventies and eighties coincided with the collapse of the golden age in education. What had for decades been regarded as a public good that enhanced the collective American workforce, produced an informed citizenry, and was therefore the responsibility of the state soon came to be understood as a private "product" that was instead the purview of individuals acting within educational "markets." Between 1980 and 1985, the Reagan administration—supported by neoliberal southern Democrats—slashed spending on higher education by nearly 25%,[98] cutting a billion dollars out of Pell Grants and other grant aid.[99] State budgets for higher education have also dramatically declined during the hyper-capitalist reordering. In the seventies, states subsidized 65% of the costs of college, but by 2013, states covered only 30% of college costs.[100]

Absent high levels of public investment and state subsidization, the zombie forces in the higher education "market" have sent tuition costs soaring over 1000% since the seventies. Students have gradually been pushed to accept larger and larger bank-based federal loans for college, initiating a trend toward ballooning student loan debt financed in part by Wall Street, which totaled an all-time high of $1.5 trillion in 2019.[101] Whereas the average cost of a four-year institution was $5,160 in 1984, it skyrocketed to $25,409 by 2014.[102,103] In 2017, for the very first time, public colleges and universities in most states received a majority of revenue from student tuition rather than from government appropriations, reflecting how the state's faltering commitment to public education in a neoliberal era has pushed an enormous burden onto individuals and families within "markets."[104] There are, of course, also racial disparities in the accrual of debt, with black college graduates owing $7,400 more on average than their white peers ($23,400 versus $16,000).[105]

So too has the zombie market produced the scourge of for-profit colleges—including the infamous Trump University—that deceive students with false promises and provide shoddy educations while loading young people with massive debt. This exploitative business model has disproportionately hurt minorities; indeed, nearly half of for-profit undergrads are students of color, while 95% of black students took out loans, and 75% who did not complete their program defaulted.[106] Another troubling manifestation of the zombification of higher education in the American dementia era is the recent emergence of so-called university income share agreements. In these arrangements, investors, including wealthy alumni, hedge funds, and so forth, are fronting students tens of thousands of dollars for their tuition, with recipients then owing back a significant percentage of their earnings during the first decade after graduating. In this way, students become "tactical investments" within a rather vulgar futures market—one that privileges young people who pursue STEM educations with greater earning potential.[107]

Our current higher education crisis is a direct result of unleashing the beast of the free market to colonize a social good we used to regard in more egalitarian times as a free (or nearly free) resource collectively accessible to all Americans. Now, college is largely the province of the well-off, and those from lower classes who wish to seek educations often emerge from universities locked into a twisted form of modern debt peonage that limits their freedom of choice across the lifespan.

Ultimately, what the decline of the golden age under neoliberal regimes from the Carter administration forward has meant is that—much like improvements in vascular health—the trend toward more years of education that we've observed over the past several decades may soon be leveling off for future cohorts of elders nearing retirement age. Whether this will have an appreciable effect on dementia rates for future graying generations remains to be seen, but given the findings in the population revelation studies, it is a pattern we and epidemiologist colleagues like Langa and Brayne will be tracking.

CONCEPTUAL PROGRESS: FROM COGNITIVE RESERVE TO POPULATION RESERVE

What we *do* know is that the dual force of (1) improved vascular health and (2) increases in total years of education appears to have been broadly protective against dementia at the population level, and that social democratic policies implemented across the mid-20th century have dramatically—if unceremoniously—influenced both preventive factors for brain health. It is straightforward why improved vascular health is beneficial to an intricately vascularized organ like the brain. But why can something like education have such a drastic effect on dementia rates, and what might that mean for us in the present and future?

Let's start at the level of common sense.

Education is aimed at increasing problem-solving skills, and receiving greater quantities of quality educational experiences can make us wiser as individuals. Not only does schooling predispose us to behave in healthier ways across our lives (avoiding immoderate tobacco/alcohol use, staying physically active, maintaining a balanced diet, adhering to treatment of vascular risk factors like diabetes, and so on), but the credentials, status, and wealth traditionally associated with formal education can confer material advantages, encompassing consistent access to healthcare, more satisfying and intellectually stimulating jobs, access to more nutritious foods and diets, safer and less stressful living and working situations, networks of intelligent friends and colleagues who support lifelong learning and reinforce healthy behaviors, less likelihood of living near factories or major roads or highways and other sources of deleterious environmental exposures, and so forth. Education also does more than simply install skills to groom people for jobs in a meritocratic market—it nourishes the soul; exposes us to beautiful, diverse, and varied ideas and experiences; and develops us as human beings as we learn who we are, where we came from, what the world is, the nature of virtue and ethics, and thus our lifelong orientation in the pursuit of purposeful social goals.[108] The values, emotional intelligences, social skills, curiosity, self-actualization, quest for meaning, and sense of responsibility to others that schooling feeds (across STEM fields and the arts and humanities alike) may be critical to whether one remains adaptive and resilient to brain aging over the course of his or her life.

Aside from the range of psychosocial benefits that confer cumulative advantages to the well educated, scientists have also studied the effects of education at the neurobiological level. While much about the brain remains mysterious, it is theorized that intellectual enrichment enhances the brain's anatomical substrate by directly growing or strengthening neurons as well as glial (support) cells and synapses and lowering levels of beta-amyloid and tau at the synapses. This capacity for the brain to *structurally* change in response to stimulating material environments and experiences (like learning) is, as you may recall from the discussion of digital brain-training gadgets last chapter, called *neuroplasticity*. Other researchers believe that the benefits of education to the brain are more the result of optimizing *function* (physiological) rather than raw structure. This theory posits that forging more functional neural connections throughout the brain across our lifespan—a likelihood made greater if we are fortunate to have access to formal schooling—may enhance the later adaptability of the brain in the face of diffuse structural-neurologic decline. Such functional connectivity might allow for the compensatory recruitment of alternative neural pathways to work around those that may be lost due to small strokes and other microscopic neurodegeneration as the brain ages.[109]

As the late neurologist and writer Oliver Sacks poetically reflected in his ruminations on this protective phenomenon, "If the brain is to stay healthy, it must remain active to the last: wondering, playing, exploring, and experimenting right to the end . . . [L]earning is possible throughout life, even in the presence of cerebral aging or disease."[110]

While the exact effects of formal and informal education on the brain remain a black box of sorts, scientists currently describe the protective dynamic of learning under the catchall term *cognitive reserve*. Itself a metaphor, the current hypothesis of cognitive reserve holds that intellectual stimulation across our lifespans can, through the mysterious confluence of the abovementioned psychosocial, structural, and functional benefits, render our brains more cognitively resilient to the neuropathologies that accumulate with age and normally contribute to cognitive challenges. Thus, the material circumstances in which we age across the lifespan are critical to our brain health.

Recall the landmark findings from the Nun Study touched on last chapter, which helped establish that older people who are cognitively and functionally healthy can tolerate a high burden of neuropathology on their brains (plaques, tangles, small strokes, Lewy Bodies, and so on) without showing decline. This protective effect—this supposed *cognitive reserve* drawn from being a beneficiary of more years of schooling—is ostensibly playing a major role in buffering the relatively well-educated elders in the population revelation studies against the effects of age-associated cognitive decline.

There is, of course, a flip side to cognitive reserve. Just as the benefits of being educated accrue, so too do the consequences of *not* having access to formal schooling. Scientists have found that people with lower socioeconomic status (SES) and less education exhibit less-organized functional brain networks and reduced cortical thickness (gray matter) compared with higher SES individuals.[111] Multiple studies have observed a relationship between lower levels of early life cognitive ability and higher risk of dementia.[112]

Although the mechanisms are admittedly complex, this observed dynamic holds up across cultures. Our colleague Eric Larson, a co-author on the 2016 *Journal of the American Medical Association* study with Langa, partnered with a Taiwanese research team to look at the cognitive well-being of a generation of people who lived on subsistence farms on Kinmen, a remote island off the coast of China, where the median length of formal education was just one year. Residents of the island, endowed with less overall cognitive reserve because of the smaller dispensation of state-provided education, tended to manifest dementia symptoms between ages 60 and 65—almost a whole decade earlier than control populations in the mainland who lived where universal education was provided by the state.[113] Again, education is but a single variable in this complex story of brain health and dementia rates over the last half century, but it appears to be an important one.

Bridging to Population Reserve

Cognitive reserve represents a tremendously exciting, if imperfect, theory about the benefits of education for the brain. Nonetheless, we have also come to believe that it has some fundamental conceptual shortcomings that limit our thinking about protecting brain health.

Unsurprisingly, in our neoliberal era, which has spawned a vast, multibillion-dollar marketplace of memory, there has been a tendency to talk about building cognitive reserve in individualistic terms—that is to say, helping *consumers* gain reserve through particular rituals of enlightened market-based self-care. While our personal behaviors are an important aspect of prevention, excessive individualism and consumerism have too often guided our zeal for preventing Alzheimer's toward brain-training technologies, super foods, smart drugs, self-help books, and other heavily marketed products that compete for our attention around the pretense of "building reserve" for ourselves, by ourselves. We, as atomized subjects within the free markets unleashed during a hyper-capitalist era, have thus come to understand dementia prevention as if it were reducible to the sum of individual consumer choices we make over our lives in the service of crafting a more resilient brain. But framing prevention as a matter of individual consumption habits spares us from having to consider through a historical (and evolutionary) lens the ways in which the current political-economic organization and the structures of power in our societies ought to be fostering cognitive reserve not just at the *individual* but more importantly at the *population* level.

When we think more deeply about how to best build cognitive reserve to resist Alzheimer's, we are led away from the notion that we are self-actualizing monads in markets and back to the powerful historical wisdom that the most effective prevention exists, not in the form of pills, consumer products, or lifestyle habits, but as material changes to our political economy and improvements in public health that "treat" society as a whole and take us collectively in the direction of a more egalitarian governance strategy. The contribution of numerous mid-20th-century social democratic policies to moving the needle on later risk for dementia are a crowning example of why *resisting Alzheimer's* is best regarded as a moral imperative to improve the health and well-being of everyone, chiefly by using societal structures, institutions, and policies to reduce historic socioeconomic inequalities.

When a concept like *cognitive reserve* is flawed, humans, as thoroughgoingly narrative creatures, must invent new concepts that better facilitate our thoughts, values, and actions. In this case, we wish to offer a variant of the concept that we call *population reserve*. By shifting our notion of *reserve* from individual brains to the wider population (and even to smaller collective units like communities), this new construct instantly delivers a moral charge demanding a broadened mindset about prevention. Understanding the critical lessons of our evolutionary history as human beings, it exhorts us to reorient our political economy around collective interests, purposes, and goods—to think in a more egalitarian way about how shared equitable investments in infrastructure, education, health services, and social welfare, which unambiguously benefit brains and bodies, can mitigate our most deleterious and ubiquitous risk factors and give whole generations—especially those currently in the lower strata of our grotesque contemporary hierarchies—the best possible chance at sustaining long-term cognitive health. Lucky for us, the population revelation studies from the United States, Norway, Sweden, Canada, the UK, and France provide a clear egalitarian blueprint to follow in using our representative democracies to build population reserve moving forward and promote greater societal resilience to the neurologic, cognitive, social, and environmental insults so common in the neoliberal era.

POPULATION RESERVE AND THE 21ST-CENTURY RESISTANCE

"So we beat on, boats against the current, borne back ceaselessly into the past." This timeless poetic line by F. Scott Fitzgerald at the close of *The Great Gatsby* also captures our current predicament in the Alzheimer's field, where we press forward with great scientific ambition and industry investment, seeking the salvation of a technical fix, but have invariably been borne back to the wisdom of the 20th-century postwar social democratic consensus that preceded our current era of American dementia.

Ironically, a common refrain by neoliberal proponents hostile to Keynesian economics and the New Deal during the Reagan years asserted,

"The solutions of the thirties will not solve the problems of the eighties."[114] And yet, within the microcosm of the contemporary Alzheimer's field, we have come to see that the most effective solutions to resisting the syndrome appear to be *intimately linked* with social democratic governance strategies that emerged in the postwar era, addressing structural poverty (and racism) and creating a gentler, more equitable and inclusively prosperous society. That we who are concerned about brain health should be most impelled in the direction of ameliorative political-economic and public health policies that engineer structural changes is perhaps an unanticipated turn of events within a field organized around the hyper-capitalist promise of technical and individualist solutions in the marketplace of memory—but it is hardly surprising. As Rudolf Virchow, the 19th-century German physician and the father of social medicine, argued, "Politics is nothing else but medicine on a large scale."

So as the boat of our aging and increasingly stratified and unequal country pushes forward into turbulent waters, what "political medicine" might we administer to the 300+ million people aboard who are all susceptible to brain aging and dementia? The two major patterns we've established (vascular health and education) are signposts from the past that point ahead at several obvious social democratic policies to pursue in our current cultural milieu.

Solving the "Shocking and Inhumane" Healthcare Crisis

In the United States, it goes without saying that a key part of the solution to building population reserve involves the state finally joining the rest of the developed world in providing universal health care for all citizens. As mentioned above, unlike every other country examined in the population revelation studies, all of which have long guaranteed health care for all citizens, the United States maintains a mixed public-private insurance system that is leaving more than 30 million Americans uninsured[115] and an additional 40 million-plus underinsured and facing high deductibles and other related costs that deter them from receiving the care they need.[116] As a result, 33% of American adults go without recommended care, seeing a doctor when sick, or filling a prescription versus only 7–8% of people in the other population revelation countries.[117] As of 2019, the average family health insurance policy was nearly $21,000 per year, and an individual policy approximately $10,000.[118] The country's health is flagging, with life expectancy moving in reverse in the 2010s, and the improvements in vascular health noted through the late 20th century beginning to level off.

As far back as the sixties, Martin Luther King spoke of the urgent need to embrace universal health care to achieve a more just and equitable society, proclaiming, "Of all the inequalities that exist, the injustice in health care is the most shocking and inhumane."[119] Besides the obvious moral dimension to ensuring coverage and security for all citizens, the data on dementia trends suggest that, inasmuch as universal access to care would help millions more people live healthier lives across decades and prevent and manage vascular risk factors that significantly affect risk for Alzheimer's syndrome, the realization of universal coverage (including dental and vision) that is free at the point of service (no copays, fees, deductibles, or premiums) could make an additive population-level contribution to lowering future rates of dementia. Such an achievement would also neutralize a major source of stress, anxiety, and precariousness in peoples' lives (recall from chapter 1 the finding by the Federal Reserve that 40% of adults don't feel they could cover a $400 hospital bill without going into debt or selling something).[120] In short, transitioning away from private insurance to a single-payer health system would be a key structural lever for brain health—a means of efficiently treating the population and building greater reserve.

Democratizing Higher Education and Vocational Training

Another intriguing and rather obvious structural lever moving forward is universal free higher education at public universities. As Larson has argued, because of the powerful, if nebulous, buffering effects of cognitive reserve, spending a federal dollar on education may ultimately deliver a more protective benefit for dementia than spending a dollar on healthcare.[121] Thus, creating another "golden age" in this century—especially at a time when many young Americans are losing faith in the financial and social value of a high-priced college degree inflated to absurd proportions by the zombie economy—could precipitate the same population reserve benefits we have witnessed in cohorts of older Americans who enjoyed the fruits of mid-20th-century investments in higher education. This would hardly be revolutionary, but would be a return to the midcentury egalitarian belief that public education is a right that does not arbitrarily end for citizens after high school. As Noam Chomsky has argued, "Rich and poor countries can do it, the United States itself did it when it was a much poorer country—there's no reason why that can't happen right now."[122]

Making four-year college, community college, and vocational training free for young people at all income levels would be a major contributor to 21st-century brain health. But why stop there? It would also be beneficial to eliminate fees for all further education and vocational courses for adults. Such a system, paid for by simply increasing progressive taxation on the top 5% of earners and on corporations, could educate young people and adults in a changing economy shaped by increasing technologization, automation, and shifting needs (renewable energy and caregiving, for example), while also enabling lifelong learning opportunities. The realization of such social democratic policies could make a major uptick in the protective total years of education that whole generations carry forward over time, which we know are protective—not only against dementia, but also against "diseases of despair."[123]

Such holistic approaches to brain health promise to scale population reserve beyond even what Western countries like the United States managed to accomplish in the mid-20th-century's golden age. And such infrastructure could also go beyond these instrumental benefits and help mitigate the deepening sense of being left behind that people (especially those without higher education) have felt as neoliberalism has ravaged cities and small towns across the country, eliminating and outsourcing countless formerly middle-class jobs, upwardly transferring wealth, retrenching the welfare state, and contributing to the deaths of despair that are a defining crisis of our hyper-capitalist age.[124] Making major investments in education would also help reverse the unjust, untenable, and societally unhealthy predicament where many states in the United States spend as much public money on prisons as on higher education.[125]

Although we are a wealthy country that could quite easily afford universal health care and higher education, we will face formidable challenges in realizing a fairer, more just, equitable, and dignified world. And yet, there is growing hope. Universal health care, or Medicare for All, now polls with consistent majority support in the American public. Although such landmark legislation to cover all Americans within a single system using progressive taxation faces major structural challenges (due in no small part to vigorous opposition from big pharma, the insurance industry,[126] Wall Street, medical societies, and other modern "elites" who sit high in our hierarchy and profit from our current medical-industrial complex), Medicare for All is gathering national momentum. So too is the current proposal to make public college tuition-free, which is projected to cost about $80 billion a year.[127] Given that Congress typically raises the annual defense budget by this sum,[128] King's prophetic warning in his "Three Evils of Society" speech, "A nation that continues, year-after-year, to spend more money on military defense than on programs of social uplift is approaching spiritual death," is as relevant now as it was in 1967, at the height of the Vietnam war.[129,130]

Ultimately, the policies that will move the needle on dementia rates are eminently possible. We have a major opportunity to enact the "revolution in values" prescribed by King, to take us in the direction of a more compassionate society that also creates the material conditions to help us build collective brain health and resist Alzheimer's syndrome. After all, the neoliberal policies of the last several decades are not chiseled into stone; they are human decisions, and decisions can be changed.

We must be bold in thinking about how the many deficiencies in our current political-economic, social, and environmental systems are driving illness rates. Instead of being transfixed on single-mechanism drugs and infatuated with our own enlightened consumption and lifestyle changes within the marketplace of memory, energy is best spent applying pressure in our national, state, and local politics to act on known risk factors entangled with poverty, inequality, racism, war, and other population-level forces. After all, in addition to the major patterns described above, we have no shortage of evidence-based information on what will lower risk for dementia across the lifespan. It has been estimated that between 20%[131] and 33%[132] of dementia cases might theoretically be preventable if we collectively do a better job of

- expanding access to childhood education and supporting lifelong learning;
- increasing physical activity;
- improving diets;
- further reducing smoking, vaping, and e-cigarette rates[133];
- managing diabetes, hypertension, cholesterol, and obesity;

- effectively treating depression and substance abuse;
- improving workplace health;
- preventing head injuries (war related and otherwise);
- treating hearing loss; and
- ensuring opportunities for social engagement and supportive care as we age.

Tellingly, at the 2019 international Alzheimer's conference, the most excitement surrounded not a drug or vaccine, but rather research showing that people who have the resources, financial security, and freedom to make lifestyle modifications—exercising 150 minutes per week; eating a high-quality diet; engaging in mentally stimulating activities at least twice a week; not drinking more than one glass of beer or wine per day; not smoking—may reduce risk for dementia even in the face of other risk factors, including genetics and pollution.[134] Put simply, upstream primary prevention has the largest effect on reduction of later dementia occurrence and disability, and we need to ensure that everyone has the ability to take advantage of resources that most benefit brain health.[135]

We can act to lower our collective dementia risk, but it will require a different set of political choices. Reordering our political-economic reality to treat our shared risk factors at the population level—not to mention to support human flourishing—should be a societal imperative, as stringing together social democratic victories in multiple areas will create the conditions that will gradually build population reserve and reduce current and future risk for dementia. Historically, governments (that is, the ruling elite) have not felt compelled to pursue more egalitarian policies until dire circumstances like the Great Depression and world wars tore apart the fabric of society and created crises of survival. Failing government action, we can still act as cities, states, neighborhoods, universities, faith institutions, workplaces and unions, creating a stream of changes in the direction of our values so that more people can live dignified and fulfilling lives than is possible in a society needlessly riven with deep inequality, poverty, hierarchies, and the random cruelties and misfortunes they engender.[136] Remember, *we*, as an engaged citizenry, are our best hope for brain health, and a strategy to resist Alzheimer's must be built on the premise that a more egalitarian organization of society is the material foundation for better brain health and collective cognitive well-being.

SEEING OZ IN TECHNICOLOR: THE ANIMATING FORCE OF AN INTERGENERATIONAL ETHIC

The historical examples we have shared about mid-20th-century social democratic state actions and their profound downstream benefits contain even subtler lessons for brain health. Chief among them is that the actions that deliver the greatest cognitive benefits to society rarely offer instant gratification but are instead realized across the space of decades. Indeed, a US policymaker who, in the 1940s, would have known that greater access to education through the GI Bill would contribute to dementia reduction by the 2000s may have had a tough time selling the longitudinal benefits of policies of such legislation in his day. And yet, the results of increasing access to schooling so powerfully underscore why an intergenerational ethic must be an animating force in brain health.

Fundamentally, such an ethic demands that we advance beyond our own individualism, self-interest, and generational solipsism and make collective investments outside the marketplace of memory that will benefit the bodies, brains, and spirits of current and future generations over time. It also demands that we conceive of the various forms of Alzheimer's not as a single "disease" affecting elder individuals but as a syndrome that develops over long timespans, the risk for which begins in the womb and is modifiable based on the sum of insults and protective measures people are subjected to across the course of their lives,[137,138] which are intimately linked to the political-economic organization of society. As Carol Brayne has told us in personal correspondence, "We must move away from an individualized approach, manifest in the focus on investment in disease mechanisms, when there is *'barn door'* evidence that population approaches are having a major impact." Carol is particularly concerned about the generational imprint of neoliberalism on the ability to think collectively. For her, "the younger generation in most societies have now been fully marketized and subject to individualized approaches, including their education. Most do not have the prospect of security in their lives—whether family, employment, or environment. When these generations grow older, they seem unlikely to have the same collective sense that has been manifest across time since the Second World War, and this could move us back to less humane approaches to vulnerable populations." Thankfully, generational attitudes toward social democratic values appear to be starting to trend in a more positive direction, and we are hopeful that they can continue to overpower the "amnesia" of the American dementia era and come to define the future.

Ultimately, learning to behave toward our brain health with a selfless intergenerational ethic organized around collective responsibility resembles the dramatic shift to technicolor in *The Wizard of Oz.* When we extricate ourselves from the dull, narrow-minded individualism and consumerism fostered by our hyper-capitalist age, we will operate in a more humane realm wherein brain health can be conceptualized across lifespans, in terms of our children, grandchildren, and neighbors, and with an imperative to improve our interdependent societies as we act to protect our brains. From ensuring that the youngest in our communities are guaranteed nutritious foods and safe drinking water, opportunities for learning, safe neighborhoods, quality healthcare, higher education, and low levels of daily stress—all risk factors we explore in greater depth in chapters to come—we can create societal conditions that optimize not only our own cognitive well-being but also the brain health of future generations. We are a society that split the atom, mapped the genome, sent men to the moon, and closed the hole in the ozone—acting to promote brain health across the population should be no big deal!

CONCLUSION

George Orwell is best known for writing famous allegories, like *1984* and *Animal Farm*, that warn of the dangers of totalitarianism. But pigeon-holing Orwell as an "antitotalitarian" writer is only half the story, as the author was also deeply committed to promoting democratic socialism.[139] In an essay, "Why Socialists Don't Believe in Fun," the Englishman wrote how he had been deeply affected by the Spanish Civil War and other events in the midthirties. For Orwell, this "turned the scale and thereafter I knew where I stood. Every line of serious work that I have written since 1936 has been written, directly or indirectly *against* totalitarianism and *for* democratic socialism." In Orwell's eyes, democratic socialism was worth fighting for because it was a political system that, as we have seen, fundamentally allowed human beings to thrive: "a world in which human beings love one another instead of swindling and murdering one another."[140]

Similar to Orwell's epiphany in the midthirties, the 2007-8 Great Recession and the dawning realization that we live in a country with grotesque levels of poverty and disparities in wealth, income, and resources has served as a wakeup call for a new generation, reminding us of deep historical and evolutionary lessons about the damaging effects of inequality and the need to take better care of one another. And while the demented neoliberal order is now one of the main forces requiring our resistance, social democracy remains no less an urgent goal now than in Orwell's time. Careful consideration of brain health in a larger historical context underscores the importance of societal organization around egalitarian social democratic principles as a humanizing, health-promoting force that acts to mitigate the public health disaster of inequality.

In the face of repeated drug failures, studies revealing a trend toward lower dementia rates in multiple countries have established beyond reasonable doubt that the most powerful "brain health intervention" exists in the form of structural changes that "treat" whole populations, improving the health and well-being of *everyone*, regardless of class, race, gender, or creed, and increasing exposure to societal resources that protect myriad brains across the lifespan.[141] The effects of social democracy—so clearly imprinted on the population revelation data showing a decline in dementia rates—provides an organizing narrative to help us think about the most effective means of collectively improving our society in ways that reach beyond reduced dementia risk. As Langa told us, "Our challenge is to create a social milieu that supports peoples' brains across the lifespan and lowers risk for dementia. Instead of 'solanezumab,' we should ensure that kids grow up in safe, unpolluted neighborhoods with good schools to which they can walk. That is the 'intervention' that will decrease dementia risk."

As scientists, we believe we must let data guide our actions, and the population revelation studies represent some of the most important evidence to emerge in the Alzheimer's field in decades. It is often said that the simplest definition of *wisdom* is *acting on knowledge*. And even despite all the damage civilization has imposed on human health over the last 12,000 years, it does confer one advantage over hunter-gatherer communities: we can leverage the immense power of the centralized state to coordinate large-scale actions—based on both evidence and an ethos of social solidarity—that benefit whole populations. Fundamentally reorganizing our societal structures, institutions, and policies to bring us into greater alignment with the egalitarianism of our hunter-gatherer heritage has proved to be the wisest and most effective strategy for improving population and brain health and is where our energy must be most applied as we seek to move beyond the era of American dementia. As the ancient Greek tragedian Aeschylus wrote over two millennia ago, the challenge of civilization remains, even in our current epoch, "to tame the savageness of man and make gentle the life of this world."

Of course, in our day, universalizing access to health care, higher education, and public health resources are fairly intuitive strategies to accomplish this goal while fostering brain health, and we can and should support the growing movements around these and other wise policies. But what if there are other not-so-obvious levers of enlightened collective resistance capable of improving the cognitive well-being of whole populations? In coming chapters, we consider other aspects of our political economy (environmental policy, minimum wage, and so on) that we don't normally talk about when we talk about Alzheimer's. We start this journey in the most unlikely of places—a pediatrician's clinic located within a farmers' market in downtown Flint, Michigan.

5

Flint *Still* Doesn't Have Clean Water

What the Lead-Poisoning Tragedy in Michigan Means for Alzheimer's

Every child who enters Mona Hanna-Attisha's pediatric clinic in Flint, Michigan, leaves with a subsidized subscription for fresh fruits and vegetables. That's because the Hurley Children's Center is not your average medical institution—it is a one-of-its-kind clinic housed within a thriving farmers' market in the heart of the city, right next to Flint's central bus stop. "It's just a ridiculously awesome idea," Hanna-Attisha, who is better known to her patients and the larger community as Dr. Mona, told us. "When we decided to co-locate the clinic with the farmers' market, we had no full-service grocery stores in Flint, so the clinic was able to directly address food security issues."

The market and clinic form the epicenter of an emerging health corridor in this hardscrabble Rust Belt city of 100,000 residents, who live with an outlier poverty rate over 40% (just under 60% for children[1]), endure high crime rates, and can expect to live an average of twenty years less than people in more affluent neighboring suburbs. But Flint is resilient, and within the market, one detects the underlying pulse of the city and its people. More than 100 vendors offer not only the locally grown produce that ends up in the bags of Hanna-Attisha's young patients, but also meats, breads and other baked goods, wines and cheeses, an art gallery, a café, Middle Eastern and Mexican groceries, and flower and craft vendors. Market goers enjoy free chef demonstrations, live music, and entertainment from storytellers, comedians, and local authors (figure 5.1). Less

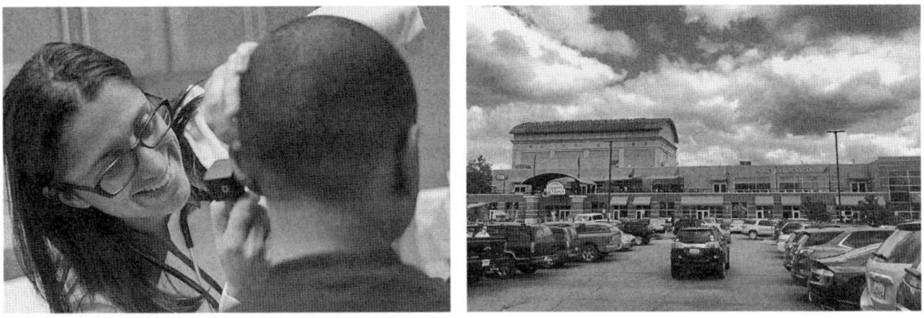

Figure 5.1. Mona Hanna-Attisha (*left*) and the Flint Farmers' Market and Hurley Children's Center (*right*).
Source: Left, courtesy of Michigan State University; right, courtesy of Karianne Martus.

than a mile away from the bustle of the market, the Flint River quietly meanders southwest, running through town before emptying into the Shiawassee River.

It was this river that vaulted Dr. Mona—most reluctantly—into the national spotlight. In the summer of 2015, Hanna-Attisha, a clinician-researcher affiliated with Michigan State University's College of Human Medicine, grew concerned when longtime friend and colleague Elin Betanzo, a water expert with the EPA, suggested during a summer barbecue that she look into the lead levels of Flint's children. A year earlier, the city had switched its water source from Lake Huron to the Flint River, and the Hurley Children's Center had treated young patients with rashes while fielding complaints from parents who reported cloudy, foul-smelling water flowing from their taps that they nevertheless had to use for baby bottles, sippy cups, and baths. Betanzo, who had worked in Washington, DC, in the first decade of this century during the city's lead crisis, stressed that changing the source and treatment methods of water alters the way it reacts with pipes as it flows into peoples' taps. "Lead was in the DC water for years," she told Hanna-Attisha. "More lead than you could imagine. More lead than I want to think about."[2]

As a scientist, Hanna-Attisha began examining the EMR blood lead data her clinic routinely collected on its young patients, comparing blood samples before and after the city had switched its municipal water supply in 2014. She analyzed the results of 1,746 children age 5 and younger from Flint, and 1,670 children from outside the city limits (lead-level data collection for children age 1 to 2 are a state-funded part of public health surveillance programs). What the results showed was that before the water switch, 2.1% of Flint children suffered from elevated blood lead levels; after the switch, that rate nearly doubled to 4%. In the areas where the water lead levels were testing the highest—in the downtown zip codes—Hanna-Attisha and her team observed an exponentially greater increase in children's lead levels (10.6%). Outside the city limits, there were no observed changes.

When a pediatrician sees even *slightly* elevated lead levels in children, the alarm bells go off. A well-known neurotoxin that has poisoned human communities for literally thousands of years, lead induces oxidative stress throughout the body (analogous to a process of internal rusting) and can, in doing so, have dramatic, deleterious effects on human health, damaging cells, proteins, and genetic material and disrupting nearly every organ system. Within the body, lead also possesses the particularly destructive ability to mimic calcium and zinc—elements that are essential to nerve conduction, reproductive processes, and the activation and mediation of many other basic physiologic functions.[3] When lead reaches the brain, its calcium mimicry disrupts neuronal development and causes an asymmetric release of neurotransmitters. This, in turn, can induce impulse-control problems, diminish the ability to respond to social and environmental stimuli, and undermine processes related to learning and memory.

For those affected, the real-world harms resulting from these microscopic processes can be devastating. Early life lead exposure has been linked to increased criminal behavior and incarceration[4,5]; lower IQ and reduced educational attainment over the lifespan[6]; early life pregnancy, aggression, and criminal behavior in youth[7]; worse labor-market outcomes; increased susceptibility to substance-abuse issues; and vulnerability to lifelong patterns of antisocial behavior that suppress upward social mobility.[8,9,10,11,12,13,14,15,16] On a neurobiological level, early life exposures have been linked to long-term abnormalities in the hippocampus and cerebral cortex, and with disrupted neuronal development, myelination, and neurochemical processing.[17,18] Children have greater vulnerability to lead because their bodies absorb more than adults, and their developing tissues and organ systems are less able to withstand the pervasively toxic effects of lead. "If you were going to put something in a population to keep them down for generations to come," says Hanna-Attisha, "it would be lead."[19]

With so much at stake for her young patients throughout the city, Hanna-Attisha double and triple checked her data, with the urgency to act growing by the day. In late September 2015, she donned her white coat and held a press conference at the pediatric clinic,[20,21] stressing the need to take immediate action and punctuating her argument by holding up a baby bottle filled with Flint's discolored water. Hanna-Attisha's claims were met with a swift rebuke from state officials, who tried to discredit her scientific work and undermine concerns voiced by Flint residents. She was called an "unfortunate researcher" who was "causing near hysteria"; but she knew the numbers didn't lie. "We were attacked just like the residents were attacked and the moms and the activists and the pastors and the water experts were attacked," Hanna-Attisha told us. "I was scared, and at times I felt absolutely sick, but I also knew we were right. And we fought back with science, hard evidence, and finally the house of cards began to fall."

Within weeks, state officials began reversing their position and acknowledging that the data were correct. Finally, news began surfacing that the city had in fact switched its water source to the Flint River in a cost-saving maneuver without putting in place proper corrosion control—a service that would have cost only about $100 a day. As Hanna-Attisha and her fellow activists had been saying, the highly corrosive water from the river—estimated to be about 20% more corrosive than water from the Great Lakes—was causing the erosion of lead pipes, joints, and fixtures and resulting in lead leaching into the drinking water of Flint residents, including upwards of 12,000 of its children. The city soon switched its water source back to Lake Huron in October 2015. But the damage to residents and the city's underlying infrastructure had already been done.

Today, because of the vast network of corroded pipes caused by the switch, Flint *still* doesn't have clean drinking water, and residents are reliant on filters and bottled water. If we are to truly understand Flint's plight, it is essential to apply the political-economic lessons of the previous chapter and evaluate how our brains are fundamentally shaped by the structures, institutions, and policies that influence our destinies from birth. By viewing brain health as embedded in historical, social, and institutional circumstance, subject to specific material forces, we can begin to see how the lead disaster and its cognitive consequences are intimately linked to deep, pervasive inequality associated with the neoliberal era, which has caused a public health crisis reaching far beyond Rust Belt Michigan and into many of our communities in the United States. In the spirit of viewing brain health as a collective endeavor and the result of our commitment to taking care of one another, it is critical that we see how the work Hanna-Attisha and her colleagues are doing inside and outside their remarkable clinic represents a living example of how we can resist the political-economic damage wrought by decades of hyper-capitalism and effectively "treat populations" to emerge healthier, more resilient, and with greater collective reserve.

THE HUMAN COSTS OF NEOLIBERALISM

In 1989, filmmaker Michael Moore released his first major documentary *Roger & Me,* set in his hometown of Flint. The film depicted the decline of the city's working class in the wake of General Motors (GM) CEO Roger Smith's decision to close several plants in Flint and outsource thousands of jobs to Mexico, where workers could be paid 70 cents an hour. This maneuver allowed GM to sidestep unionized labor and domestic regulation, maximize shareholder profit, and also shift resources to new growth industries such as weapons manufacturing.

The structural conditions that enabled this turn of events was, of course, facilitated by hyper-capitalist policies fixated on economic growth, productivity, efficiency, and higher profit rates, and brokered by none other than Wall Street in an era of financialization. Both political parties, including the Democrats, who, as we know, began abandoning their New Deal roots in the "pivotal decade" of the 1970s, have facilitated Wall Street deregulation, tax cuts on corporate and financial elites, and antiworker trade deals that have made it easier and easier for companies to ship jobs abroad from places like Flint to the developing world.[22] As former Wall Street-trader-turned-journalist Chris Arnade has written in his 2019 book *Dignity,* which explores through photography and personal stories the lives of people in "forgotten towns" like Flint, these financialized policies have purposefully engineered capital disinvestment, which has caused towns to become hollowed out, denuded of middle-class jobs, racially segregated, and increasingly despairing and drug ridden.[23] Meanwhile, as factories shuttered and jobs moved to countries with cheaper and more exploitable labor pools or were transitioned to robot automation, shareholder and executive pockets have swelled.

In Flint, gutting the GM employee base beginning in the seventies was especially reprehensible given the transformational victories the plant's workers had achieved decades before, in the nascence of the postwar social democratic consensus. In winter 1936, factory workers had occupied GM car plants in Flint for 44 days, holding sit-down strikes and demanding better wages and working conditions. They established a powerful union—the United Auto Workers (UAW)—and helped forge a "grand bargain" with management, putting in place a living wage, guaranteed healthcare, housing, schools, and pensions for all workers. In the prosperous postwar consensus period, when US political institutions were heavily regulating, taxing, and managing capitalism on a tight leash under the Keynesian/New Deal political-economic order and forging a more equitable balance between labor and capital to grow a robust middle class, GM was the country's largest employer and paid its workers what would be, in today's dollars, about $50 an hour with benefits.[24] Hanna-Attisha's father, an immigrant who had relocated his family from Iraq, was an engineer who designed custom metals for GM cars ("*Zinc*, not lead!" as Dr. Mona now makes sure to emphasize) and was a beneficiary of the UAW's bargaining during the city's burst of midcentury prosperity. "We came to the US as refugees, very much in search of the American dream, and for my family it became a reality," said Hanna-Attisha.

Indeed, when Flint was at the height of its powers in 1955, 80,000 GM jobs were located in the booming city. Yet, the gradual offshoring of labor throughout the neoliberal era, engineered by Smith and other GM executives as a strategy to maximize capital profits and sidestep unions in the United States, has reduced that number to around 8,000 today, thinning out the local labor market and severely reducing waged employment even while generating record wealth for the company. As Flint's economic health has rapidly declined, poverty has festered, with unemployment levels at double the national average (10%), median household income ($25,242) less than half of the average in Michigan ($51,063), and soaring rates of crime and housing foreclosures.[25,26] Moore's film poignantly captured this urban blight, showing door-to-door evictions; depicting the brazen, desperate crimes taking place in the city each day; detailing the "white flight" of the upper classes into surrounding suburbs; and memorably featuring one Flint resident who was scratching out a living by selling and breeding caged rabbits in a business branded Pets or Meat. Such dark vignettes are the inevitable biproducts of a hyper-capitalist zombie economy, in which unleashed corporate power systemically treats workers in places like Flint as costs to be eliminated. In doing so, capitalists successfully wrestled back large portions of the wealth and power that unionized workers at GM and elsewhere had won for working people starting in the 1930s.

Flint's Shock Doctrine: Crisis in an Age of Austerity

Simply put, the desperate material conditions sown by deregulated free market forces in Flint and throughout the state of Michigan laid the groundwork for the lead-poisoning crisis in the 2010s. Specifically, cities like Flint that have suffered plummeting public revenues throughout the American dementia era have, in turn, been made to adopt strict "austerity" measures that enforce fiscal discipline by cutting state and municipal services. Under austerity regimes, social democratic services like environmental regulation, social welfare programs, employee protection, quality education, and infrastructure that had been considered foundational in the American social contract since the New Deal era's predominance in the thriving mid-20th century[27] all became potential victims on the zombie economy's fiscal chopping block.

Flint's already desperate decades-long decline grew even worse when the Great Recession of 2007–2008 swept through the heartland like an economic tornado. While the federal government dipped deep into the Treasury to bail out Wall Street and the auto industry (including GM) with trillions of dollars in corporate welfare, states received relatively little such help. As Michigan further tightened its belt during this "austerity crisis," state lawmakers implemented tax cuts for businesses and began using sales tax collections to replenish state budget holes rather than fulfill statutory revenue-sharing promises to local communities.[28] This resulted in Flint actually losing an additional *$60 million* of annual revenue from the state.[29] Then, in 2010, when Rick Snyder—a former CEO of Gateway computers and a darling of the ascendant Tea Party movement—was elected with a mandate for even deeper fiscal discipline, it intensified the climate of austerity for struggling cities like Flint, whose budgets were already being starved at near bankruptcy.

Snyder's administration made the market-fundamentalist pledge to run Michigan like a business, and one area where they immediately slashed costs was the state's regulatory agencies. When the Michigan Department of Environmental Quality (MDEQ)—a critical body in charge of environmental regulation and detection of environmental hazards (including drinking water quality)—was placed on the chopping block, the Snyder administration lopped off spending where they could. A 2010 federal audit reported that MDEQ had been beset by budget cuts, staffing issues, and reduced resources—starved to the point of no longer being functional as a regulatory agency.[30]

In 2011, the gerrymandered state's legislature forced through a law (PA-436) allowing sitting governors to appoint "emergency managers" for cities like Flint that were subject to strict fiscal discipline. Unlike traditional political offices, the position of emergency manager is not democratically elected, is accountable to no one but the governor, and can override elected officials, break union contracts, sell off public assets, privatize public functions, and otherwise run cities like private businesses.[31] In this way, the viceroy-like position inherently violates the principle of local self-governance and self-determination. According to a Civil Rights Commission report about Flint,[32] *half* of Michigan's black residents have at one time lived under an emergency manager.

Astute readers might recognize the phenomenon of emergency managers as a prime example of Naomi Klein's "shock doctrine," which refers to techniques neoliberal politicians have used in places like post-Katrina New Orleans to rapidly implement market-friendly austerity policies during moments of crisis and emergency.[33] Indeed, in October 2013, as a paralyzing fiscal crisis gripped the municipality of Flint, governor Snyder unceremoniously installed a man named Darnell Earley as the city's fourth emergency manager and charged him with ramping up painful but "necessary" austerity "shock treatments" for the city.

Earley combed through Flint's municipal budgets for ways to further trim costs. When he reviewed the city's water situation, he calculated that switching the source from Lake Huron to the Flint River (and thereby overriding an arrangement in place since 1967) could cut around $2 million per year. While there were precautionary warnings about the corrosiveness of the river water (the stripped-down MDEQ is reported to have inexplicably disposed of samples it had collected demonstrating dangerously high lead levels[34]), the city and feeble regulatory agency failed to carry out full and comprehensive safety tests and thus approved the water source transfer without putting corrosion control in place.

This systemic institutional failure traced a through line back to Roger Smith's ruthless gutting of Flint's manufacturing base in the eighties and through recent decades of bipartisan neoliberal governance, which dismantled New Deal protections and facilitated loss of jobs, historic wealth disparities, urban decay, historic recession, and austerity regimes, ultimately producing the social and infrastructural conditions wherein lead particulates leaching from old piping and into Flint's drinking water reached over 880 times the actionable federal level of 15 parts per billion and entered the developing bodies and brains of the city's children.[35] As if lead poisoning wasn't enough of a scourge, the switching of Flint's water also caused an outbreak of infectious disease, including deaths from Legionnaires' disease, and has led to high rates of miscarriage and infertility in the city.[36]

In another cruel twist that underscores how embedded Flint's current situation is within the unhealthy institutions and circumstances of the neoliberal era, while the city continued sourcing its water from the Flint River in the wake of the crisis, GM, which had realized the city's river water was corroding auto parts in its factories, had reached an agreement in October 2014 to switch *its* water source back to Lake Huron.[37] While clean water flowed into factories owned by a wealthy multinational corporation that had just been bailed out by the government, the city's poor residents were being sent water bills for lead-laced toxic sludge they could not safely drink or bathe in.

This, in itself, is dark and dystopic.

But to add insult to injury, residents were infuriated by the Obama administration's desultory handling of the crisis, which was not formally declared a state of emergency until 2016, two years after the switch of the city's water supply began poisoning residents. Later that year, Obama staged a highly scrutinized press conference in Flint, where he sipped from a glass of water allegedly from Flint's supply, and glibly deemed it "drinkable." As Michael Moore tweeted after Obama's press conference, "I'm sorry to tell you your visit is too little too late . . . Sir, they've been poisoned for two damn years . . . Every child here now has some form of permanent brain damage."[38] To make matters worse, during Obama's second term, his Department of Defense used Flint as a staging ground for urban warfare exercises to train soldiers readying for overseas deployments in how to operate in urban environments. Without informing the public, the army inflicted loud explosions and hovering military helicopters on terrified residents.[39]

Such an undignified predicament has left Hanna-Attisha and Flint residents feeling justified fury at the political establishment but also a sense of social abandonment that cuts deep. As Ariana Hawk, a Flint resident whose children had been exposed to lead-laced water, told the *Detroit Free Press*: "We get treated like . . . we don't matter."[40] Indeed, the almost unfathomable inhumanity of the crisis in Flint has inscribed not merely a lasting physical cost on its citizens but also a deep psychological trauma that will be felt for generations to come. "This is not just a lead crisis; it is a lot more than that," Hanna-Attisha told us. "The crisis itself is a trauma. Being a part of this betrayal, the anxiety, fear, and guilt—just having that toxic stress can lead to more chronic diseases. You can think of it as a population-wide PTSD, and that, in and of itself, can have consequences."

People often ask Hanna-Attisha why she, as a pediatrician, has remained such a vocal public critic of the political-economic milieu that has imposed the mantle of austerity on cities like Flint. She has taken to responding with one of her favorite quotes: "Pediatricians are the ultimate witnesses to failed social policies." She elaborated:

> It's often in our exam rooms where we see the consequences of these policies. In Flint, it was austerity-driven policies—the cutting of resources to cities, cutting revenue sharing, cutting services and programs and public health protection—that created the situation we are seeing in our clinics. The biggest lesson we've learned here is *you can't run government like a business or put a price on public health!* If you want clean water and clean air, *that costs money*, and it comes with a different kind of philosophy, not austerity. It's not about minimal compliance but maximal protection. Our public health protections show how much or little we value our children.

When we shared with Hanna-Attisha the finding that millennials increasingly have a more favorable opinion of social democracy than capitalism, she laughed and said, "Well, thank god, there's hope!"

"A THOUSAND FLINTS": THE PERSISTENT SCOURGE OF LEAD IN OUR COMMUNITIES

In Flint's former era of 20th-century prosperity, it was often said that "America is a thousand Flints."[41] Sadly, this statement remains true—though not in the way it was originally intended.

Indeed, as singularly tragic as the situation in Flint has been, the problem—quite horrifyingly—extends far beyond central Michigan and into many cities and towns across the country that have lead service lines and have similarly been pushed to the brink of collective endangerment by decades of hyper-capitalism, financialization, and austerity regimes. In fact, in 2016, Reuters examined neighborhood-level blood lead testing results across the country, finding 2,606 census tracts and 278 zip code areas in which the percentage of children with a blood lead concentration greater than 5 mcg (the federal limit recognized as "safe" by the government) was higher than rates during the peak of the crisis in Flint, which doesn't even rank among the "hotspots" of lead poisoning in the United States.[42] America is truly a thousand Flints, and worse, it seems.

"Every week, I get an email or contact by another city or school district that has found lead in its water, and it's no surprise because we *do* have lead in our water," Hanna-Attisha told us. "As a nation, we were so in the arms of the lead industry that we didn't restrict lead from plumbing until 1986 from our pipes and not until 2014 from our brass fixtures. Brass could still have lead in it until *2014*! And so of course there's lead in our solder and other parts of our plumbing, and when people test water, they're gonna find lead. This is the legacy of the profit-driven lead industry that ignored science and fought regulation to get their product into gas, paint, and plumbing."

The Reuters database is searchable,[43] and we encourage readers to explore how their local communities are faring. Personally, it was jarring see that the percentage of elevated lead levels in the Cleveland neighborhood I (Danny) grew up in were 15.6%, five percentage points higher than the worst testing areas of Flint. Also upsetting was that the neighborhood where the Intergenerational School, an elementary school cofounded by Peter in 2000, which invites people with dementia to mentor inner-city children (see chapter 10), was located in a region of Cleveland where *43%* of children are testing positive for elevated lead. As the *New York Times* reported in 2016, when 14.2% of children throughout all of Cleveland tested positive for elevated lead in their blood, it was twice the percentage of Flint's kids at the time.[44] This threat looms over the country like a gathering storm, particularly in working-class communities that have been hollowed out and abandoned by the neoliberal zombie economy.[45]

In addition to poor socioeconomic conditions being a clear risk factor for lead exposure, an unavoidable dynamic of environmental racism is at play. Childhood exposures are disproportionately higher in black youth, and black and Hispanic neighborhoods show extremely high rates of lead toxicity compared to white neighborhoods, with the situation being relatively worse for blacks on the whole.[46] Certainly this was the case in Flint, a poor, majority black city. In recent years, however, this cruel expression of systemic racism—which some have referred to as "the new Jim Crow"[47]—has manifested in our culture in other tragic ways.

In 2015, Freddie Gray, a black 25-year-old Baltimore man, died in police custody after sustaining a fatal spinal cord injury when he was handcuffed and transported in the back of a police van. Gray's death launched riots throughout the city that drew national attention, and his name is still invoked in ongoing protests against police violence and systemic racism. One little-discussed biographical detail about Gray, however, was that he had suffered from acute lead poisoning in his youth,[48,49] with his exposure occurring in the Sandtown-Winchester row housing where he'd grown up. Beyond lead that was present in the neighborhood's drinking water, Gray had been doubly exposed by interacting with lead-laced paint that peeled from the walls of his low-income project housing. In a 2009 deposition, part of a lead-poisoning lawsuit Gray's family brought against the property owner, Freddie described the dilapidated home he grew up in: "There was a big hole when you go up the steps. There was a couple of walls that wasn't painted all the way, peeled . . . and like the windows, paint was peeling off the windows."[50]

For decades, paint manufacturers used lead as a cheap pigment and additive to decrease drying time and make paint more durable. While the neurotoxin was banned for interior use in 1950 and for all residential uses in 1978, the danger still looms in older neglected housing, where lead-based paints are deteriorating into paint chips and toxic dusts that are inhaled or ingested by naturally curious children like Gray, who seek out sensorial interaction with their environment (paint chips can be particularly dangerous for children because lead acetate is sweet to the tongue).

As Hanna-Attisha preaches, *no* levels of lead are safe, and the CDC (conservatively) holds that anything higher than 5 mcg can damage a child's cognitive development. And yet, when Gray was merely 22 months old, his blood carried an astounding *37 mcg* of lead. This tragic predicament extended across Baltimore, where the Coalition to End Childhood Lead Poisoning estimates that nearly 30,000 Baltimore kids in Gray's generation had been poisoned.[51] Given lead's devastating cellular activity within the developing human body, such exposures place a lifelong imprint on those who suffer them, including on their cognitive development. In Gray's case, the effects are obvious: he had been diagnosed with attention-deficit disorder in his youth; didn't graduate from high school; was often suspended; and had been arrested more than a dozen times, including his final brush with police custody that lead to his death.

While it is perhaps reductive to attribute all Gray's problems to lead poisoning and to subordinate the myriad aspects of intractable poverty and structural racism that also impinged on his life, it is undeniable that his early life lead exposures, due to his brain and body being embedded in particular political-economic circumstances, contributed to diminished cognitive functioning, school performance, ability to focus and think, greater aggression, and impaired self-regulation, all of which culminated to some degree in his tragic demise. Gray's life came to an untimely end in his midtwenties—but what if he had lived longer? How might this exposure have affected his brain health in later decades? And what does this mean for the children of Flint, Baltimore, Cleveland, and elsewhere who have been subjected to such high levels of lead so early in their lives?

LEAD AND ALZHEIMER'S SYNDROME: APPLYING THE FRAMEWORK OF COGNITIVE AND POPULATION RESERVE

While a direct link between early lead exposure and Alzheimer's risk is not strongly established (owing mostly to difficulty in study design over decades), we know that exposure to the neurotoxin has long-term ramifications for cognition. Studies have established that early life exposure to the heavy metal can reduce the birth and survival of new neurons (especially in the hippocampus, a region critical to memory), shorten the length of dendrites that span between neurons (compromising communication), and perhaps even alter the expression of genes related to amyloid production.[52] Researchers in New Zealand recently examined a cohort of more than 1,000 children exposed to lead poisoning in the early 1970s, finding that early life exposure was associated not only with lower cognitive function and socioeconomic status at age 38 but also with declines in IQ and downward social mobility.[53] Other studies have shown that higher bone lead levels (a marker of cumulative lead exposure over the lifespan) are associated with a greater decline in cognitive performance later in life.[54,55,56,57]

Given the good deal we know about the role of vascular risk factors in Alzheimer's syndrome, it is further worrying that studies have strongly established that lead exposure—even if just in childhood—can induce late-life hypertension, arteriosclerosis, atherosclerosis, thrombosis, and cardiovascular disease.[58] In fact, researchers have estimated that if average blood levels of lead could be cut in half for the US population, the annual number of heart attacks would fall by nearly 24,000, and incidence of cardiovascular disease would drop by over 100,000.[59]

These worrying links between early life lead exposures and late-life risk for Alzheimer's syndrome demand that we think about Flint, Freddie Gray, and our broad lead epidemic across the United States through the prism of *cognitive reserve*. Recall from last chapter that this is a theory based on the observation that intellectual stimulation across our lifespans—for instance through increased exposure to formal schooling—can make us more cognitively resilient to the neuropathologies that accumulate with age, leading to cognitive challenges. *Reserve* is built on a biological substrate that is not entirely clear to scientists but likely involves both structural (for example, brain size or number of neurons, synapses, and support cells) and functional factors (increasing efficiency of neural circuit function or the recruitment of other compensatory neural circuits that can function despite diffuse damage from vascular, inflammatory, and other brain insults).

Insofar as we know that lead is toxic to cells and synapses, is a major risk factor for cardiovascular disease,[60] is disruptive at the molecular level in ways that lower IQ, creates disinhibition, and causes other behavioral patterns reducing academic attainment, limiting social mobility, and increasing the risk of incarceration, it is logical to surmise that *childhood exposure to neurotoxins* would, at the point of exposure and over the course of time, *weaken the biological substrate* (that is, the cognitive reserve) *that buffers the brain against cognitive decline and dementia as we age*. Put otherwise, by reducing the number of neurons, synapses, support cells, and neuronal networks in a person's brain and altering the vasculature that effectively—if somewhat mysteriously—builds reserve over time, those who are poisoned will logically be *less able* to resist the accrual of normal pathologies of brain aging and thus have a shorter threshold for converting into Alzheimer's syndrome than those who have been embedded in circumstances more favorable to building strong reserve from youth forward.

Tragically, this depletion of cognitive reserve is part of the legacy of Flint and the thousands of other American communities where children like Gray are being exposed to unsafe levels of lead every day. As Philip Landrigan, a pediatrician renowned for his work on lead exposure, has said, "Even at the very lowest levels of exposure, we know that lead erodes a child's IQ, shortens attention span, and disrupts their behavior. We know when we do follow-up studies that children exposed when they were kids are more likely to be dyslexic, have behavioral problems, and get in trouble with the law. There's no question about that."[61] There are already concerning warning signs in Flint, where state researchers have noted a drop in third-grade reading proficiency from 41.8% in 2014 to 10.7% in 2017—a decline significantly worse than the state's average.[62]

Even with the marginal progress that has been made in removing lead from environments in recent decades, the amount found nowadays in adults remains 10 to 100 times higher than people who lived in the pre-industrial era (700-1000 years ago).[63] Thanks to the dramatic scale of this problem, we must again think of the crisis as threatening the cumulative *population reserve* of our nation across whole generations. Drawing on this concept helps us reflect more deeply about the long-term societal costs of the catastrophe of widespread lead poisoning—not only greater aggregate risk for heart disease and dementia, but also risk for higher crime rates and incidence of violent crime, a continued bloating of the prison-industrial complex, and a body politic less able to think critically and challenge entrenched wealth and power in our era of historic inequality.

For this reason, we continue to urge advocacy groups like the Alzheimer's Association to recognize that they have a *moral obligation* to take on the national lead crisis as a core priority. An organization committed to healthy brain aging ought to be outraged about widespread lead poisoning and advocate for testing and aggressive abatement strategies in US cities, especially since lead is being revealed as present in drinking water across the country. But frustratingly, no mention of lead or the crisis in Flint can be found in any Alzheimer's Association materials. Even so, there is hope for resisting our lead crisis, and we don't need to resign ourselves to the random senseless cruelty imposed on us during the era of American dementia. Imagining how we might progress beyond neoliberalism to build a healthier society with healthier institutions brings us back to Hanna-Attisha's clinic in downtown Flint.

How We Can Resist: A Resilient City

In thinking about the daunting decades-long challenge ahead for Flint, Hanna-Attisha has been quoting Frederick Douglass a lot lately: "'It's easier to build strong children than repair broken men' . . . that is absolutely the philosophy we're pursuing here," she says.

Not unlike our vision for pursuing healthy brains through the attainment of a healthier society and more humane social democratic institutions, Hanna-Attisha is less focused on "fixing" the dauntingly complex problem of lead poisoning and is instead marshaling all available resources and reorganizing the political-economic realities of Flint in the service of building lifelong resilience in the city's children. Within a climate of neoliberal austerity that has stripped away the aegis of social democratic protections from a vulnerable population like the poor residents in Flint, while unleashing the savagery of global free markets and austerity (that is, death by politics), she is using the crisis as a chance to actualize her dream of building a model public health program that nevertheless surrounds the city's children with every possible evidence-based intervention to promote their development and mitigate the impact of their lead exposure. It is a project with clear echoes back to the great bargain that GM's workers were able to achieve during their 1936 factory occupation, which brought greater security, solidarity, and inclusive prosperity to generations of Flint's workers and their families. Now, in 2020, Hanna-Attisha, an intergenerational beneficiary of the great bargain, is leading the charge to weave together a protective tapestry of resources, services, and programs around today's children, which includes

- free childcare centers
- universal preschool
- family nutrition counseling programs
- expanded school health initiatives
- breastfeeding education for young mothers
- social work home visitation and family support
- early literacy programs

- 24-hour access to mental health care
- health care for all through Medicaid expansion

In this way, the lead crisis is fueling a kind of reverse shock politics—seizing on a catastrophe as an opportunity to *restore* social democratic principles and institutional humanity to a community ravaged by neoliberalism and austerity, and thereby systematically initiating long-term population-level actions to influence the social determinants of health, which will not disappear even if the city's infrastructure is miraculously fixed and drinkable water is flowing into peoples' homes. "Basically, what we're putting in place for lead exposure are simply things that all cities need," Hanna-Attisha told us.

Of course, the partnership between the Hurley Children's Center and its farmers' market neighbor is key to promoting nutrition as a means of directly helping children and families. Not only can greater access to healthy foods high in vitamin C, calcium, zinc, magnesium, iron, and antioxidants decrease the absorption of lead and reduce the oxidative stress it induces in the bodies of Flint's children, it also lays the groundwork for better lifelong nutrition and thus vascular and cognitive health. In addition to making sure every child walks away from a doctor's appointment with a written prescription for subsidized market produce and nutritional counseling, Hanna-Attisha's clinic is partnered with the federal Double Up program, which provides Supplemental Nutrition Assistance Program (SNAP) beneficiaries with a one-to-one match to purchase healthy, locally grown fruits and vegetables. When Flint parents make a fruit, vegetable, or milk purchase, they effectively receive double the amount of the expense back from SNAP, which can then be used to buy healthier foods. As of 2018, the program was reaching approximately 40% of SNAP households in Flint, and store owners have been doubling their inventories of fruits and vegetables to keep up with consumer demand.[64]

This multifaceted, bottom-up approach to "building strong children" can serve as a model for communities whose youth are dealt an unfair hand, whether through environmental exposures or other traumas born of structural poverty, racism, and neglect. In this way, Flint uniquely and paradoxically serves as a microcosm of our era's most destructive problems *and* our capacity to evolve, adapt, resist, and set up more egalitarian institutions that engender greater community resilience and reinforce our responsibility to and for one another. Recall the lesson from last chapter: Universal public health programs and societal infrastructure = brain health. "I'm so excited that we're finally able to put in place some things our kids have needed for decades," said Hanna-Attisha. "And the other piece of it that energizes me is to share these best practices with other communities that may also be struggling with lead, poverty, violence, or other adversity that messes kids up for their entire life course trajectories." For Dr. Mona, such collective-minded actions are how we begin shifting from the neoliberal misapprehension that resilience is purely an "individual trait" to a broader concept that, in her words, "describes a community—and society—that cares for everyone."[65]

Evidence shows that early intervention programs for exposed children, such as the one Hanna-Attisha is developing in Flint, which focus on lead remediation, nutritional assessment, medical evaluation, and public assistance referrals, can have a major influence on "righting the ship" to optimize academic and behavioral outcomes as well as quality of life. For perspective, as scholar Fredrik deBoer has argued, while the overall cost to treat the 5% of US children estimated by the CDC to have high lead exposure is $20 billion ($5,288 per child), the F-35 fighter plane is projected to cost taxpayers more than 72 times that amount over its lifespan. "Ultimately," argues deBoer, "our lead problems are a matter of political will. What we need is a muscular federal policy to combat this problem, funded with public dollars."[66]

A National Response to the Lead Crisis

We obviously concur with deBoer's assessment that, in our market-fundamentalist era, we need to relearn to think about an active role for the state in redressing systemic problems and building collective resilience. Given the ubiquity of lead in our country's drinking water, it would not be far fetched to declare the whole nation a Superfund site (a term the US government uses to refer to any land that has been contaminated by hazardous waste and poses a risk to human health or the environment). The vast reach of the lead epidemic across the United States is a direct result of choices made during the neoliberal era that have shifted wealth into private hands and away from public investment in protective programs, services, and infrastructure. Federal funding to maintain public water and sewer systems has declined 74% since the 1970s. Whereas in 1977 the federal government spent $76.27 per person (in 2014 dollars) on water services, by 2014 that support had fallen to $13.68 per person.[67] Such austerity-minded cost cutting has, as Hanna-Attisha described, put cities like Flint and the thousands of census tracts with even higher rates of elevated lead "in this reactive, near-bankrupt state where they can't even provide basic services like water, public health, and infrastructure."

Politicians often talk about "big infrastructure projects," and this evokes imagery of high-speed trains, new roads, and orange construction barrels. But given the current predicament whereby the United States has essentially become a Superfund site of a thousand Flints, we ought to "think big" in terms of replacing our country's toxic water infrastructure so that *no* children are exposed to *any* lead when they drink water from a faucet or water fountain. In this age of great but disparate prosperity, we should ask why we are not able to forge a whole workforce committed to surveilling lead levels, creating abatement teams to safely remove it from homes, soils, and workplaces, and replacing aging lead-based piping.

For a country that has built the largest empire in world history, with more than 300,000 military personnel abroad stationed in over 800 bases in 80 countries[68] (at a cost estimated at $300 billion annually[69]), there would seem to be opportunities to redeploy and reskill our troops to assist in this sort of domestic disaster relief. Effectively, such an initiative could redirect a portion of military personnel stationed abroad into a civil defense force to provide lead abatement, install filtration systems, and replace national lead-based infrastructure (lead service lines still connect the plumbing of over 6 million known homes to water mains under the street).[70] Few institutions in our country garner the respect and trust of the public as much as the military, which encompasses such diverse scientific, technical, and engineering expertise, making them an ideal partner to lead on-the-ground efforts. A small portion of the budget for our seemingly endless foreign wars (not to mention even a partial repatriation of the money corporations and wealthy elites illegally stash in overseas tax havens) could easily cover the annual costs of such a program. It is a rather bracing gut punch to consider that while our country's drinking water infrastructure has crumbled at home, putting tens of millions of Americans at risk for lead exposure, the United States has since 2001 spent $6.4 trillion on wars abroad in the Middle East and Asia.[71]

Perhaps we should continue taking inspiration from the New Deal and think bigger as we seek escape velocity to exit the American dementia era. Creating a civil defense force for lead safety would be a powerful connective thread back to the Works Progress Administration and Civilian Conservation Corps, which provided gainful, purposeful employment to millions of Americans after the Great Depression and enriched civic culture in ways still present and visible today.[72]

Absent such a major state investment, lead will continue plaguing our communities, degrading bodies and brains, and lowering population reserve. Just in Flint alone, replacing the more than 15,000 lead service lines in the city is estimated to cost more than $60 million (note that this is the same amount Flint lost in annual revenue sharing from the state in the wake of the Great Recession,.as well as an amount nearly equal to Bill Gates's donation to Alzheimer's drug development discussed in chapter 3) and take up to 15 years.[73] In a country that annually spends $700 billion on military-related expenditures, is currently bombing over half a dozen foreign countries, and remains every bit the "greatest purveyor of violence in the world" that Dr. Martin Luther King assailed in his 1967 "Three Evils of Society" speech, it is not clear why finding dollars to properly address the domestic crisis in Flint and elsewhere should be so vexing. King warned of how endless war had created a "malady within the American spirit" and urged that, as a result of this debasement, the nation's "soul becomes totally poisoned." Considering today's situation in Flint and elsewhere, this statement seems, quite tragically, to be both literally and figuratively true.

While rising to the monumental challenge of lead abatement would affirm our common humanity and egalitarian commitment to our collective well-being as we build population reserve, there are also clear economic benefits to treating populations by removing the heavy metal from our water, homes, and public spaces. A 2017 report by the Robert Wood Johnson Foundation and Pew Research estimated that for the babies born in 2018, if blood lead levels were kept to zero micrograms per deciliter, the benefits would amount to $84 billion.[74] The report's five key findings were as follows:

1. Removing leaded drinking water service lines from the homes of children born in 2018 would protect more than 350,000 children and yield $2.7 billion in future benefits, or about $1.33 per dollar invested.

2. Eradicating lead paint hazards from older homes of children from low-income families would provide $3.5 billion in future benefits, or approximately $1.39 per dollar invested, and protect more than 311,000 children.
3. Ensuring that contractors comply with the Environmental Protection Agency's rule that requires lead-safe renovation, repair, and painting practices would protect about 211,000 children born in 2018 and provide future benefits of $4.5 billion, or about $3.10 per dollar spent.
4. Eliminating lead from airplane fuel would protect more than 226,000 children born in 2018 who live near airports, generate $262 million in future benefits, and remove roughly 450 tons of lead from the environment every year.
5. Providing targeted, evidence-based academic and behavioral interventions to the roughly 1.8 million children with a history of lead exposure could increase their lifetime family incomes and likelihood of graduating from high school and college and decrease their potential for teen parenthood and criminal conviction.

We have precedent for the widespread public health effects that might be realized in conjunction with widespread lead removal. From 1922 to 1975, thousands of tons of lead were used annually as an additive in gasoline to enhance engine power.[75] In turn, gaseous lead was expelled from the exhaust of cars and settled into the soils and sediment in and around roads. Under the muscular Clean Air Act, however, lead was phased out of the country's petrol between 1975 and 1985, dramatically reducing the environmental burden of lead from vehicle exhaust and dropping collective lead levels in our blood by more than 80% (figure 5.2). In 1976, the average American child's blood lead level was 13.7 lg/dl, but by 1991—thanks to regulation—it had fallen to 3.2 lg/dl. Removal of lead from gasoline spared as many as 3.4 million children from growing up with hazardous concentrations of the toxic metal in their bodies,[76,77] underscoring just how environmental protections can make an immediate and profound impact on public health.

The conversion to unleaded gasoline—a move fiercely opposed by the auto and lead industries and politicians at the time—may be one factor

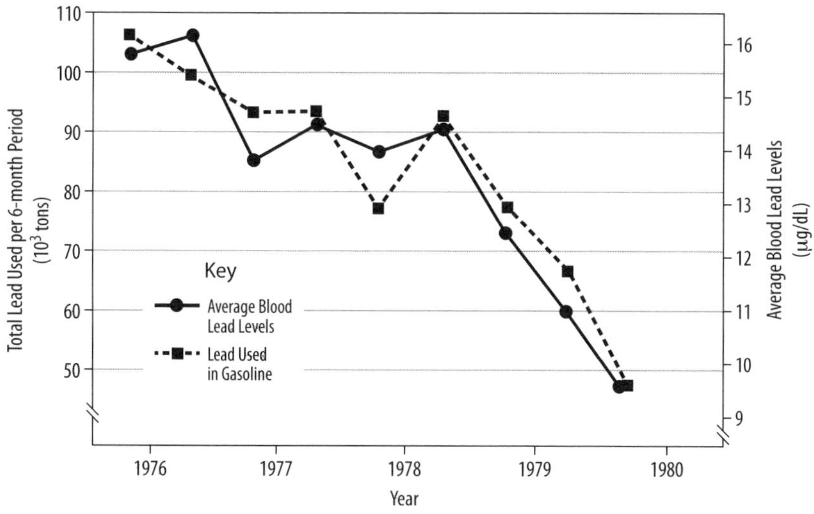

Figure 5.2. Average blood-lead levels versus lead used in gasoline
Source: Adapted from the U.S. Environmental Protection Agency.

that helps explain the reduction of violent crime since the 1970s (figure 5.3),[78] an uptick in population mean IQ by nearly 5 points,[79] as well as the falling rates of dementia in the United States and elsewhere that have been documented in the *population revelation* studies.[80,81] Obviously, these findings are only correlations and not evidence of causation (it would be ethically impossible to conduct a controlled experiment that intentionally exposed some but not all participants to lead), but the removal of a major neurotoxin from human environments has clearly been to the benefit of our species.

In the 1970s, before neoliberalism had fully unleashed domestic and global markets, the United States was the first nation in the world to begin regulating lead out of paint and gas. As we have moved into the 2020s, the Trump administration sought to aggressively reduce regulations and environmental protections that are "burdensome" to big industry but crucial to the provision of clean water for the masses.[82] Do we have the courage to act on the available evidence (and, more importantly, our moral convictions) and use the state as an instrument to treat populations and bring about even greater public health benefits in the 21st century? At this point, what excuse do we have? How many more Flints are necessary before we say "enough"?

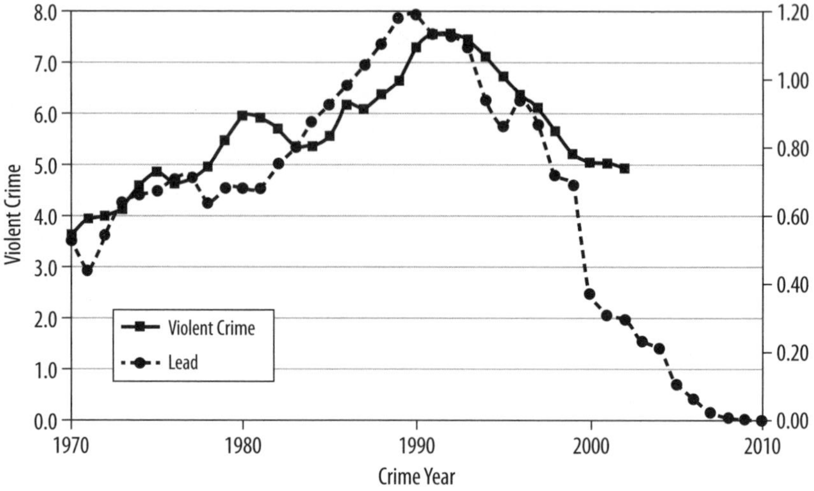

Figure 5.3. Violent crime and lead.
Source: Adapted from a graph by Jessica Wolpaw Reyes.

CONCLUSION

At times, the onset of the COVID-19 pandemic has felt like watching the Flint crisis in fast forward. Both situations exposed the failure of austerity politics, crumbling infrastructure, the incompetence of neoliberal governments, vast inequality, and—perhaps most of all—the consequences of hyper-capitalism placing the growth of the market over the needs of people. Yet, while crises like the ones we've experienced in quick succession over the last decade often evoke terror and panic, they also reveal a unique capacity to create solidarity between human beings and mobilize collective actions and material investments in our shared destinies. In today's world, when something like an epidemic threatens to unleash widespread devastation, we see the possibility for a change in tone from neoliberal individualism, atomization, austerity, and alienation to collective responsibility for domestic and international public health, and an acknowledgment of the inherent connectedness of our species. In the United States, for instance, the coronavirus created unique conditions in which millions of protestors filled the streets to protest systemic racism and demand more fair and just treatment of black citizens.

With respect to brain health, we are facing down yet another "invisible enemy"—a national lead epidemic—and vested powers continue pushing to weaken the EPA's regulatory power over clean water[83] and let groundwater contamination escape regulation under the Clean Water Act.[84] However, in the spirit of Occupy, leaders like Hanna-Attisha in Flint are providing a blueprint for how we can pull together as a collective force to address the crisis while making our society safer, more humane, resilient, and equitable in the balance of power and resources, and less victim to the triple-pronged evils of poverty, racism, and war. With a surge of political will and popular courage, and a bold commitment to reorganizing our society and its institutions around social democratic principles that put people over profits and guarantee universal rights to health care, education, clean water, and other public goods, we could achieve domestic progress that would protect our children for generations, promote brain health for millions, and further lower collective risk for Alzheimer's syndrome, among countless other health benefits. Those of us who—like Mona Hanna-Attisha—wish to pursue human flourishing and oppose injustice, pain, and suffering may draw inspiration from philosopher and novelist Albert Camus, who in his famous allegory *The Plague* wrote, "All I say is that on this earth there are pestilences and there are victims—and as far as possible one must refuse to be on the side of the pestilence."[85]

To donate to Flint's children, visit the Community Foundation Greater Flint website, www.cfgf.org. To read more about Mona Hanna-Attisha and her leadership in responding to the Flint crisis, see her 2018 book *What the Eyes Don't See* (New York: One World).

6

#PoorLivesMatter

Fighting Poverty to Resist Alzheimer's

In late October 2012, Superstorm Sandy began brewing in the warm waters of the Caribbean. In a matter of days, the storm matured into a massive hurricane that swept north, battering the East Coast of the United States with heavy rains, gusting winds, and surging flood waters. Thousands were left without homes, electricity, or public transport, once again touching a nerve of deep social inequity in a way that stoked peoples' sense of indignation at the political-economic order.

While Occupy Wall Street's tent village had been evicted from New York City's Zuccotti Park earlier in the year, within days of the storm's landfall, 16,000 Occupy supporters had rapidly mobilized in the coastal Northeast as part of an #OccupySandy operation. Working with churches and community organizations, the group helped open medical clinics, deliver food and supplies to people in need, visit homes to conduct mold remediation and repair damage, and assist those affected in receiving proper help from the government.[1] Occupy's labor working group—99 Pickets—supported efforts to mobilize low-wage workers who had lost pay (or jobs altogether) because of the storm.[2]

Just a month after Sandy hit, in front of a McDonald's a mere five miles north of Zuccotti Park, 200 New York City (NYC) fast-food workers went on strike. In addition to protesting their treatment during Sandy, these workers—many of whom were earning the federal minimum wage of $7.25 per hour—demanded higher pay and the right to unionize.[3] Like the superstorm itself, the movement continued gaining strength throughout the next year, and, as we saw in Flint, the crisis became an opportunity to build working-class solidarity and make demands for a healthier society and more supportive structures and institutions. On April 4, 2013, hundreds more workers went on strike in NYC, staging the largest single-day demonstration in the history of the fast-food industry.

The timing of this second strike was symbolic—held on the solemn 45th anniversary of Martin Luther King's assassination in Memphis in 1968. Despite mounting death threats and increased FBI surveillance due to King's criticism of US militarism and Western capitalism, he had visited the Tennessee city to support striking municipal sanitation workers, nearly half of whom worked full time but required welfare benefits to survive because they were so poorly paid. A day after delivering his rousing "I've Been to the Mountaintop" speech in support of the workers, King was tragically slain under suspicious circumstances at the Lorraine Motel. Unbowed, the Memphis sanitation workers persevered to win the wage increases and union recognition they sought.

Thanks to the dominant rise of the neoliberal order in the decades after King's death, the world of the fast-food protesters who took to the NYC streets after Sandy in 2012 looks equally as despairing as that of the sanitation workers, if not worse. Despite the fast-food industry pocketing combined annual global revenue of $570 billion,[4] the mean wage for front-line workers is $18,600 (about $8.69/hour)—lowest of any industry in the United States[5,6]—and employees make an average of 1,200 times less than industry CEOs.[7] As a result of the epidemic of low-wage pay in the industry, one in five families with a member holding a fast-food job live below the poverty line. Recalling the struggles of the sanitation workers in Memphis, an estimated 87% of fast-food workers don't receive health benefits through their employer, and over half are enrolled in at least one public assistance program.[8,9]

That the day-to-day struggles and exploitation of our low-wage workers remain as desperate now as when Dr. King joined the picket lines in Memphis in 1968 is dispiriting. And yet, there is a pulse of resistance within the national fast-food workforce. The McDonald's uprisings spawned by Sandy's devastation went on to spark a strike wave among fast-food workers in Chicago, St. Louis, Milwaukee, Seattle, and even in Flint. Now, the protest has expanded to more than 300 cities on six continents under the banner of the Fight for $15—an antipoverty movement that one can well imagine King championing were he still with us today—and has helped galvanize a record strike wave, resulting in 2018 seeing the most organized worker actions in 35 years.

As we have seen in Flint and elsewhere, socioeconomic marginalization is linked with greater late-life risk for dementia,[10,11,12,13] and the material impoverishment unleashed by the neoliberal order works through insidious causative pathways to inscribe damaging effects on the brains and bodies of the 99%. In this chapter, we continue examining these pathways, looking primarily through the lens of the fast-food workers who are rising up as part of the Fight for $15 movement as a representative slice of the working poor, who labor at the lower reaches of the massive hierarchy of contemporary America. Thinking about the systemic challenges faced by low-wage workers who subsist in the poverty conditions wrought by the unleashed beast of hyper-capitalism can help further illuminate the social determinants of health that affect brain aging for all of us (especially the most vulnerable) and can further identify areas where we must intervene as a society to challenge power, build institutions that foster a more inclusive prosperity, and treat whole populations to build collective reserve. In doing so, it will also be useful to consider ways in which poverty pushes people into professional niches where they assume greater physical risk for neurodegenerative disease. In a spirit of solidarity (and empathy), let's put ourselves in the shoes of our fellow citizens who toil in the American fast-food industry.

NUTRITION

"I'm not trying to be a millionaire working at Taco Bell, but I do want the basics. I don't want to have to sacrifice breakfast to buy a Metro Card."
—CHAD TALL, Taco Bell

"I've got to be making choices: putting food on the table, paying the bills, and paying rent."
—ALVIN MAJOR, KFC

America, land of abundance and the cradle of fast food, faces a most confounding national nutritional crisis.[14,15] Thirty-seven million US citizens—over 11% of the population—were food insecure during 2018,

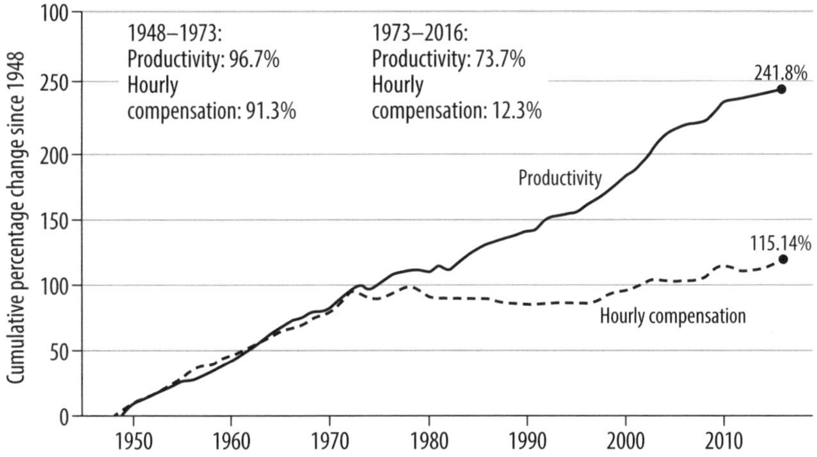

Figure 6.1. Since the emergence of neoliberalism in the 1970s, hourly compensation for workers has failed to track with rising productivity.
Source: Adapted from the Economic Policy Institute, December 12, 2018.

meaning that they and those in their households lacked access to enough food for an active, healthy life.[16] A startling one in seven Americans living in our "land of plenty" currently rely on a food bank (organizations that are, themselves, prominent symbols of hyper-capitalism[17]), with nearly half being from families with full-time wage earners, a reflection of just how much wages have stagnated under decades of neoliberal reordering of the economy. As wealth has transferred upward, workers have been asked to do more while receiving less compensation (figure 6.1).

In a stroke of cruel irony, reliance on outside support to achieve basic food security often befalls workers in the fast-food industry, who receive an annual average of $1.04 billion in food stamp benefits and commonly make use of food pantries. So ubiquitous is this form of *corporate welfare* that McDonald's even offers its low-wage employees a McResource phone line to facilitate underpaid employees registering for public assistance.[18] While the company resists paying all workers a living wage, it nevertheless has offered a recent disgraced CEO an exit package upward of $42 million.[19]

As reflected in the lament of both fast-food workers quoted above, paltry wages and scarce benefits create a precarious day-to-day existence that makes it *virtually impossible* to adhere to the types of diets that we know are protective against dementia. In general, the life-course eating patterns that have shown consistent benefit for brain health are those broadly aligned with the diets of our hunter-gatherer ancestors, which predated the disastrous shift to agriculture we examine in chapter 4. There is a cottage industry commodifying such diets, but perhaps the most evidence-based model is the so-called Mediterranean diet, which is an umbrella term for an eating pattern defined by a high intake of vegetables, fruits, cereals, and nuts; moderate intake of fish and alcohol; and low intake of dairy products, red meat, and processed products (such as fast food). While randomized controlled data are more limited, retrospective studies have consistently shown such diets—which are mostly plant based; contain high levels of fiber, vitamins and minerals, antioxidants, phenolic compounds, and unsaturated fatty acids—to be associated not only with lower risk of cognitive decline, dementia,[20,21,22,23,24,25,26,27,28,29] and the pathology of Alzheimer's syndrome,[30] but also with reduced risk of cardiovascular disease[31] and diabetes,[32] which are major companion risk factors for dementia and age-related frailty.[33] Even more recent studies have shown that a hybrid of Mediterranean-like diets and low-salt diets (perhaps better known as DASH, or dietary approaches to stop hypertension) exert a more powerful protective effect on cognitive function and reduced dementia risk, again confirming the intuitive benefits of diets that benefit the highly intertwined brain and vascular system.[34,35] Mechanistically, healthier cardiovascular systems can over time contribute to better cardiometabolic health and brain perfusion, neuronal function, energy metabolism, and beta-amyloid processing, thereby helping fortify cognitive reserve.[36]

For millions of people who prepare our nation's fast foods, poverty not only precludes the possibility of achieving such lifelong patterns of healthy eating but also nudges them toward low-cost, highly processed, starch- and sugar-heavy junk foods, which are calorie dense and nutrient deficient. As in Flint, *food deserts* (areas lacking full-service grocery stores and supermarkets, where it is difficult to purchase healthy foods) are present throughout the country, particularly in low-income urban areas. Mona Hanna-Attisha calls Flint a "food swamp" because of not only the paucity of healthy foods, but also the surfeit of low-cost, heavily marketed junk foods that are—out of necessity—daily sustenance for the working poor. Such is the nutritionally impoverished food environment many of our low-income citizens, including frontline fast-food workers, must navigate daily: one dominated by transnational corporations whose business model is dependent on enticing the public to consume high-margin processed foods that cost little to produce.[37]

We know that the consequences of poor diets shaped by both economic and food insecurity can make an imprint starting early in life as our brains and body systems develop—even in utero. In fact, similar to lead exposure, low birthweight caused by fetal malnutrition, among other factors, is strongly associated with reduced cognitive test scores, attention deficit hyperactivity disorder, lower schooling attainment, lower earnings, and higher rates of social welfare program participation.[38,39,40] Low birthweight has also been shown to put people at greater risk for vascular illnesses decades later in their lives, which affect the vast underlying system of vasculature that keeps our brains healthy, oxygenated, and detoxified.[41] Perhaps unsurprisingly, studies have linked lower minimum wages to increases in low birthweight babies.[42] Increasingly, research is demonstrating that the microbiome—the massive ecosystem of bacteria, viruses, and fungi that live in our intestinal tract and can be weakened or strengthened by the quality of our diets (and other lifestyle factors)—may have a role to play in modulating neural, immune/inflammatory, endocrine, and metabolic pathways that affect our aging brains across the lifespan.[43,44,45,46,47,48] Plant-based, Mediterranean-like diets have, quite unsurprisingly, also been shown to be most beneficial to the health of our microbiota.[49]

Until we address the unconscionable poverty and exploitation engineered by the imbalanced structures and institutions of the neoliberal era and provide a decent standard of living to all Americans, poor nutrition—and the resulting inflammation, oxidative stress, insulin resistance, impaired vascular health, and weakened microbiome—will continue to plague our country's poorest citizens to the long-term detriment of millions of aging bodies and brains. Indeed, it is a fundamental sign of our American dementia that we forget the past and do not have the forethought to invest for the long-term through population-level prevention.

STRESS AND DEPRESSION

"I have always needed two jobs. You basically need two jobs to survive working on low wages. I [am] so tired . . . If I [take] a break I would go to sleep, so I work straight through."

—FRAN MARION, Popeyes (and janitor)

"It is so depressing. You put a smile on because you're in customer service and you have to. But on the inside it really breaks you down when you're always at work but you're always broke. With [$15 minimum wage] I could walk with my head held high. No more crying at night. Because you can't cry in front of the kids because they'll know something is wrong."
—AKILAROSE THOMPSON, McDonald's

In chapter 4, we examine the stunning *population reserve* finding that dementia rates have been on the decline in the United States and elsewhere. Yet, these dropping rates are not equally distributed across the board. Researchers have found that African Americans over the age of 65 are two times and Latin Americans one and a half times as likely to develop Alzheimer's as Caucasians, with these trends expected to continue in future decades.[50] People of color are, of course, disproportionately employed in low-wage service jobs, including the fast-food industry, where 23% of workers are black and 20% are Latino.[51,52,53]

The reasons for this unbalanced racial distribution are complex. Yet research suggests that one major variable has an outsize influence on risk for historically disadvantaged groups, in addition to their having been subjected to inequitable access to higher education across the mid- to late 20th century: the *frequency of stressful experiences* suffered across the life course. Researchers have found that a single major stressful event—which they defined as "being fired from a job, the death of a child, growing up with a parent who abused alcohol or drugs, or experiencing combat"—is equal to about four years of cognitive aging, and that African-Americans endure over 60% more of such events than Caucasians over their lifetimes.[54]

Of course, stress-related illnesses on the whole have increased across the board during the American dementia era, with one study finding that between 1983 and 2009, rates of stress rose by 18% for women and 24% for men.[55] A Gallup poll of US workers found that 31% of those surveyed were either somewhat or completely dissatisfied with their levels of on-the-job stress, which was up three percentage points from the previous year and eight points from before the Great Recession. Correspondingly, there has been a fourfold rise in antidepressant medication use in the United States between 1988 and 2008.[56] Researchers have shown that stress has a greater effect on health in countries that are more strongly neoliberal (like the United States and the UK) than those that are more strongly organized around social democratic principles (Scandinavian countries). The biology of chronic stress may help explain the *Spirit Level* findings shared in chapter 4, which established that less egalitarian societies are almost always less healthy societies in every objective measure.[57,58]

So what are the mechanisms of poverty-related stress on the body and brain? While adaptive in the short term, stress can over time cause elevation in adrenaline, cortisol, and other stress hormones; chronic inflammation; muscle tension; blood vessel constriction; and increased heartbeat, all of which can—like poor nutrition—affect brain cells and the overall health of the vascular system. Scientists refer to this as the *allostatic load*—a measure of the microscopic wear and tear that chronic stress exerts on the body. Of course, chronic stress related to poverty and precariousness (worrying daily about paying bills, feeding kids, safety, and so on) also creates a "bandwidth" problem in the brain that diminishes cognitive function, reduces brainpower necessary for navigating other aspects of life,[59] and results in neurologic changes, such as less-organized functional brain networks and reduced cortical thickness.[60] Researchers have suggested that people exposed to sustained day-to-day hardship chronically operate at a diminished cognitive level akin to losing a night of sleep.

Depression has also long been associated with greater risk for cognitive aging, linked to specific structural changes in the brain (smaller hippocampal volume; abnormalities in the frontal lobes, caudate, and putamen; and increased deposition of plaques and tangles). Of course, both stress and depression also affect the vascular system. Researchers have recently found that the trauma and fallout from the Great Recession worsened overall blood pressure in American adults, reversing the decades-long improvements we describe in chapter 4.[61]

As reflected in the comments of the fast-food employees above, for the working poor—who so often lack job security, benefits, and predictable scheduling, and who harbor daily worries, anxieties, and resentments related to their relative powerlessness and lack of representation in the workplace—the context of day-to-day poverty can impose a heavy cognitive and psychological load that exacts commensurate physical costs "under the skin."[62] In an era when a stagnant minimum wage has failed to keep up with inflation and rising productivity, when unions have been steadily weakened by the 1% and their political allies, and when more and more people work on temporary contracts without full benefits, many are made to suffer daily indignities in relative powerlessness vis-à-vis management without the prospect of material improvement. Such chronically precarious circumstances have led some to term the modern workforce the "precariat."[63] Indeed, the indignity of having a persistently low and unstable social position can leak into emotional lives, which can become, quite literally, *toxic* over time—a reality that is quite comprehensible in the context of our evolution from small egalitarian bands that carefully regulated the formation of hierarchies. Studies consistently associate job insecurity with numerous adverse outcomes, including worse mental health, high blood pressure, higher rates of smoking, and unhealthy diet.[64] Researchers have established that internalizing a sense of unfairness in one's workplace puts employees at higher risk for coronary events.[65,66] In 2020, when the COVID-19 pandemic hit, we saw in real time the stress on "essential" workers who were either laid off or forced to assume exponentially greater risk and day-to-day stress than those with "nonessential" jobs and greater material security.

Another toxic, underexamined pathway through which poverty-related stress affects the brain is sleep disruption. Such a daily state is particularly problematic for shift workers and those in the precariat who, like Fran Marion above, are forced to work multiple jobs to piece together an even marginally livable income. Increasingly, sleep research is showing how essential consistent, quality, unobstructed sleep is to brain health. When we lapse into deep sleep, the brain's glymphatic system goes to work, with waves of cerebrospinal fluid flowing rhythmically through the brain, cleaning up metabolic waste that has accrued through the day.[67] Disrupting that process through sleep deprivation can downregulate the glymphatic system, leading to the buildup of toxic cellular detritus that can damage and impair the brain over time.[68]

Ultimately, until we achieve more fair, equitable, and democratically managed workplaces and address the unfettered free-market beast that—in the American dementia era—exposes the working poor to cruel and random indignities, the deprivations, chronic stress, and depression intermingled with poverty will continue leaving their indelible toxic marks on millions of aging bodies and brains.

SUBSTANCE ABUSE

"It's just stressful and really frustrating. It creates this push and pull within you that you really want to—but often can't—resolve. And in trying to cope with these fake feelings, I've turned to things I'm not proud of and don't admit to everyone."
—DONNA ABBOTT, McDonald's

One of the disturbing public health findings to emerge in recent years is the earlier mentioned rising number of what researchers call "deaths of despair," which have been increasing nationally, especially among the white working class and people out of the labor force who lack college education, but increasingly across racial, ethnic, and gender lines, as well as in cities and suburbs.[69,70,71]

As we touched on earlier, these deaths are often caused by self-harming behaviors involving suicide, drugs, and alcohol, born largely of grinding socioeconomic circumstance. They have become such a deep-seated problem that in the middle of the last decade they reversed, in part, previously rising average life expectancy in the United States.[72] Unavoidably, the underlying malaise causing such deaths is intertwined with the neoliberal political-economic order (powered by Wall Street), which has since the 1970s purposefully shipped quality jobs overseas; allocated capital away from industries that previously employed millions of middle-class Americans; created more hostile labor markets with fewer permanent jobs, which are low paying and include minimal (or no) benefits; reduced upward mobility (with skyrocketing costs for higher education); weakened social support (for example, decreased access to quality health care and mental health care); and enacted austerity measures that dismantled safety nets and funding for social infrastructure. For millions of Americans, such deteriorating conditions caused by the acid bath of neoliberal governance across the decades have fostered growing feelings of stress, disillusionment, precariousness, and a toxic resignation that prospects for the future will not improve—particularly for those with less education and lower socioeconomic status.[73]

Essentially, our zombie economy has created an underclass that is regarded by the free market as expendable, disposable, and nonessential. Whereas even in a caste system like India's, the lowest members of society (untouchables) retain an ostensibly meaningful role within the social hierarchy, in hyper-capitalist societies, members of the precariat (especially those without formal educations who struggle to find a place in today's service- and knowledge-based economy) exist on the razor's edge of job loss and total dislocation. Celia Vargas, a former cleaner in Trump International Hotel Las Vegas, captured the plight and precarity of the modern working class in a statement about her boss, Donald Trump: "We don't matter as workers or as human beings. For Mr. Donald Trump we're just a number."[74]

As the Fight for $15 has shown, the political-economic conditions that drive the underlying pain, distress, and social dysfunction rendering people more susceptible to addiction and substance abuse than ever before are also strongly manifest in the fast-food industry. According to the Substance Abuse and Mental Health Services Association, food service workers have the highest rate of drug use, with an estimated 17.4% of employees abusing substances.[75] As Donna Abbot and Celia Vargas reflect above, low-wage jobs in modern service industry workplaces can foster inhospitable and downright humiliating daily environments, which render employees more vulnerable to self-medication through substance abuse. Such self-destructive behaviors can range from overeating and smoking to more serious drug usage, such as alcoholism—all of which can directly damage the brain and vascular system, increasing risk for all types of dementia.[76,77] Indeed, poverty has consistently been shown to increase prevalence of smoking and alcohol abuse, and lower minimum wage has been associated with higher rates of smoking among low-income workers.[78,79]

It is perhaps a sad indictment of the deep injustices and cultural mood of our time that turning to painkillers (opioids)—drugs that effectively suppress pain receptors in the brain—happens to be a major form of coping with despair for people in our country. The defining drugs that humans covet in particular eras for existential escape—for instance, LSD and barbiturates in the culturally turbulent sixties, ecstasy and cocaine in the yuppy eighties, or painkillers today in an era of lethal despair—point us toward societal questions that demand answers.[80] Thus, we must focus not only on the substances that are killing people and damaging their bodies and brains, but, more critically, on what is systemically driving such widespread—and utterly unnecessary—accrual of pain and despair, especially for society's most dispossessed. Nor must we ignore the abjectly "demented" situation in which the Sackler family, which owns Purdue Pharmaceuticals (the manufacturer of OxyContin), has profited off the despair epidemic to the tune of $13 billion.[81]

PHYSICAL ACTIVITY

"I work downtown in a beautiful community, but then I come home to a neighborhood where I can't even take my kids to the park without worrying about a dangerous situation. Everyone's trying to get over on the next person because of what they don't have, and what they can't afford and what they can't do."

—KRYSTAL MAXIE-COLLINS, McDonald's

Above, we considered how modern dietary patterns and nutritionally impoverished food environments accessible to the working poor are mismatched with our ancestral heritage as hunter-gatherers who survived on diverse diets. Just as this evolutionary disconnect can make us more susceptible to chronic diseases that affect the brain over time, the bodies we have inherited from our hunter-gatherer forebears—which are adapted with unique morphological traits (such as long femurs, Achilles tendons, ability to regulate our body temperatures through perspiration) that enabled our ancestors to walk and run long distances in search of shared sustenance—are built to move but often subsist in modern home and work environments that drastically limit our physical activity.

For the working poor in the fast-food industry and elsewhere, the demands of the modern workplace and general exigencies of life in the precariat often preclude having sufficient time or resources for any meaningful exercise. As Krystal Maxie-Collins so poignantly expresses above, living in poorer neighborhoods that present more immediate dangers and lack social infrastructure like parks, pools, walking trails, markets, and gardens, further discourages people from exercising in ways that would offer biopsychosocial and brain health benefits.[82] Indeed, while there has been a significant decline in the absolute risk of cardiovascular events among high-earning US individuals over a recent 15-year period, these same improvements have not been observed among those with much lower incomes. Worsening rates of heart health over the last decade and a half among adults at or below the poverty line is a trend owed as much to lack of exercise as poor diet and implicates larger structural failures in the neoliberal era that are stacked against the working poor.[83]

Thanks to the intimate connection between vascular and brain health that we've seen throughout the book, one of the great truisms in the Alzheimer's field is that "What's good for the heart is good for the head," and countless studies have established exercise as a primary means of improving brain health and reducing dementia risk[84]—even as little as a one-hour walk three times a week,[85] or more than 4,000 steps a day.[86] In addition to improving vascular health throughout the body and brain, we also know that exercise—whether it be isometric routines, strength training, aerobics, or flexibility maintenance—increases brain-derived growth factors, which can yield new neurons and synapses, improve the health and integrity of the brain's white matter,[87] and increase neuroplasticity[88] and semantic memory.[89] Studies also consistently suggest that the location of the physical activity may be key, with outdoor, nature-based workouts conferring even greater benefits (for example, better mood, improved sleep, reduced obesity, better recovery from surgery) than indoor exercise.[90,91]

That the complex circumstances of poverty are impinging so profoundly on opportunities for physical activity across the course of the lives of people like Maxie-Collins ought to be a major focus for the Alzheimer's field—especially when there is such an abundance of data recommending the benefits of exercise for brain health.

FORMAL EDUCATION

"I know with $15 an hour, if it started tomorrow, I would only have to work one job then I would have an opportunity to go to work and then go to school."
—TERRENCE WISE, Burger King and McDonald's

As we know, education is a social resource that—through not yet fully understood mechanisms—builds *cognitive reserve*, which can extend the thresholds at which our aging brains convert to states of dementia.[92] Perhaps even more than access to health care, universalizing free higher and vocational education is likely to have a profound effect on the country's overall *population reserve*. Yet, given the runaway costs of our hyper-capitalist higher education system, which has come to treat college as big business and a market commodity rather than a civil right, poverty is a major barrier to quality education for the working poor. In the United States, only one-third of children whose parents are among the bottom 10% of income earners go to college. When children's parents are within the top 10% of earners, however, that figure reaches 90%. Such structural imbalances are, in part, how poverty and class invisibly, and inexorably, reproduce themselves to perpetuate durable societal hierarchies.

Other structural issues related to poverty reduce the odds of disadvantaged students gaining access to formal higher education. Significant gaps in skills (such as reading, math, self-control) between children with high versus low socioeconomic status can be observed as early as kindergarten, and these discrepancies persist through life.[93,94] Moreover, because of the way we fund our schools, poorer districts have weaker tax bases and thus generate less revenue for educational infrastructure, while also featuring higher student-teacher ratios; these districts suffer from diminished resources in ways that reduce educational quality that might otherwise prepare students to flourish in college, earn living-wage jobs, and derive the attendant myriad brain health benefits across the life course.

The high cost (and decades-long manacle of debt) associated with college in our "demented" neoliberal era and the pressing financial need for many youth to join the workforce right out of high school pushes many poor teenagers into low-wage labor. The need for the precariat to work multiple jobs to attain a livable income to support families—a reality voiced by Terrence Wise above—impose fundamental limits to accessing higher education. As a result, the cumulative cognitive reserve of the working poor is suppressed by the circumstances of their lives that impose barriers to formal education. For many like Wise, a $15 per hour (or higher) minimum wage—not to mention a guarantee of universally free higher education or vocational training—would provide the material foundation to make college a possibility and thereby allow more people the opportunity to strengthen the complex substrate that buffers us against dementia risk later in life, as well as obtaining a protective factor that significantly diminishes risk for despair-related deaths. Until we address this pernicious aspect of poverty and make higher education and vocational training a human right, millions will continue to be arbitrarily denied access to resources that could materially improve their lives (and society).

TOXIC EXPOSURES

"The managers at the store constantly push us to work fast . . . I've been repeatedly burned on the job . . . I see workers at the store getting burned all the time. This is exactly why workers at McDonald's need a union so we can have a voice."

—BRITTNEY BERRY, McDonald's

In 2015, the Fight for $15 conducted a national survey among fast-food workers, finding that 87% have suffered an injury on the job in the past year, including 78% with multiple injuries.[95] Burns are most common, with 4 of 5 workers experiencing them over the last year, while also reporting cuts, falls, injuries from lifting, and assaults.[96]

Other sectors of the hyper-capitalist zombie economy beyond fast food provide occupational hazards that are even more directly dangerous to the brains of low-income employees. For instance, laborers in conventional agriculture (farmers, farmworkers, ranchers, migrant workers, and so on) suffer from more pesticide-related health problems than those in any other occupation in the United States. Besides being potentially carcinogenic and damaging to the endocrine system, eyes, lungs, skin, and nervous system, pesticide exposure has also been linked with increased risk for dementia[97,98] and poorer IQ performance.[99,100,101] Researchers have also found elevated levels of common insecticides in brains of patients with AD diagnoses.[102]

Emerging industries like hydraulic fracturing (or *fracking*) for natural gas have raised major concerns about neurologic risk for both industry employees and community members who work and live near open fracking sites. While the practice has been fully banned in other countries, like France and Scotland, for its health risks and contributions to climate change, the United States currently allows drilling and fracking operations. At present, there are 1.2 million wells, with 20,000 new sites being opened annually.[103] Just as in Flint, Baltimore, Cleveland, and elsewhere with respect to lead, there is an environmental justice element to fracking that is interlaced with poverty. For decades, studies have shown that drill sites, wastewater disposal wells, and pipelines have been disproportionately permitted in areas with higher proportions of people of color and residents living in poverty, and that these communities have disproportionately suffered the effects of the air, soil, surface, and groundwater contamination related to the profiteering practice while not enjoying proportional local benefits.[104,105]

Research has also shown that the existence of fracking wells introduces environmental pollution (for instance, airborne particulates, ozone, organic/radioactive materials, exhaust from mechanical equipment, and the approximately 1,200 truck deliveries needed for every fracked well[106]) that degrades local air quality and subjects workers and local populations to a range of harmful exposures. Studies have linked well sites with exacerbations of asthma and respiratory illness,[107] as well as with greater incidence of headaches, migraines, sinus infections, fatigue,[108] and cancer.[109,110]

More apropos to risk for dementia, it is increasingly clear that the brain and central nervous system of the developing fetus are especially vulnerable to frequent maternal exposures to environmental pollution related to fracking. In 2017, scientists who analyzed 1.1 million births in Pennsylvania from 2004 to 2013 found that mothers living within 3 kilometers of a fracking site were more likely to give birth to infants with low birthweights (which dispose people to lower cognitive performance and increased risk for vascular disease), and congenital problems were more pronounced for those who lived geographically closer to active wells.[111] There is also concern that the practice of injecting acidic fracking fluids into the earth may cause greater leaching of heavy metals like manganese and mercury—which, like lead, are known neurotoxins associated with greater risk for dementia—into drinking water.[112] Of course, the very act of fracking puts frontline workers at risk for a host of occupational injuries, including falls, high-pressure accidents, and explosions that can cause traumatic brain injuries.[113]

In addition to fracking, air pollution (from cars, power plants, forest fires, and so forth) is a growing concern as a risk factor for dementia that disproportionately affects children and low-income residents living in crowded urban environments.[114] Several studies have recently suggested that airborne particulates from polluted air—roughly 1/30th the diameter of a human hair—can enter the lungs and pass into the bloodstream (or even bypass the blood-brain barrier altogether by infiltrating the olfactory bulb through the nose),[115] over time causing systematic inflammation throughout the body, damaging brain tissue and the vascular system and putting people at greater risk for heart attacks and strokes,[116] undermining cognitive development,[117,118] and predisposing people to higher risk for dementia.[119,120,121] A 2018 study in London found that people disproportionally exposed to air pollutants released by fossil fuel combustion were significantly more likely to develop Alzheimer's syndrome,[122] and a similar association has been observed in Taiwan[123] and in the United States.[124] Researchers have also linked 15 years of Medicare records for 6.9 million adults ages 65 and older to the EPA's air-quality-monitoring network. They found that in areas with higher compliance to air quality standards, older people developed Alzheimer's diseases at lower rates than peers in areas lacking regulatory safeguards. The team estimated that enforcing the EPA's stricter air quality standard likely resulted in 140,000 fewer people living with dementia by 2014, at a savings of $163 billion.[125]

High-density urban areas—places where the majority of fast-food jobs exist—are more at risk for airborne exposures because asphalt and concrete prevent the wind from dissipating particulates. Researchers have found plaques and markers of inflammation in brains of children and young adults in Mexico City, which has one of the worst air quality indexes in the world.[126] Comparisons of brain tissues show more pronounced markers of inflammation, oxidative stress, and plaques and tangles in residents of polluted-air cities compared to residents of relatively clean-air cities. Moreover, children in Mexico City and Boston, another polluted-air city, have performed poorer on measures of intelligence and short-term memory, and MRI scans and autopsies on otherwise healthy children who died in auto accidents or other traumatic events have revealed higher incidence of abnormal lesions in the prefrontal areas of their brains.[127] Air pollution is also linked with other complications, like low birthweight and general disruption of infant lung and brain development.[128]

Such realities make it all the more despairing that, in the early 2020s, the Trump administration has aggressively pursued the *four D's* of neoliberalism (deregulation, decreased taxation, decreased social programs, deunionized labor), including rolling back protections that lowered air-polluting emissions.[129]

TRAUMATIC BRAIN INJURIES: WHERE THE THREE EVILS OF POVERTY, RACISM, AND MILITARISM COME TO A HEAD

On the Battlefield

Traumatic brain injuries (TBIs) have become one of the defining medical conditions of the early 21st century. In addition to being a risk for workers in the volatile fracking industry, TBIs have entered mainstream discourse because of the so-called war on terror waged by successive US presidents in the wake of 9/11, which has created combat theaters in Iraq, Afghanistan, and elsewhere. Modern warfare often involves exposure to improvised explosive devices (IEDs), capable of inflicting tremendous concussive force that can cause the brain to move violently inside the skull, damaging cortical tissue and subcortical structures, precipitating vascular injuries, and damaging long axons interconnecting brain regions in ways not yet fully understood.

Consequently, TBIs have become the "signature wound" of the seemingly endless war on terror, accounting for 22% of casualties and 59% of blast-related injuries.[130] To say nothing of the countless innocents in non-hostile foreign countries, like Iraq and Afghanistan, who have been maimed or killed by our armaments, an estimated 350,000 US military personnel have experienced TBI, and many veterans have returned home suffering both neurologic and psychological damage from head injuries.[131] Similar to the insidious effects of lead, TBI can alter the brain's structure and function, expediting brain aging processes,[132] and research across cultures has increasingly demonstrated that one or more TBI can significantly increase long-term risk of developing dementia.[133,134,135,136,137,138,139,140,141,142] Studies on veterans from past wars—namely World War II[143] and Vietnam[144]—have found evidence of more rapid cognitive decline in soldiers who suffered head injuries compared to soldiers without such injuries.[145] As with neurotoxin exposure in children, this decline is likely because TBI materially weakens one's cognitive reserve, leaving the brain less resilient to age-related processes (neuronal loss, oxidative stress, inflammation, altered glucose metabolism, vascular damage, and so on) over time and increasing the threshold at which one would convert to cognitive dysfunction in the face of underlying neurodegeneration.

On the Playing Field

So too have TBIs become a crisis for major contact sports like football, where players, like troops in modern warfare, are at risk for both sudden concussive and repeated subconcussive blows to the head. The phenomenon of brain trauma being correlated with dementia has been studied since the 1920s. Early researchers focused on symptomatic boxers, who were labeled with a condition then called *dementia pugilistica*, and deployed terms like *goofy* and *slug-nutty* to describe the effects of blows to the head. In 1949, a British neurologist published a paper on *punch-drunk syndromes* in boxers, referring to the condition as *chronic traumatic encephalopathy*, or CTE.[146]

In the 21st century, more robust inquiry into the link between TBI and CTE has expanded beyond just boxing (a sport where the literal goal is to induce brain damage in one's opponent via knockout) to other athletes engaged in contact sports, like football, who have been found to be at higher risk for CTE. In 2005, neuropathologist Bennet Omalu was tasked with an autopsy of former Pittsburgh Steeler football player Mike Webster, who had died with severe cognitive dysfunction at age 50 while living homeless in his truck. While Webster's brain looked normal to the naked eye, Omalu insisted on fixing it for microscopic autopsy. Upon examination, he famously found *diffuse tauopathy*—essentially the widespread existence of tangles—in the former offensive lineman's brain tissue. It seemed that repetitive trauma from tens of thousands of head-on collisions in the trenches had started a cascade of events in Webster's brain, which had caused tau to go awry and damage the integrity of his brain cells in a way reminiscent of that particular feature of Alzheimer's syndrome.

As dramatized in the 2015 film *Concussion,* wherein actor Will Smith played Omalu, the billion-dollar corporate juggernaut of the NFL actively suppressed preliminary data correlating TBI with greater dementia risk. Three years after Omalu's autopsy of Webster, however, Boston School of Medicine launched the Center for the Study of Traumatic Encephalopathy, which has been banking brains of former athletes and developing a deeper understanding of the neurologic consequences of TBI.[147,148,149] Their data overwhelmingly show that TBI—caused by single concussive traumas and repetitive subconcussive injuries—put contact sport athletes at risk for CTE and related long-term cognitive complications. In 2017, the group shook up the sporting world when they released data showing that 110 of 111 brains of former NFL players, including Webster, showed signs of CTE.[150]

Robert Stern, who directs the center, believes the repetitive nature of head trauma overwhelms the brain's natural metabolic clearance systems, leading to loss of integrity of the blood-brain barrier, leakage of proteins, chronic inflammation, and diffuse tauopathy, particularly in the depths of the brain's folds (the *sulci*). This cumulative damage can cause changes in mood and behavior, sadness and depression, apathy, short-fuse temper and impulsivity, anxiety and agitation, as well as poor episodic memory, executive functioning, attention issues, Parkinsonism, gait disturbance, and impairment in activities of daily living. So far, the center has established this pathology in hockey, rugby, boxing, pro wrestling, bull riding, soccer, military veterans, and contact sport athletes as young as 17.

Indeed, the age of first exposure to football appears to affect later-life impact as well. Former NFL players who started playing before age 12—when the brain is undergoing a key period of development and maturation—were observed to have worse executive function and memory loss, smaller brain volumes, and more depression, apathy, and executive function problems later in life.[151] Youth with more cumulative head impact exposure but no concussions had more changes in white matter after only one season of play.[152] Stern is highly critical of youth football, telling us in a lecture at Penn State: "It doesn't make logical sense to drop kids at a playing field to hit their heads over and over again during periods of extensive brain growth and maturation." Even more bluntly, Omalu has argued that allowing children to play football "is the definition of child abuse . . . [I]f your child plays football, there is a 100% risk exposure."[153]

Poverty and Brain Injuries

So how does poverty associated with our era of neoliberal dysfunction fit into this story? As one might suspect, those with lower status in our socioeconomic hierarchy are more inclined to enter vocations in which they assume greater physical risk for TBI. Research evaluating the history of US military enrollment has found that the all-volunteer force continues to see overrepresentation of the working and middle classes, with fewer incentives for upper-class participation.[154] Researchers found that those with lower family income are more likely to enroll than those with higher family income, and that communities hit by trade shocks and the overall consequences of free trade in the neoliberal era have seen enrollment surges (the military even sends more recruiters to these areas).[155,156] In this way, the vast poverty and income inequality sown by zombie hypercapitalism over the last four decades have consistently increased the exposure of poor and socially disadvantaged groups to neurologic damage from TBI, which will broadly increase risk for dementia later in life.

Put simply: the working class disproportionately suffers from the imperial misadventures and endless war that are a prime derangement in our era of American dementia.

A similar class and race dynamic is at play in football, which regularly produces many collegiate and NFL players hailing disproportionately from impoverished backgrounds. An analysis of US census data has shown that the NFL is increasingly being represented by players (approximately 70% of whom are black,[157] in a league with no black owners) who were born in counties with poverty rates higher than the national average.[158] The prospect of escaping the privations and precariousness of poverty for million-dollar contracts, endorsement deals, and fame will continue to be a powerful incentive driving people from lower socioeconomic brackets to play a violent, dangerous game, which begins exposing them to long-term neurologic damage before they're even old enough to drive. This class dynamic is only going to increase as wealthier parents pull their children out of football for fear of long-term injuries. Just over the last decade, we've seen the number of high school athletes playing tackle football drop by more than 75,000 players.[159]

HOW WE CAN RESIST

Organize to Raise the Federal Minimum Wage

For the well-being of our bodies, brains, and collective society, we must make structural changes to address the widening inequalities in income and wealth that define our era. In 2019, 2.2 million working people were paid the federal minimum wage of $7.25 an hour or less. Approximately another 23 million people were paid between $7.25 and $11 an hour. Nearly half (42.4%) of working Americans made less than $15 per hour.[160] There are deep gender and racial gaps in earnings as well. Women make up more than half the total workforce earning less than $15 per hour despite being a minority of the workforce overall, and 53% of black workers and 60% of Hispanic workers make less than $15 per hour.[161] This racial wage gap has worsened over time relative to white workers.

As a result of these structural issues, where so many workers lack a federally enforced living wage of $15 an hour or more, tens of millions of people in this country spend their careers in the precariat, earning poverty wages, particularly minorities. Meanwhile, the annual Wall Street bonus pool alone is consistently larger than the *annual year-round earnings* of all 3.3 million Americans working full time at the federal minimum wage, which has been inexplicably frozen at $7.25 per hour since 2009. In all of US history, this represents the longest stretch without a minimum wage increase.[162] Because of this stagnation, since 1968, the federal minimum wage has lost a stunning 31% of purchasing power, again underscoring the material pinch on the lives of the working poor.[163] It is perhaps unsurprising, then, that research has shown a strong link between lower minimum wage and higher risk for suicide. In fact, research published as part of the *British Medical Journal* group has recently suggested that between 1990 and 2015, raising the minimum wage by $1 in each state might have saved more than 27,000 lives, and an increase of $2 might have prevented more than 57,000 suicides.[164]

Thankfully, there is a clear blueprint for how to mitigate this problem and thereby support societal and brain health: pass a federal minimum wage of at least $15 with provisions to link future rises to productivity, inflation, median earnings, or consumer price index. As we've established, spanning high periods of growth during the social democratic consensus of the postwar era, increases in minimum wage tracked with worker productivity, creating a robust middle class in the United States that shared the growing prosperity of the broader economy. Had trends continued to match productivity rather than being stifled by the neoliberal reordering ascendant in the seventies, minimum wage workers would be approaching $20 per hour (figure 6.2).[165,166] Seen in this light, the current aspiration to raise the wage floor from the paltry $7.25 it's been stuck at for a decade to $15 would seem a relatively modest demand.

In the not-too-distant future, we will reckon with the reality that a significant portion of American jobs may be replaced by artificial intelligence (AI) and automation[167] (even AD diagnosis is, in part, being shifted to

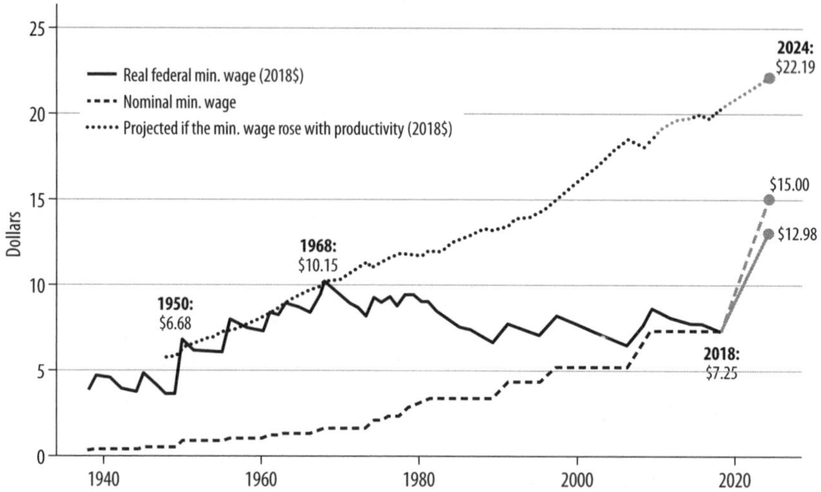

Figure 6.2. What minimum wage would look like today had it kept up with the rowing economy.
Source: Adapted from the Economic Policy Institute, July 24, 2017.

AI[168]). There is growing support for a federal jobs guarantee that would furnish work with a minimum salary above the poverty line for anyone seeking employment. Similar programs have been implemented in India and Argentina to reduce poverty and stimulate economic growth.[169] They also have an antecedent in the United States with the Works Progress Administration and Civilian Conservation Corps—the post–Great Depression programs that created jobs when the national unemployment rate reached 25%, causing FDR to propose a Second Bill of Rights, which included "The right to a useful and remunerative job."[170] One can imagine modern-day public works projects aiming labor at a multitude of contemporary societal exigencies: infrastructure improvement, the widespread integration of green energy, ensuring universal services (for example, childcare, elder care), school maintenance, local self-sustaining agriculture (food production), healthy food preparation (preparing and delivering medically tailored meals), waste management and redistribution (composting), artistic and cultural contributions, and so forth. Such work could provide purposeful and dignified labor and a living wage for workers, make workers more resilient to economic shocks like those caused by COVID-19, and create jobs aimed at promoting planetary health. We explore this possibility in greater detail in the next chapter, when we discuss the Green New Deal, and in chapter 9, when we explore the rising phenomenon of age- and dementia-friendly communities.

Ultimately, any measures to fight poverty would strengthen population reserve. Any progress, however, will mean resisting the impulses of the zombie economy to eviscerate public sector jobs, weaken unions, and defer to unbridled markets as a panacea. Given the lingering dominance of the American dementia era, there will be strong arguments in opposition to such programs, but aggressive social democratic action makes sense in not only *moral* but *economic* (Keynesian) terms. When jobs are created, the consumption and demand from additional workers produces a multiplier effect, which results in more jobs in other sectors of the economy. Moreover, a living wage can transition people living below the poverty line away from collecting traditional welfare, as well as increase the tax base. But mostly, guaranteeing a living wage for honest work ought to be a basic moral obligation we provide in a just and healthy society in the 21st century.

Support the Fight for $15 and Organized Labor

In 2019, Pew Research Center reported 67% support for raising the national minimum wage to $15 per hour.[171] Nonetheless, in an aggressively neoliberal era, when we must brace for federal inaction from the political class, who serve the interests of the 1%, people can still mobilize at state and local levels to push minimum wage in a fairer direction. Since its post-Sandy inception in NYC in 2012, the Fight for $15 has won a string of important victories and started a drumbeat for a more dignified wage that is echoing well beyond the fast-food industry. As of 2019, there are now $15-per-hour statewide minimum wage laws in seven states (and growing),[172] and more than 40 cities are moving toward that standard by 2022.[173] For full-time workers, this translates to an annual salary of about $31,000—hardly a king's ransom but enough to live on (for now).

Some corporations have even started to realize that raising their wages is good business. In 2017, Target became the first low-wage chain to announce it would raise its pay floor to $15 an hour in 2020[174]—their argument being that it would help attract and retain talent in a competitive retail sector. Such actions expose claims from corporate lobbyists, politicians and others who have staunchly argued against the feasibility of a living wage as empty, self serving, and ultimately cruel. Todd Carmichael,

CEO of La Colombe Coffee, has put it well: "Unless you pay your employees a nonpredatory living wage that keeps people and their families above the poverty line, you don't deserve to be in business."[175]

Collectively applying pressure on businesses and elected officials to help people live a more dignified and less precarious life (and, in doing so, lowering cumulative risk for dementia) is a critical way to contribute, and the Fight for $15 provides a powerful mechanism for resistance. Of course, improving minimum wage is only half the battle; we must also support the right of workers to form unions for leverage and negotiating power against companies that effectively view them as dispensable labor widgets. Over the last 50-plus years of neoliberal regimes, organized labor has been summarily weakened. In the 1960s, when King joined the sanitation workers in Memphis, one-third of US workers belonged to a union. Today, that number has dwindled to around 10%,[176,177] compared to Scandinavian social democracies like Norway, Denmark, and Finland, where the percentage of workers covered by union contract stands at 70%, 84%, and 93%, respectively.[178] In Germany, company boards are legally required to include workers, an arrangement that helps to curb inequalities within organizations, ensure better working conditions, provide greater control over work schedule and wages, and mitigate feelings of worker disempowerment. In the United States, a reliance on employee-based health care makes it extremely difficult to unionize, much less strike, and capital dominates the landscape and sets self-serving terms of employment.

When workers have more organization and leverage, income growth across the whole economy is more equal (according to the Bureau of Labor statistics, union workers earn 22% more on average than nonunion workers).[179] When they lose that structural power, income inequality and wage gaps expand. This fact was recognized by no less than Ronald Reagan, who, in 1980, before attacking unions in practice during his first administration, said, "Where free unions and collective bargaining are forbidden, freedom is lost."[180] Such proworker organizations are critical not just to protecting the material interests of the working class but also to ensuring safe, healthy, equitable workplaces that reduce stress and depression, support healthy lifestyles, and promote biopsychosocial well-being. Without unions again becoming a political force, it is difficult to imagine much cultural progress in resisting poverty and corporate power.[181]

A higher minimum wage will make enormous and pervasive impact in peoples' lives that will redound to better brain health as well as survival. As Matthew Desmond, author of the book *Evicted,* has eloquently written in the *New York Times,* "A $15 minimum wage is an antidepressant. It is a sleep aid. A diet. A stress reliever. It is a contraceptive, preventing teenage pregnancy. It prevents premature death. It shields children from neglect."[182]

Improve Local Food Systems

Given the broad food insecurity in our country, we can act in our communities to strengthen and grow local food systems for ourselves and our low-income neighbors. One of my (Danny) most rewarding community projects has been being part of a team that started a farmers' market at our hospital. These organizations—which numbered only a few thousand in the nineties but have grown to nearly 10,000 today—can be a powerful platform for supporting local efforts to mitigate the effects of poverty and to improve public health. In Hershey, we have had our market registered with several federal food stamp programs—SNAP and the Senior Farmers Market Nutrition Program—which expand access to fresh local produce for low-income community members (and are, resultingly, constantly placed on the neoliberal chopping block in Washington, DC).

I have also worked with Penn State medical students to launch programs that provide low-income, food-insecure patients at our hospital with "prescriptions" for fruits and vegetables that can be redeemed at several farmers' markets throughout our region. Students pair with families as "mentors" and meet them at the market over the course of multiple visits, learning the family's background, nutritional knowledge, and eating habits and helping them shop for foods and learn simple preparation techniques.[183,184] Slowly, our program has grown to include vulnerable groups in our region, including women living in transitional housing and resettled refugee families in Central Pennsylvania (figure 6.3).[185]

The success of these programs has led us to start a community garden on our hospital campus with over 200 plots—several of which donate thousands of pounds of produce each year to food-insecure populations in our community. Markets and gardens are relatively inexpensive pieces of community infrastructure that can directly provide material benefit to those for whom poverty is a major barrier to healthy eating.[186] They also

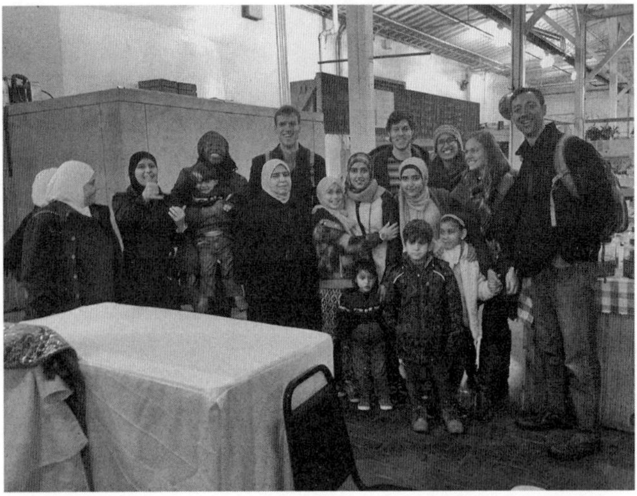

Figure 6.3. Medical students with Syrian families at a Harrisburg, Pennsylvania, farmers' market.
Source: Photograph by Daniel George.

undercut corporate control of our food supply, mitigating food deserts and food swamps, supporting the growth and sale of local fruits and vegetables, and increasing access to produce free of pesticides and herbicides. Perhaps most important, such spaces can serve as cultural, artistic, and political epicenters that more tightly bind us in self-contained, resilient communities with shared destinies, reducing the alienation and despair felt by so many. Hospitals, schools, churches, community groups, and other local advocates should increasingly "occupy" markets and gardens, growing their presence in our communities while making special effort to make them accessible to the food-insecure poor. As we know, eating a healthy balanced diet is a form of "vaccination" against chronic disease, and so too can food—one of the universal threads of humanity—be a starting point for a deeper moral commitment to one another.

Evolve the NFL

There is a scene in the film *Patton* where US General George S. Patton watches his soldiers wage battle in North Africa during World War II. As artillery shells burst like fireworks around him, Patton ruefully intones, "God help me, I do love it so." Such a sentiment almost perfectly captures the draw that we and many others feel to football. As former players and (recovering) fans, there is a certain aesthetic to a collective physical struggle of football that we cannot deny. But at this point, it is beyond any shred of doubt that contact sports like football *directly* cause greater risk for CTE and dementia.

Put otherwise, we have arrived at a point where we know that playing contact sports like football—as a professional or an amateur—exposes players to some degree of brain damage, often diffuse damage that affects peoples' executive functioning and susceptibility to impaired decision making over the course of their lives (for example, drug use, aggression, suicide). As with Alzheimer's, despite the innovation fantasies of neoliberalism, there appears to be no technological, market-driven solution to make football safer.

Given the self-interest at play with owners, players, TV networks, corporate sponsors, and others who profit from the cash cow of pro and amateur football, while treating players—disproportionately from impoverished backgrounds—like disposable commodities, the NFL and NCAA are clearly zombie entities that will impose only incremental changes on themselves without addressing the underlying fact that the structure of the game is what's wrong.

One school of thought suggests that by removing or modifying[187] the most dangerous elements of football (punt and kickoff returns, helmet-to-helmet contact, and the like), we can salvage the sport. Another school of thought rejects the proposition that a high-speed contact sport as inherently dangerous as football can be rendered safe through the alchemy of rule changes. Indeed, while small tweaks to protect players have been implemented across the past decade, concussions in the NFL have actually increased in recent seasons.[188]

Tellingly, the number of Americans reporting they are fans of pro football has dropped from 67% in 2012 to 57% in 2017,[189] with 90% of fans agreeing that head injuries represent a problem in the sport.[190] Personally, we believe the safest eventual outcome would be for the NFL to transition into high-level flag football. Such an evolution would retain the fundamentals of the game—using intricate schemes to score and defend—while succeeding in nearly removing the head from play. The finesse, athleticism, and complex strategy of football would remain, but there would be only minimal physical contact and head trauma, similar to the NBA. As fans, we could watch world-class athletes joyfully playing an offense-oriented game with dramatically less toll on the physical and mental health of players. Ideally, such a league would become the template for the new NFL as well as collegiate and amateur football.

Clearly, such an idea would draw the rebuke of many Americans. But football stripped of outright violence and related head trauma would still be a beautiful sport, perhaps even more so than the current game marred by the weekly sight of players (whose careers last, on average, 3.5 seasons) convulsing, stumbling off the field disoriented, and being knocked out cold by hits that literally injure the brain and increase material risk for dementia. Flag football with world-class athletes would be like expanding the exhilarating NBA game to a larger field of play. The ascendant popularity of the NBA, MLB, and even soccer in recent years would suggest that we perhaps overestimate our national lust for violence and understate our appreciation for beautiful games. There would even seem to be a role for the Alzheimer's Association to play in this major public health initiative—perhaps by supporting youth flag football across the country, especially in urban and rural poor areas.

Campaign against Militarism and Assist Our Veterans

The incalculable injuries suffered in Iraq, Afghanistan, and other modern theaters of war will be a sad legacy of militarism across the 21st century. Even so, the military-industrial complex first identified by Dwight D. Eisenhower continues unabated, and for the last two decades of the war on terror, which started with George W. Bush and grew under Barack Obama (who expanded Bush's two wars to bombing and drone attacking seven countries), the United States has spent $250 million *a day* on war.[191] Militarism and corporatism are intimately connected, and this dysfunctional symbiosis of the zombie economy will continue driving the United States into martial conflicts that kill, maim, and injure human beings and loot our public coffers until we as a citizenry confront it.

Doing so is urgent. Even beyond the untold number of brain injuries suffered by veterans in the war on terror, we are beginning to see that soldiers who fought in combat zones are increasingly affected by painkiller addiction, drug abuse, and related deaths of despair.[192] Global militarism effectively feeds domestic crisis.

We can find resistance at all levels. For instance, in May 2019, dock workers in Genoa, Italy, refused to load electric generators onto a Saudi

Arabian vessel that also carried military weapons and armaments. Union leaders who organized the efforts said, "We will not be complicit in what is happening in Yemen," referring to the Saudi's US- and EU-backed assault on its southern neighbor.[193] Protestors had also previously blocked the ship from loading weapons in France.

In addition to such grassroots resistance to militarism, we must demand nonimperial platforms from our politicians that fundamentally change a global order sustained by armed conflict and corporate power, as well as supporting candidates who commit to fighting wars on poverty rather than wars for US imperialism, foreign regime change, and corporate revenue.

So too must we take care of our troops who have been maimed and injured, particularly with the invisible TBIs that have such devastating consequences for servicemen and women. Coincidentally, according to the Economic Policy Institute, if we succeeded in raising the federal minimum wage to $15 per hour, nearly 2 million US veterans would benefit.[194] We can also help by lending our time and talents to veterans. Try reaching out to VA hospitals, many of which are eager to match your interests with their assignments and activities. There are organizations that connect volunteers with opportunities. For instance, Disabled American Veterans' Voluntary Service Program asks volunteers to transport vets to and from medical appointments and to visit hospitalized veterans. So too can lawyers offer services pro bono in the National Veterans Legal Services Program, and for those with backgrounds in psychiatry, psychology, or counseling, the Coming Home Project is a nonprofit organization that provides compassionate expert care, support, education, and stress-management tools for veterans and their families.

CONCLUSION

In 1968, just before Martin Luther King's death, he led efforts to organize a Poor People's Campaign to promote economic justice for poor Americans of all races—the original #PoorLivesMatter movement. The goal of the initiative was to visit the nation's poorest towns and hamlets, interrogating poverty, raising awareness of what King called "a kind of social insanity which could lead to national ruin,"[195] and eventually building a large multiracial coalition that would occupy the National Mall in Washington,

DC. There, those gathered en masse would pressure Lyndon Johnson's administration and Congress to allocate $30 billion to full employment, a guaranteed annual income, and increased low-income housing.

King and his fellow leaders toured poor cities across the country to drum up support for the campaign. In March 1968, the group made one of their first stops in Marks, Mississippi, a small Delta sharecropping community located in the heart of the state's poorest county. Upon visiting a ramshackle school that housed a Head Start daycare center, King encountered a roomful of children whom he observed were "wide-eyed and silent . . . virtually all were underweight, a condition that lent a special poignancy to their enormous eyes."[196] King and his fellow leaders looked on as the teacher set about feeding her undernourished students a meager meal. The Reverend Ralph Abernathy, one of King's most trusted confidants, who would go on to take the mantle of leadership after King's assassination, recalled how this experience touched something deep within his fellow reverend: "There was one apple. And they took this apple and cut it into four pieces for four hungry waiting students. And when Dr. King realized that that was all they had for lunch, he began to cry. The tears came streaming down his cheek. And he had to leave the room."[197]

It is hard not to be moved by such a story, particularly since 43 million Americans (13% of the population) and over one-third of American children still live in poverty.[198] We watch as our government facilitates the upward transfer of wealth and uses austerity policies to dismantle safety net programs, like Head Start, that give children (and their developing brains) a fair fighting chance, rendering the United States into what the Stanford Center on Poverty and Inequality identifies as "a clear and constant outlier in the child poverty league."[199] Indeed, the "social insanity" King railed against has continued growing into a full-fledged "dementia."

While our predicament is, in itself, morally repellent, in this chapter we've also examined how the context of poverty created and deepened by neoliberalism and its zombie economy is *actively driving* individual and societal risk factors for brain aging. Confronting the depths of immiseration due to our country's derangement and reordering our institutions around more humane principles is a moral mission that naturally aligns with the goals of resisting Alzheimer's syndrome. By probing deeper into how we can address the structural problems that drive and sustain poverty, we will also pursue a society that will better support the health of our bodies and brains, reducing risk for dementia. Indeed, there is little doubt that the reductions in dementia risk we have observed in the United States and elsewhere in recent years have been linked to the more egalitarian political-economic circumstances enjoyed by elders who came of age in the mid-20th century and benefited from sustained exposure to a fairer, more equitable, and protective society with less widespread poverty. As King said in 1965, "Call it democracy, or call it democratic socialism, but there must be a better distribution of wealth within this country for all of God's children."[200]

Just as in the sixties, there is gathering momentum for a healthier society, and it has found footing in the Occupy encampments in Zuccotti Park, in the rubble of Superstorm Sandy, in Flint, Michigan, in the Fight for $15, in the wave of teachers strikes, in the emergence of social democracy as an electoral force, in the Black Lives Matter movement, and in countless other places where people are pushing back to some degree against neoliberalism and the societal structures and institutions that promote systemic poverty, racism, the war economy, and environmental devastation. Our challenge will be to resist by making population-wide changes in public policy and public health that will lower and remove known and suspected risk factors across the life course. Put simply: *Poor. Lives. Matter.*

7

Turning Up the Heat on Global Warming

The Neurologic Costs of Climate Change

While driving to the grocery store a few years ago, during a stretch of work at Baycrest Health Center in Toronto, Canada, I (Peter) looked up at the sky and felt a bolt of fear. Never before had I seen a more threatening landscape, with gusty winds and dark clouds rolling overhead. After shopping for a few minutes, I stepped back outside to find torrential rains whipping around me in all directions. But the adventure had only just begun.

At the time, I was staying at a mixed assisted-independent living residential tower on Baycrest's campus—in a sixth-floor apartment normally occupied by elder residents. By the time I finished unloading my groceries, the rain was falling in buckets, and though soaked to the bone, I breathed a sigh of relief to be home. Little did I know that in the basement below my apartment, quickly rising waters were overtaking the building's transformer. In one high-voltage burst, electricity was lost, and I found myself in the dark with more than a hundred elder residents.

Frailer folks were quickly evacuated to a nearby hospital, and the rest of us to a hotel. While everyone in the community pulled together, there was much distress about spoiled food, recovering difficult-to-obtain medicines, and confusion about what would come next. After spending a week as low-level "climate refugees," we finally returned home.

Elder residents in other cities affected by disastrous weather events like Superstorm Sandy, Hurricane Katrina, and Hurricane Harvey have not been so lucky as we were. Nearly half of the people who died during

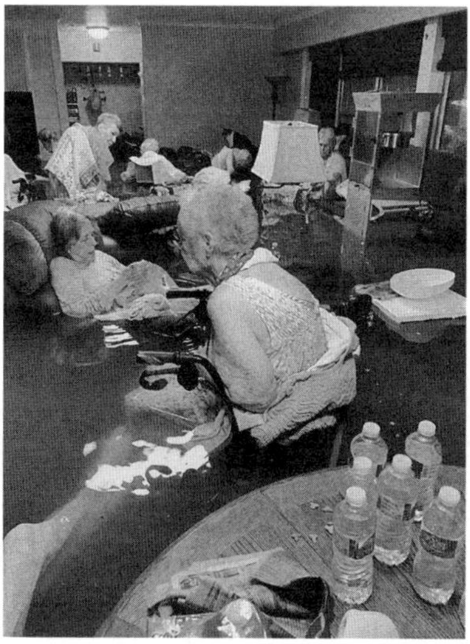

Figure 7.1. When Hurricane Harvey made landfall in Houston in August 2017, a record 57 inches of rain led to massive flooding throughout the city, affecting residents in residential care homes, including La Vita Bella in nearby Dickinson, Texas. Waters in the facility rose to five feet, and when the owners couldn't get anyone to help, they posted the photo to Twitter, eventually prompting attention from the national guard.
Source: Photograph courtesy of Trudy Lampson.

Hurricane Katrina in 2005 were 75 or older,[1] and when Sandy hit the East Coast in 2012, nearly half of those who died were over 65.[2] Five years later, Hurricane Harvey produced a record 57 inches of rainfall in Houston, paralyzing rescue efforts and forcing elders around the city to survive in place. A jarring photograph taken in the city's La Vita Bella nursing home, where residents sat neck deep in water for more than eight hours, waiting for help, has become one of the defining images of our global warming era (figure 7.1).

In an age of intense climate change, the simple lesson is this: people with dementia and others who have dependency, including children and the poor, are exponentially more vulnerable to environmental disasters. As our atmosphere further warms, we can expect to see disproportionate suffering in these populations. Yet so too will new physical, biological, and ecological threats associated with changing climates alter the circumstances that materially affect the health of *all* our aging bodies and brains. Climate change has already rendered the future of civilization an open question. Our window for acting is relatively short, and in that time, we will need to rewire our brains, reckon with our collectively "demented" behavior, and initiate *drastic* changes in our society if we are to reverse environmental breakdown and its myriad consequences.

Indeed, the basic facts underlying the science of climate change are settled, so much so that people along the political spectrum have accepted the premise of global warming. According to a 2018 poll, 71% of Americans (86% of Democrats and 52% of Republicans) believe global climate change is caused by human activities[3]—this even though corporate TV networks (CNN, Fox, MSNBC) largely ignore the topic because it doesn't net big ratings.[4] The *Wall Street Journal* op-ed page no longer disputes climate change, and even *The Economist*, perhaps the preeminent neoliberal publication of our time, admits that if the zombie economy continues to allow fossil fuel companies to go forth with their plans, the earth will be unfit for human survival.[5,6] Speaking of fossil fuel companies, ExxonMobil, which for decades denied the dire realities of climate change in the face of extant scientific evidence, now publicly states on its website, "We believe that climate change risk warrants action and it's going to take all of us . . . to make meaningful progress."[7] While President Trump has been in a minority of contemporary climate change deniers, the *Fourth National Climate Assessment* put out by 13 agencies during his administration warned of "cascading impacts that threaten our economy, national security, essential services, and health and well-being."[8]

The peril we are facing is clear. Now the question is, what do we do about it?

In this chapter, we examine why we are in this predicament. What does it say about the frankly *suicidal* nature of growth-obsessed hyper-capitalism and the necessity for social democracy and international coordination around shared existential goals as a rebalancing force? What are the neurologic and other health costs of a rapidly changing environment? And as we think about healthy brains and healthy societies, how can we adapt our local, and most essentially *global*, communities to address and mitigate the consequences of changing weather patterns, while meeting the needs of vulnerable citizens—including elders, children, and the poor—to ensure a safe, secure, equitable, and sustainable future?

ECOLOGICAL BREAKDOWN IN A GROWTH-ORIENTED CULTURE POWERED BY FOSSIL FUELS

Modern humans have tended to take our environment for granted. After all, the dominant economic system of the American dementia era—capitalism—has conditioned us to objectify nature and see ourselves as separate from the biosphere rather than part of it. As philosopher and ecologist Aldo Leopold wrote last century, "We abuse land because we regard it as a commodity belonging to us. When we see land as a community to which we belong, we may begin to use it with love and respect."[9] The underlying logic of a capitalist system, however, fundamentally requires just the opposite: perpetual increases in extraction, production, and consumption and an alienated view of nature as an exploitable resource. Not only do the runaway patterns of consumption associated with capitalism not improve our lives (happiness and well-being indicators[10] have been falling since the dawn of the neoliberal era in the seventies), they are also systematically destroying our ecologic home.

The burning of fossil fuels, factory farming of animals, clearing of forests, as well as the growth of road networks, expansion of the US military's imperial footprint, and other practices associated with constant escalating extraction, production, and commodification of resources from the earth, have transitioned untold amounts of carbon dioxide, methane, and other greenhouse gases from the ground into the atmosphere, causing the planet to rapidly warm. As the gases have permeated the environment, temperatures have risen precipitously, with 2015-18 being documented as the hottest recorded years on earth since 1850.[11] While warming accelerates, ancient ice sheets, tundra, and permafrost melt; ocean waters warm, rise, and experience shifting currents; and wind patterns alter, in sum creating "weird" and volatile patterns of weather all around the globe in the form of droughts, floods, heat waves, wildfires, and superstorms that imperil human beings from New Orleans to New Jersey to Houston to Toronto.[12] Fittingly, our era of American dementia has rendered weather weirding as our new "normal."

We have now put so much greenhouse gas into the atmosphere that civilization itself is existentially in question. In 2018, the UN Intergovernmental Panel on Climate Change (IPCC) issued a jarring report warning of a mere *twelve-year window* in which global warming must be halted, beyond which even half a degree will initiate climatic feedback loops that significantly exacerbate catastrophic drought, floods, extreme heat, and poverty for hundreds of millions of people.[13] Failing to curtail the increase in global temperatures at 2 degrees Celsius or below, the IPCC warns, will result in a planet that is mostly unlivable by the end of the century. With every report, we see rising concern and shorter windows for action. In fact, some pessimistically believe, but with some justification, that we may be too late to prevent major environmental catastrophes.[14] Positive feedback loops—(for instance, melting ice and decreased reflection of the sun's rays and release of methane from various sources)—may accelerate warming and create discontinuous events that cause even more major disruptions than we are seeing today.

With both political parties beholden to a capitalist power structure that is driving us toward species extinction, neither has led on climate change, instead kowtowing to the corporate interests of the fossil fuel industry, which funds and helps paralyze the political process in our deadly status quo. How deep is the problem of political corruption? Even in November 2018, with the world in the throes of climate change and the dire recent warnings issued from the IPCC looming over us like swirling storm clouds, former president Barack Obama still saw fit to publicly brag about the record oil production that occurred under his administration during an event at Rice University in Houston: "You wouldn't always know it," Obama told residents of the very city that had been hammered by Hurricane Harvey and its deluge of rainfall a mere 15 months before, "but [production] went up every year I was president. Suddenly America's like the biggest oil producer and the biggest gas [producer]—*that was me, people!*"[15] (Coincidentally, Obama largely dithered on climate change during his eight years in power and also has the legacy of unleashing the largest fracking and fossil fuel expansion in US history, opening 10 million acres of public land to oil, gas, and coal corporations, and expanding 100 million-plus more acres of offshore drilling in the Arctic and Gulf of Mexico.)[16] Both the Republican and Democratic National Committees continue to accept fossil fuel donations to this day, despite urgent warnings from the IPCC, darkly symbolizing the stranglehold that industry has on our politics and planet over and above the common good.

The ruling class's fealty to a capitalist political-economic system and the fossil fuel industry foundationally powering and perpetuating it has set in motion geologic forces that will be difficult to halt or reverse. And as developing countries industrialize and provide more material security for their populations, billions more human beings become absorbed into a global capitalist system. Some believe our species' impact has become so profound that we have entered a new geologic epoch, called the Anthropocene (epoch of man). Others have perhaps more appropriately called this age the Capitalocene to recognize capitalism's primary role as the driving force behind humanity's outsize effect on the climate. Bill McKibben, climate activist and founder of the organization 350.org, has made the apt suggestion that we start naming hurricanes and storms after giant multinational corporations (Hurricane Exxon Mobil, Superstorm BP, and so forth).[17] Just as we've done in linking Alzheimer's with the political-economic structures and forces of neoliberalism, let's explore this destructive connection a bit more.

Capitalism: The Engine of Global Heating

Carbon dioxide levels have certainly fluctuated slowly over millions of years. But human beings, in ramping up our extraction of stored energy from living forests and the fossil remains of dead organic matter in the form of oil, coal, and natural gas, have accelerated the increase in carbon dioxide levels in the atmosphere—most aggressively after the Industrial Revolution began in the 18th century.

Prior to the Industrial Revolution, climate perturbations over time were largely explained by natural causes, such as changes in solar energy, volcanic eruptions, and natural changes in greenhouse gas concentrations.[18] Yet, as the Industrial Revolution spread through Europe and the United States, transforming manufacturing processes, accelerating the growth of populations, and ushering in the emergence of modern capitalism and its perpetual cycles of production, consumption, and growth, the tide of human activities organized en masse by this new economic system has been the dominant cause of that warming.[19] By burning fossil fuels to power our growing industrialized civilization, we have collectively unleashed massive amounts of greenhouse gases (carbon dioxide, methane, nitrous oxide, fluorinated gases), which had been stored in the earth for hundreds of millions of years, into the air around us.[20] Thus liberated by our economic activity, these gases linger, trapping heat like a spherical greenhouse and contributing to the gradual warming of the planet and an increase in unpredictable weather events, like the storms that turned New Orleans, Houston, and Toronto into deadly water worlds.

This global greenhouse effect has not been linear since the Industrial Revolution. Researchers have identified another phenomenon in modern climate change—the so-called great acceleration of the mid-20th century—a period of rapid industrialization following World War II, driven by the carbon-fueled competition between the United States and the Soviet

Union. Not only is this period associated with precipitous rises in carbon dioxide and temperature that altered our earth-system metabolism, it was also witness to massive extinctions and growth of invasive species. Amazingly, three-quarters of carbon emissions in the entire history of humanity have been produced since 1968.[21]

When Peter was born, in 1949, there were 2.5 billion people on the planet; now, we approach 8 billion. The positive feedback loops among increasing energy extraction, food production, rising consumers, and more environmental destruction have hurtled us headlong toward climate destruction. Had the baby boomers and silent generation listened to the early warnings, we would have had decades more time to act. Instead, we have lost enormous ground during the great acceleration, a period defined by short sightedness, greed, and inaction in business and government.

Of course, accelerating changes in greenhouse gas emissions and weather patterns have also coincided with the global dominance of multinational corporations and the rise of Wall Street, which has underwritten the rapid expansion of cash cows like big coal, big oil, and big gas. In the quest for short-term profits, corporations have set up global operations engineered for constant growth, fueled by combustion energy, and, in the process, have ramped up atmospheric carbon while decimating ecosystems as they have carried on with business as usual. In fact, research has shown that just 100 companies have been the source of *more than 70%* of the world's greenhouse gas emissions since 1988.[22]

At times, corporate ecological damage has been explicit and horrifically visible in catastrophes like BP's Deep Horizon oil spill in the Gulf of Mexico in 2010 or the earthquakes and flammable tap water caused by the fracking industry and dramatized in documentaries like *Gasland*, but most destruction happens in the rather banal day-to-day pursuit of short-term corporate profitability. Greenhouse gas emissions have simply been the price of doing business in a global economy wedded to fossil fuels. Such is the logic of the zombie economy.

Of course, corporate activities despoil the environment in even more insidious ways. Levels of toxic metals in water and air—for instance, mercury and particulates from coal-fired power plants—contribute to multiple health problems such as brain, lung, and organ damage. Mercury exists in organic and inorganic forms and has been listed by the WHO as one of the top ten chemicals of major public health concern[23] (despite this, the Trump administration moved to loosen regulations on mercury and other air pollutants from coal and oil plants in 2020).[24] Air pollution more generally occurs in many forms and not only warms the atmosphere but also causes health problems in several ways. Exposure to airborne particulates is increasingly being linked to dementia risk.

Further, industrial products derived from oil (such as plastics and polymers) have led to the accumulation of inorganic waste products that escape normal patterns of environmental degradation and recycling. Plastics are beginning to dominate the ecosystems and waterways with dramatic consequences for their pervasiveness. Grossly visible plastic islands float in gyres in oceans and lakes. Animals that consume this water-borne plastic, for instance, sea-faring birds and fish, can be directly harmed when their stomachs are unable to function as a result of ingesting our indigestible waste.[25] Invisible to the naked eye, partially degraded plastics from microscopic spheres are becoming ubiquitous in our food and even in the Mariana trench, where animals living at the lowest point in our ocean are being found to have corporate-derived plastic pollution in their guts.[26] Chemicals associated with some plastic production, such as bisphenol A (BPA), can leach out and damage the endocrine systems of animals, including us.[27] Such endocrine disruptors can mimic natural hormones, such as estrogens, and may be associated with human problems such as fertility. We still do not know why average male sperm counts have fallen dramatically,[28] but environmental toxins like BPA are a likely cause.

We reviewed the potential brain health impact of fracking last chapter. Of course, another major harm of fracked earth is the release of methane gas as a byproduct of drilling, often through leaks in the pipes and equipment; intentional venting or burning (flaring); and emissions associated with trucking and transport operations. About one-half of a recent massive increase in methane emissions has been attributed to shale gas operations. Methane itself is a major cause of climate change, as it is 80 times more potent in its effects on greenhouse warming than carbon dioxide in the first twenty years after it is released. Many countries in Europe and states in the United States are banning fracking at the same time that the Trump administration, like the Obama administration before it, pushed for more gas fields to open.[29,30]

In the deregulated, growth-obsessed environment of our hypercapitalist era, corporations have essentially imposed these damaging visible and invisible externalities on the natural environment in the name of growth and profit for the 1%, and the rest of life on earth must now deal with the consequences. This demented behavior accelerated under the Trump administration, which in its first two years alone rolled back 84 environmental regulations concerning air pollution and emissions, drilling and extraction, infrastructure and planning, toxic substances and safety, and water pollution.[31]

Beyond despoiling our natural environments and playing a central role in facilitating deadly carbon flows into the atmosphere, corporations have made massive investments to protect their wealth and preserve the conditions that have allowed for its continued accumulation. Indeed, in the neoliberal era, corporations have wielded immense, almost totalizing power over our political, economic, and environmental systems and have been slow to adapt to the urgency of climate change, particularly when such adaptations have threatened their ability to maximize shareholder value.

As powerful corporations have realized that their bottom lines will be affected by the necessary societal response to climate change, they have not only bought off both political parties to stave off regulation, but also sought to obfuscate public debate by sowing misinformation about climate science. In a landmark report published in the *Proceedings of the National Academy of the Sciences* in 2019, researchers found that "organizations with corporate funding were more likely to have written and disseminated texts meant to polarize the climate change issue." This paper empirically highlights "the actual social arrangements within which large-scale scientific (mis)information is generated, and the important role private funding plays in shaping the actual ideological content of scientific information that is written and amplified."[32]

In short, the very logic of contemporary hyper-capitalism—pursuit of endless growth and profit—is *the* primary engine that has driven our changing climate over the last several centuries, from the Industrial Revolution through the great acceleration to today. As Naomi Klein has argued in her 2014 manifesto *This Changes Everything*,[33] it is impossible to acknowledge the full scope of climate change without implicating the perpetual extraction, production, and consumption that capitalism demands and the behavior of industries (and politicians) that have protected their financial interest above the public good. These contradictions inherent in capitalism have, in turn, produced a crisis of survival. In an era of ecological breakdown, we are going to need to change the basic rules undergirding our zombie economic system so that it no longer requires exponential fossil fuel–powered growth, which is driving our society into dire straits and putting our most vulnerable at great risk.

Inequity and Migration

The global domination of capitalism has not only damaged the environment but has also precipitated growing income and wealth inequality between those who control capital and those who don't. In recent decades, the economic inequity between the haves and have-nots has swelled, with billions of people living in crushing poverty and several billionaires controlling much of the world's wealth. And the middle class is now shrinking, suffering, and growing increasingly restive and despairing in many areas of the world, where corporate power has dominated the political process. Again, it is no stretch to say that we live not in a democracy but in an *oligarchy*, where the wealthiest few—the 1% that Occupy Wall Street rallied against—hold disproportionate power over the many and are driving us toward extinction in psychotic fashion.

As I (Peter) got a taste of firsthand in Toronto, the socially disadvantaged are more affected by climate change and its consequences because they tend to live in communities more likely to be damaged by industrial waste and pollutants, and they are more at risk for flooding and other environmental forces. These violent disasters of climate change (which can no longer be considered "natural" because of the human component that exacerbates their effects) have taught us that the boundaries between environmental justice and social justice are being eliminated. Just as in Flint, where the CEOs of General Motors could ensure that noncorrosive water entered their factories while residents received contaminated water in their taps, the wealthy can afford to escape from environmental disasters and future risks. They can insure themselves against approaching calamities, relocate from their mansions or alternative homes to places not exposed to rising waters or industrial waste, or even purchase emergency evacuation plans to be airlifted to private islands with doomsday bunkers and high perimeter fences in the event of climate catastrophe or social unrest.[34,35] In a cruel twist on the biblical axiom, it seems that the wealthy shall inherit what's left of the (uninhabitable) earth.

Meanwhile, for the poor, climate change creates climate refugees—people who will increasingly need to escape from ecological disasters, such as droughts and floods, or from warfare, which itself is often related to environmental pressures or political instability. Unlike those of us in Toronto, many will lack the wealth and resources to ride out extreme storms. As we saw in Flint, the poor—and disproportionately people of color—are likely to live in areas exposed to multiple environmental risks. Water and air quality are likely to be lower; soil is more likely to be degraded and contaminated with heavy metals, pesticides, and other damaging products. And as we have seen in the past decade, in a neoliberal era marked by disparity, austerity, and precarity, climate migration creates combustible tensions in host countries where the domestic population is already suffering from declining material conditions and despair.

But where do our aging brains sit in this rather harrowing story of climate change? Let's examine this question more carefully.

AN ECOPSYCHOSOCIAL MODEL TO UNDERSTAND THE NEUROLOGIC COSTS OF CLIMATE CHANGE

While it may be somewhat of a cliché, health is an inescapably holistic phenomenon. Thus, to achieve a sense of well-being, people must not only be healthy in a biologic sense but also harmonize physical health with psychological, social, and broader ecological well-being. Brain health is therefore inseparable from these overall layers of health.

In our current "marketplace of memory," which treats us as isolated and atomized consumers, the individuated brain has been isolated as *the* organ of major concern, almost to the point of becoming a decontextualized biologic entity. Thus, rarely do discussions of brain health integrate themes of broader psychosocial well-being, much less any consideration of our warming and polluted climate. Once again, we find ourselves confined by the practical, ideological, and narrative limitations of a marketplace that is fundamentally unable to deal with the *depth* and *breadth* necessary for a proper assessment of collective brain health. We must move beyond instrumental questions at the level of biology (for instance, does a nutritional supplement or brain fitness app or tonic increase neurons and synapses?) and ponder how the built and natural environments we exist in as humans are supporting our brain health and that of others (and other species), and how those around us affect our well-being and sense of shared purpose.

This conceptual model of holistic health is often referred to as *biopsychosocial,* with *spiritual* occasionally added as a component beyond *social.*

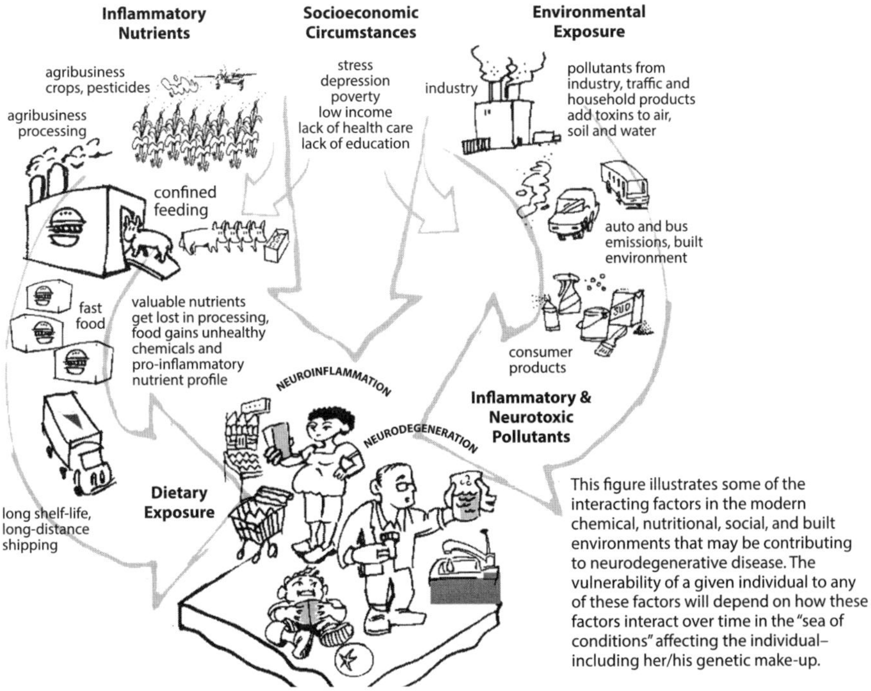

Figure 7.2. An ecopsychosocial model adds a critical *eco* dimension to the standard *biopsychosocial* model, allowing for deeper consideration of environmental exposures and broader planetary health.
Source: Adapted from an illustration by Stephen Burdick.

Despite sounding all inclusive, however, the biopsychosocial model is actually an inadequate framework for health because it fundamentally ignores the environment—the *eco*. Thus, in our formulation, we replace *bio* with *eco* in an *ecopsychosocial* model of health to signal that we must aim at greater breadth and depth in thinking about the biology of brain health in the context of broader social and ecosystems (figure 7.2).[36]

Replacing *bio* with *eco* encourages us to think of health in terms of systems and over time. The health of ecosystems themselves and the organisms in them depend on balance between energy flows in and out of the system and between multiple different cycles of inorganic molecules, like carbon, nitrogen, phosphorus, oxygen, and water. These biological systems evolve often over long intervals, with organisms adapting to the environment and one another through evolution.

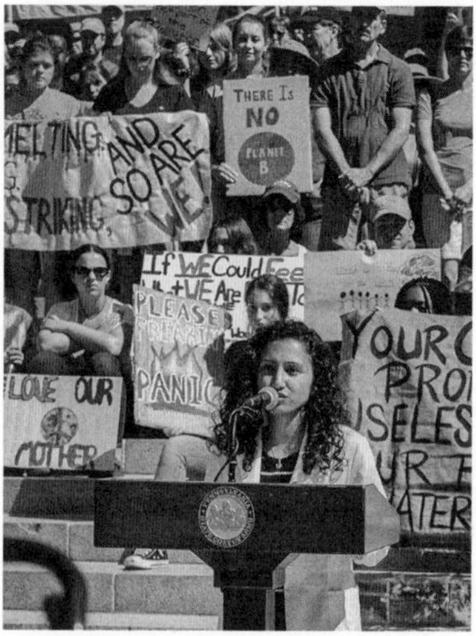

Figure 7.3. Penn State medical student Natasha Sood speaks on the Capitol steps in Harrisburg, Pennsylvania, during the global climate strike in September 2019.
Source: Photograph courtesy of Natasha Sood.

Doctors in Western biomedicine generally do not think broadly or longitudinally enough. Even at the molecular level they ignore, for example, that genes are affected by epigenetic factors at both molecular and ecosystem levels, and that genes and humans evolved over time in environments that required adaptation. Whether a gene expresses itself is regulated in the cell by methylation, histone bodies, and other local microenvironmental factors, and the manifestation of a genetic predisposition is influenced by the ecosystem in which the organism finds itself.

Thankfully, the reductionism that has defined Western medicine is beginning to change. Symbolically, the British medical journal the *Lancet* has been internationally promoting a new concept of *planetary health* for physicians to embrace, which argues that medicine must pay "judicious attention to the human systems—political, economic, and social—that shape the future of humanity *and* the Earth's natural systems"[37] (figure 7.3). To truly achieve healthy brains, we and our healers (and political representatives) must embrace this nuanced *ecopsychosocial* framework, which can help us imagine new repertoires of thinking and acting in pursuit of better individual—and more importantly, *collective*—brain health. At a time of climate catastrophe, aligning the well-being of our brains with greater planetary health is essential. Such a reframing means paying attention to complex connections and pathways. After all, the brain is the organ most vulnerable to environmental degradation, both in terms of direct threats to neural function and because of environmental damage to peripheral systems like the heart, lungs, and other organs that the brain relies on for sustained metabolic support.

In that spirit, let's apply an ecopsychosocial lens and look briefly at some of the main pathways through which our changing climate can be expected to affect our aging bodies and brains now and in the future.

BRAIN HEALTH EFFECTS ASSOCIATED WITH CLIMATE CHANGE

Mental Health

Thinking back to the stories and images shared at the outset of this chapter about elders whose very survival is threatened by severe storms, it is unavoidable that extreme climate events and general environmental deterioration will exacerbate anxiety and depression for those who are most affected and least resilient. As the *Fourth National Climate Assessment* has predicted, such events "can have lasting mental health consequences in affected communities, particularly if they result in degradation of livelihoods or community relocation . . . Populations including older adults, children, low-income communities, and some communities of color are often disproportionately affected by, and less resilient to, the health impacts of climate change."[38]

As we've seen with the superstorms and droughts of our era, traumas inflicted by these singular events are not just harmful in the moment but can impose long-term posttraumatic stress on those affected, particularly on climate refugees, who experience prolonged dislocation and who may be the target of animosity, social tensions, and even acts of aggression from societies or communities that assume their care.[39] Such social pressures can exacerbate mental health challenges. In New Orleans in the wake of Katrina, storm-related stressors doubled the prevalence of probable serious mental illness (including PTSD), which lasted for over a year.[40] Research has also shown how changes in climate have led to rises in substance use and suicide rates in India,[41] Australia,[42] the United States, and Mexico.[43] Heatwaves have been found to increase psychiatric hospitalization[44] and disrupt sleep,[45] and depression rates are eight times higher among people in flooded homes.[46] Humans, though ever adaptable, are nevertheless highly affected by extreme weather events and their fallout.

Psychologists have also noted a growing rise in anxiety related to climate change—even for people who are not directly affected by extreme climate events but still beset by feelings of fatalism, fear, and grief related to declining planetary health. A new concept of *solastalgia*, defined as "the distress that is produced by environmental change," has become such a concern that the American Psychological Association (APA) created a 69-page climate change guide to assist mental health care providers in treatment.[47] My (Peter's) mentor in psychiatry, Jerome Frank, formerly used a more common word to label these vague feelings of existential unease: *demoralization*. This word validates the APA's observation of a profoundly damaging effect from feeling that our relationship with one another, and to the planet at large, is out of sorts.

You know from previous chapters the toxic effects of chronic stress, depression, and sleep disruption on the brain, and inasmuch as climate change will expose millions more people to disastrous events or patterns of events that imperil their security, ecopsychosocial well-being, financial stability, and access to health care resources (for example, closure of hospitals, separation from medications), the deleterious effects of psychic distress on aging brains will be multiplied, with more dire outcomes expected for the vulnerable populations mentioned above, as well as people with preexisting mental health challenges.

We must prepare for a reality in which environmental destabilization will contribute to emotional breakdowns. Acute events will cause PTSD and related disorders, but the chronic inexorable decline in morale from slow but ever-increasing ecosystem and community failure will likely be more profound. Communities will have to learn to adapt locally, regionally, and nationally, as well as support one another during times of disasters, and solidarity—the core value of social democracy—will be essential to our survival, resilience, and mental well-being. Establishing safety nets and basic standards of dignity for citizens will be critical to fostering a resilient and supportive societal fabric.

Warfare

Climatic conditions have played a role in armed conflict for thousands of years. Moving forward, the magnitude and frequency of climate perturbations such as drought, diminished agriculture (production of food and jobs), and water management stress may press on existing social and economic pressures and elevate risk of violence within societies and between nations.

Recently, the US Department of Defense assessed these risks as part of its *Quadrennial Defense Review Report*.[48] Among its conclusions: "Assessments conducted by the intelligence community indicate that climate change could have significant geopolitical impacts around the world, contributing to poverty, environmental degradation, and the further weakening of fragile governments. Climate change will contribute to food and water scarcity, will increase the spread of disease, and may spur or exacerbate mass migration."[49] Throughout Africa, drought is already fomenting deadly conflicts between herders and farmers over land rights.[50,51,52,53] And conflict in the world's most devastating war zone, in Syria, which has created over a million refugees, was initially exacerbated, in part, by drought and other factors linked to climate change (as well as American imperial overreach). In the broader Middle East, there are projections that the region could see a 9% drop in water availability at 1.5 degrees (C) of warming and a 17% drop at 2 degrees,[54] a prediction loaded with troubling portent.

Armed conflict in the Middle East or elsewhere will elevate risk not only for psychological distress and PTSD but also for penetrating and nonpenetrating traumatic brain injuries (TBIs). Last chapter, we explored the consequences of TBIs on risk for dementia, learning from research on veterans from previous wars that TBIs inflict structural and functional damage that weaken one's cognitive reserve, leaving the brain less resilient to age-related processes (further neuronal loss, oxidative stress, inflammation, altered glucose metabolism, vascular damage, and so on) over time. Therefore, upstream neurologic and psychological damage wrought by conflicts affected by climate change will be felt by individuals, families, and health systems for decades beyond the initial injury.

We should also not forget that the brain is dependent on a healthy body to provide metabolic support (energy, oxygen, etc.) but also to allow it to interact with the world. Thus, war-related injuries to the body, for example, to one's limbs, can constrain the ability to move and exercise, affecting long-term vascular health and cognitive well-being and quality of life. So too are soldiers and civilians often exposed to chemicals of various kinds, for instance, the defoliant Agent Orange in Vietnam, and various neurotoxic nerve gases. The short- and especially long-term toxicities of these compounds on both brain and body are often not fully known, but—as we've seen in Syria—exposures are likely to increase with rising modern warfare.

That our current geopolitical power structure is engineering warfare in less affluent countries that has been, in part, exacerbated by climate change is a stark reminder that while the conditions driving environmental fluctuations have been largely created in one part of the world (wealthy Western nations), their consequences are overwhelmingly being felt in the bodies, brains, and communities of people living in poorer regions, who have not enjoyed the spoils of globalization.[55]

Extreme Heat

We live in an era of increasingly severe heat waves, and the IPCC estimates that more than 350 million more people will be exposed globally to deadly heat stress by 2050. The elderly and the young are always at disproportionately greater risk during moments of excess temperatures, and recent heat waves in France and elsewhere have been particularly lethal for seniors, whose bodies and brains cannot as quickly adapt to rapidly shifting thermometer readings. Excess heat—that is, hyperthermia—can induce complex metabolic changes in the brain that can cause acute central nervous dysfunction (such as combativeness, delirium, seizures, and coma) that threaten survival, as well as long-term processes (mitochondrial dysfunction, oxidative stress, neuroinflammation, impaired brain microcirculation, tau pathology, and so on) implicated in neurodegeneration and other brain diseases.[56,57]

In general, even in times of normal temperatures, dehydration is a common cause of confusion in the elderly, and this problem will be multiplied by further global heating. Beyond dehydration, a recent study has suggested that by the year 2099, even with economic growth and adaptation, 1.5 million more people will die each year around the world because of increased heat, particularly in poorer cities, where inhabitants are less able to withstand the extremes. Some areas of the world will get so hot there will be days when even a healthy young adult cannot survive without air conditioning. Our bodies cannot dissipate the heat from internal metabolism through perspiration if the outside temperature is above 130 degrees Fahrenheit, particularly if the humidity is high. Greater cumulative stress on bodies and vascular systems across lifespans can be expected to exert deleterious downstream effects on the functioning of brains and shorten the threshold at which people convert to dementia.

It is also impossible to ignore emerging data showing that lower-income neighborhoods are more likely to be hotter than their wealthier counterparts—even in the same municipality.[58] Principally, this is due to less tree cover, more concrete and heat-trapping buildings, and proximity to industrial areas and main roadways for the former. As a result, poor urban populations will be disproportionately affected by temperature spikes, and we can expect to see higher prevalence of heat-related illnesses (for example, fatal heat stroke, COPD, respiratory distress, high blood pressure, dehydration, and so forth) in socioeconomically deprived areas.

Crop Failures, Malnutrition, and Further Environmental Degradation

Of course, extreme heat also threatens food production. Malnutrition—especially when chronic and suffered early in life—can cause low birth weight, stunt normal brain development in children, and profoundly alter neurocognitive performance.[59] The outlook on this front is rather grim. As the *Fourth National Climate Assessment* projects:

> While some regions (such as the Northern Great Plains) may see conditions conducive to expanded or alternative crop productivity over the next few decades, overall, yields from major U.S. crops are expected to decline as a consequence of increases in temperatures and possibly changes in water availability, soil erosion, and disease and pest outbreaks. Increases in temperatures during the growing season in the Midwest are projected to be the largest contributing factor to declines in the productivity of U.S. agriculture. Projected increases in extreme heat conditions are expected to lead to further heat stress for livestock, which can result in large economic losses for producers.[60]

Some estimates[61] project that, by century's end, global heating could effectively reduce rice yields by 40% while intensifying levels of arsenic in cereal grain.

There is also concern about the effects of large-scale perturbations in food production on the biopsychosocial well-being of producers, as recent years have witnessed increasing prevalence of suicides, substance abuse, and self-harm (including head injuries) in farmers affected by prolonged drought and flooding conditions. Many are concerned that the combination of climate change and unpredictable growing seasons, rising populations, resource scarcity, and volatile price shocks will lead to increasingly violent and injurious food riots across the world, particularly in less affluent urban centers.

Malnutrition can take many forms, and being either underweight or overweight can cause health problems. Having a diet heavy in meats, especially red meat, can contribute to myriad chronic diseases. Much is written about diets that are better for nutrition, and much of the debates are influenced by the dirty money of the food industry. Growing evidence suggests that Mediterranean-like diets, which avoid trans fats and excessive processed sugars, while including lots of fruits and vegetables, are supportive of general and brain health, and our goal must be to develop sustainable food systems that make Mediterranean-like diets possible for everyone.

Of course, corporate concerns have taken over much of the world's food production, where the bottom line is profit and not nutrition. These companies also often grow huge swaths of monoculture crops that are less resistant to pests and changes in weather patterns. Looking for profit, they also produce proteins, such as animal meat, which have a large ecological footprint in terms of water usage and carbon and methane emissions. Moreover, animals are often raised in conditions that cause widespread suffering. Antibiotics are used to increase yields but, in the meantime, contribute to the development of drug-resistant bacteria, which can then cause human illness and death. The industry often hides their facilities so that the full scale of their degrading and dangerous practices are not visible to the public.

Small-scale farming can create agricultural ecosystems that are more responsive to local conditions and resilient to environmental conditions because of more diverse and balanced portfolios of food products. Permaculture rather than monoculture should be the watchword. All of us should support local food production produced with as few pesticides and chemical fertilizers as possible. Farmers' markets are great places to get healthy foods, interact with neighbors, and build community resilience.

Infection Patterns

Infectious disease patterns are fluctuating as a result of climate change, for instance, through the spread of vector-borne and zoonotic (crossing from animals to humans) diseases resulting from rising temperatures and unusual rainfall patterns. The pathogens from such illnesses can target the brain (for example, causing encephalitis or neuroborreliosis) and induce neurologic deficits (such as epilepsy, cognitive impairment, attention deficit, hyperactivity, and aggression). Mosquitos of different species are a common source of human suffering because they transmit viruses (dengue, yellow fever, West Nile virus, Zika virus, Rift Valley fever) and parasites (malaria).[62]

Incidence of these diseases as well as river blindness, hantavirus, Lyme disease, and other tick-borne viruses are all migrating as temperatures rise and are likely to increase their distribution within a warming climate. Many of these spreading viral, bacterial, fungal, and parasitic infections can directly or indirectly affect brain function in both an acute and chronic sense. For instance, the various forms of *encephalitis* and *meningitis* signal that inflammation of the brain itself and its outer covering are common pathophysiologic mechanisms in infections. People who have such infection-related brain damage earlier in life, and thus suffer from microcephaly, cortical thinning, or any other number of neurologic complications, may be limited in their functioning in society as a result of their early exposures and weakened cognitive reserve. Moreover, as those exposed age, their abilities to compensate in response to changes associated with normal aging or other late-life neurologic diseases may be reduced, further impairing activities of daily living. In other words, with the limited capacity of the brain to repair itself from acute injury of whatever kind, as people age, they will be more likely to cross the threshold into neurologic or psychiatric disability because of the combined effects of earlier acute injuries with the effects of aging on the brain.

Toxic Exposures

Perturbations in weather influence human exposures to environmental contaminants through various pathways. Increased temperature and humidity have been shown to have a strong influence on distribution and concentration of airborne contaminants, particularly in urban areas.[63] Increases in temperature and decreased precipitation also portend greater numbers of wildfires, which unleash massive levels of particulate matter and other pollutants into the environment. Considerable and growing data link exposure to airborne particulate matter with neurologic and vascular illnesses, including dementia.

So too can the flooding associated with the warming climate produce overflows of water into land contaminated with heavy metals linked with neuronal damage (lead, arsenic, mercury, and so on); pesticides, herbicides, and insecticides linked with Parkinson's; and industrial nitrogen and phosphorus fertilizers that have a cascade of effects in the ecosystem. When environmental disasters occur, storage facilities for toxic compounds—disproportionately located in poorer areas—are prone to leaks that can subject humans (and other animals) to acute exposures that may damage bodies and brains.

As these pollutants leach and sometimes pour into our waterways, excess temperatures and ocean acidification may increase their volatility and the bioaccumulation and bioavailability of toxins in aquatic organisms that enter the human food chain.[64] Fertilizer runoff into water supplies causes nitrification, with cascading damages that can include outcomes like toxic algae blooms. These blooms can produce neurotoxins (such as microcystins) that also accumulate in fish and seafood. Ingesting foods poisoned with neurotoxins like microcystins, which can destroy nerve tissue in mammals, can have neurologic effects like amnesia and epilepsy, as well as Parkinsonian and dementia-like symptoms. This is especially concerning given that, as crops fail because of climate change, there may be a reactive tendency to apply more fertilizer and pesticides to our fields in efforts to increase productivity, which further exacerbates the likelihood of food-chain poisoning and downstream ecological consequences in our waterways (and on our frontline farm workers).

As people suffer more environment-induced mental stress and physical illnesses, we may be tempted to use more medications. Already, the environment, especially water supplies, are full of detectable human medications, such as birth control pills, antibiotics, and psychotropic drugs, like Prozac, that affect the brain. These drugs surface at detectable levels in ecosystems because people excrete them in their urine, and they are not removed by water treatment plants.

Ultimately, while our list of climate effects on brain health is far from exhaustive, it provides a template for how we can begin thinking in an *ecopsychosocial* way about the neurologic, psychologic, and social costs of worsening planetary health driven by a warming climate. Let us now turn to the more hopeful direction of what we can do to rise to the challenges we face.

HOW WE CAN RESIST

By now it should be clear that, as with Alzheimer's itself, the myopic, demented free markets of the zombie economy will not provide a sweeping solution to a challenge like climate change that demands foresight, long-term planning, coordination, and systems thinking. Nor can we expect to profoundly shift things with lifestyle tweaks (such as biking to work), changes in personal consumption habits (buying local, going vegan, driving a hybrid car), incentivized market mechanisms (emissions trading schemes and carbon offsets), or accelerationism (the very notion that capitalism will produce a technology to save itself). While these types of solutions may be psychologically comforting—and perhaps even escapist—they ultimately divert energy and resources away from politics and collective action. Indeed, coordinated systemic changes are needed at the international level to overhaul our current sclerotic political-economic order and transform global energy infrastructure; as the IPCC noted in its epochal 2018 report, we require "*rapid, far-reaching and unprecedented changes in all aspects of society*."[65]

Given our current era of collective stultification, such a quantum leap forward perhaps sounds overwhelming. But human beings, with our capacity to learn, think, dream, create, and act as a collective force, are already defining a vision for how we can adapt as a species. Recall from chapter 4 that, while medical and technological advancement has had relatively modest positive influence on our collective health, the more fundamental factors in influencing health and survival outcomes over human history have been *changes in political-economic organization*. As we face down the existential challenge of climate change, this lesson rings truer than ever.

Sure, technology will have a role to play in adapting to climate change (particularly future technology that might efficiently remove some carbon from the atmosphere and sequester it back in the ground), but to address the problem at the scale required of us will demand bold new ideas and actions that fundamentally transform the organization of our societies and our identities—not as individuals or nations but as a global human community coordinating urgent changes together. The fight will not merely be to invest in clean, renewable, and zero-emission energy sources to forestall global heating; it will require us to engage our minds (and hearts), think beyond our current economic system (that is, the endless fossil fuel–driven growth of demented hyper-capitalism), and imagine not only new patterns of production and consumption but also ways that we can set up global structures to materially provide for all human beings. We need breakthroughs not only in science and technology, but also in our political conceptions of ourselves as creatures living within a fragile planetary ecosystem on whom our basic and ever-tenuous survival depends. For too long, fear and money have limited our thinking and contributed to our American dementia. Thankfully, things are starting to change.

Policy Solutions: The Green New Deal

In the United States, one of the most encouraging initiatives to emerge in the last several years to cultivate a broader understanding of our shared destinies as human beings is the Green New Deal (GND). This proposed legislative framework[66] has been developed by the Sunrise Movement, a youth-oriented environmental advocacy group that formed in late 2017, and was introduced as a congressional resolution in 2019. The GND is predicated on economic stimulus programs that would fight climate change by aggressively transitioning the nation to a zero-carbon economy with a renewable energy grid (via wind, solar, and geothermal, as well as wave and tidal power), replacing virtually all the coal plants and gasoline-burning vehicles on the planet, and achieving net-zero global emissions by 2050.

But the GND frames the fight against climate change not merely as a "green industrial revolution" but as a much bigger struggle inextricably linked with social, economic, and racial justice, as well as the proposition that #PoorLivesMatter. For instance, in addition to revolutionizing our energy grid, the ambitious legislation would generate up to 20 million new living-wage jobs and ensure full employment through a federal jobs guarantee. This would unleash a major workforce in sustainable energy (clean manufacturing, infrastructure, mass transit like high-speed rail, and energy efficiency, retrofitting, safe bike and pedestrian traffic), as well as bridging into areas like regional food systems based on sustainable organic agriculture, mitigating waste and pollution, sustainable forestry and permaculture, and public services (education, youth programs, child care, senior care). Beyond guaranteeing full employment, reviving our fading industrial sector (now only 12% of the GDP), and expanding tax revenue, the big vision of the GND also includes a commitment to universal health care and establishing new facets of a social safety net (such as union jobs, a living wage, affordable housing, baby bonds, and retirement funds that enable all families to save and accumulate wealth, thereby closing the racial wealth gap) that harken back to the original New Deal.

Ultimately, as with the postwar social democratic consensus in the mid-20th century, the GND aims at pushing the country toward a more egalitarian governance structure and inclusive prosperity—decarbonizing the economy as we chip away at inequality and hierarchies of race, class, and gender and work toward more inclusive prosperity. Such a cultural milieu—in which everyone is taken care of with a basic level of dignity and protection—will be necessary to reduce social tensions that will inevitably arise as climate change contracts our natural resources, compresses our shared livable spaces, and creates waves of refugees. It is also the model a more internationalist movement will have to follow to truly salvage our continued existence on the planet.

As part of this more humane, sustainable, and democratic social contract, advocates have argued that a GND will prioritize the urgent needs of "frontline and vulnerable communities"—those most susceptible to the vagaries of changing climates (that is, indigenous peoples, communities of color, migrant communities, deindustrialized communities, depopulated rural communities, the poor, low-income workers, women, the elderly, the unhoused, people with disabilities, and youth).[67] As Representative Alexandra Ocasio-Cortez, who introduced the GND resolution to Congress, has said: "We fix the pipes in Flint first. We fix the electrical grid in Puerto Rico first. And we fully fund the pensions of coal miners in West Virginia."[68]

Besides the tangible benefits of the GND for the American people, the emerging plan also represents what Martin Luther King defined as "a program of social uplift," with the potential to spiritually renew an ailing national morale caused by our overlapping crises (which, as of spring 2020, welcomed into the fold a global pandemic and economic shock).

At a time when so many are feeling precariousness, alienation, and dislocation in their lives—again, the result of decades of neoliberalism and austerity that have brought wage stagnation, the greatest income inequality in a century, declining access to health care and education, diminished organized labor, reduced socioeconomic mobility, falling life expectancy, and a spreading epidemic of deaths of despair—a national movement that can provide material security for people while ensuring the long-term survival of our species on the planet would be a welcome salve, if not a panacea. Throughout history, tragedy, loss, and warfare have tended to bring humans together en masse; now, we can perhaps find unification by fighting for our planetary health, for one another, and for a world where everyone is provided for. Such an effort will be necessary to preempt the dire circumstances we may face if we continue our current course.[69]

The GND has been called a "moonshot"—a vision even more ambitious than FDR's New Deal or the space program that landed men on the moon. In response to such charges, and with clear echoes of Mona Hanna-Attisha in Flint, Rep. Ocasio-Cortez has argued: "We have never gotten out of desperate situations in this country with a scarcity mindset. We have never austerity'd our way to prosperity, ever. It's never happened. The only way we got out of the Great Depression is through a massive injection of public investment, and also a massive expansion in public ambition and the idea of what is possible in America. We're not gonna get out of this through incrementalism. We *need* moonshots."[70]

While more than 80% of registered voters supported the GND in 2019 (92% of Democrats and 64% of Republicans),[71] passing the legislation will be one of the most difficult political fights in our country's history. Members of the political establishment have shown indifference to the vision. As former President Trump disingenuously argued in 2018, "I really don't like their policy of taking away your car, of taking away your airplane flights, of 'Let's hop a train to California,' of you're not allowed to own cows anymore!"[72] On the other side of the political aisle, Democrat Dianne Feinstein was roundly criticized in 2019 for a viral clip that showed her browbeating a group of children from the Sunrise Movement, who had visited her Bay Area office imploring her to support the GND.[73] Democratic House Speaker Nancy Pelosi has offered a similarly smug assessment, saying "The 'green dream,' or whatever they call it, nobody knows what it is, but they're for it, right?" It's almost enough to make your average person fully give in to the dismissive "OK Boomer" meme![74]

There are many entrenched members of the current establishment like the ones above—let's generously call them *climate delayers*—who drag their feet on climate change and dismissively argue that such a vision is "unrealistic," or "too expensive," or "will never pass." This message will be amplified by a corrupt fossil fuel industry with a nearly endless war chest, which will spare no expense in sowing public doubt to kill legislation like the GND.

So what does a successful political movement look like?

Because of the inextricable link between capitalism and climate change, any political formation must necessarily present a vision of the world that moves away from our current economic system and embraces democratic socialism. As the hosts of the popular satirical podcast *Chapo Trap House* have argued: "There is no reforming a system built on exploitation and nonstop, infinite growth. Socialism is the only genuine alternative to the savage, hopeless, gangster system of capitalism—an alternative that offers an actual future, one in which there are enough resources to take care of everybody and to take on humanity's challenges with a dab of dignity. That, or we'll all drown in boiling seawater. Always good to have options."[75]

In other words, if we are to solve this existential problem, all of us who care about the future of our species on the planet must work through the (rational and irrational) discomforts we have with socialism and imagine ways in which things can and must be different. As an ecopsychosocial analysis suggests, if we can't make a transition away from hyper-capitalism, not only will things get hotter and precipitate more extreme weather events, they will also get crueler, more ruthless, and more damaging to our bodies and brains—in short, more demented.

Socialism—or whatever we call a rising material commitment to one another within a healthier society—is the path forward and the road on which the GND and the future of our species must travel if we are to avoid a Mad Max–style fever dream dystopia. Embracing its principles gives us a chance to break away from the paradigms that have led us to the brink of disaster. Instead of having societies in thrall to GDP as the principal metric of economic success and having our collective fates shaped by Wall Street financiers, industry, and corrupt politicians, we can retake control of our shared destiny and structure our lives not around constant profit, competition, meritocracy, and growth but around the things we covet as sentient creatures—autonomy, health, free time, purpose, sustainability of the environment, and sense of community. As Naomi Klein has written in her 2019 book *On Fire: The (Burning) Case for a Green New Deal*,[76] we must respond to our climate emergency with *the power of human imagination* to visualize and pursue a future that is healthier and more sustainable.

Speaking of imagination, although the changes we face for our survival and societal well-being may seem daunting, we should take to heart the guidance tendered by the late (prophetic) writer Ursula Le Guin: "We live in capitalism. Its power seems inescapable. So did the divine right of kings. Any human power can be resisted and changed by human beings. Resistance and change often begin in art, and very often in our art, the art of words."[77]

Education

There is perhaps no better way to foster resistance and change what is politically, economically, and culturally possible than through education. And given the task ahead of us, we need the healthiest possible brains of current and future generations to be up to the task.

Earth sciences education and ecoliteracy should be at the core of both K–12 and higher education. Without exception, climate science must be integrated into the curricula of our children and grandchildren. Classrooms, nature centers, and museums must become intergenerational contact zones, where children, elders, and youth can learn together, particularly since multiage learning can contribute to deeper and broader understandings for students. Research has also found that children (particularly daughters!) who are educated on climate change are especially effective in influencing the views and climate concerns of their parents, particularly male, conservative parents.[78]

Students at every level should be made abundantly aware of the gravity of the challenge we face and the scale of human cooperation that will be required to meaningfully change our destiny. As Noam Chomsky has said, "I start my classes these last couple of years by simply pointing out to the students that they have to make a choice that no one in human history has ever made. They have to decide whether organized human society is going to survive. Even when the Nazis were on the rampage, you didn't have to face that question. Now you do."[79]

But as Le Guin counseled above, the challenge won't simply be met by uploading facts, logic, and reason into young minds. To advance new

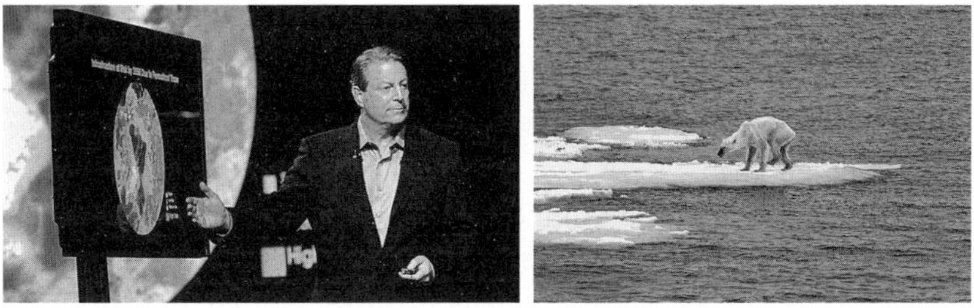

Figure 7.4. Still of Al Gore in *An Inconvenient Truth* (*left*), and a starving polar bear on melting Arctic ice floes (*right*).
Source: Left, courtesy of Paramount Pictures; right, courtesy of Kerstin Langenberger, http://www.arctic-dreams.com/.

ideas and spark generational shifts in consciousness and behavior we must disrupt the culturally ossified mental patterns that got us into this mess. This means empowering younger generations to create inspiring, subversive, transformational, and visionary artwork that can multiply rapid and substantial social progress across the species. The truth is, while much discourse on climate change is delivered via dreary apocalyptic sermon (including, we worry, this chapter), people respond best to stories, images, emotions, humor, beauty, and memes, which are the province of artists. Consider the striking emotional contrast between former vice president Al Gore delivering a PowerPoint dissertation in the film *An Inconvenient Truth* versus photographer Kerstin Langenberger's gut-wrenching *National Geographic* image of a starving polar bear on melting Arctic ice floes, which went viral across the globe in 2017 (figure 7.4).

When we reached out to Kerstin about her "photograph seen around the world," she said she was overwhelmed at how the image swept like wildfire across social media, and then kept proliferating in magazines, news productions, art projects, as the backdrop for concerts, and on election posters and flyers. As to why the image struck such an emotional chord with people, Kerstin speculated, "It touches people by demanding their empathy, and I strongly believe that this can lead to increased interest in the climate crisis as well as increased reflection on one's own impact on nature and other beings." To that effect, Kerstin also passed along a remarkable anecdote potentially linking her picture to Greta Thunberg, the Swedish teenager who has become a preeminent international advocate addressing the climate crisis. "The most interesting piece of news I received about the image," Kerstin told us, "is that, in school, Greta was confronted with a series of images of natural destruction: amongst others, that of a starving polar bear. This was the main trigger for her depression and, afterwards, the need to act and start her school strike for the climate. If that would be true, it could be counted as the greatest impact this image ever might have had."

Artists like Kerstin can produce work with visceral power across all mediums, guiding people in experiencing beauty, feeling connection and inspiration, and seeing new possibilities for cross-cultural solidarity, mobilization, and enlightened collectivism. To change the deranged cognitive patterning that got us into this predicament, beat the entrenched capitalist interests leading us to doom, and coordinate widespread adaptations, we will need to blend the left and right brain and summon up the deepest genius of our species to feel, act, innovate, adapt, and mutually care for one another. To do so, we will need artists—painters, poets, dancers, writers, and other "plugged-in" souls who have developed a deep and profound understanding of themselves, their fellow humans, the natural (and supernatural) world, and the space between.

That said, though personal enlightenment and a national plan like the GND may represent good starting points to organize initial actions against climate change, they are not enough. In fact, the United States, though the world's economic powerhouse, represents only 15% of global emissions. To solve climate change, we are going to have to imagine solutions not only beyond the individual but also beyond the nation-state. For a problem as irreducibly global as climate change, our fundamental challenge will be to think about how to transcend the structural drivers of global warming (that is, global capitalism), create solidarity and human bonds that span beyond our national borders, and globally coordinate actions that equally transition countries away from greenhouse gas emissions while guaranteeing a life with security, dignity, and purpose to all human beings. We in wealthy countries cannot demand that developing countries not industrialize—we must bring them with us. Consequently, we must find ways to build international political institutions that foster basic security and improved standards of living while decarbonizing economies. As Bernie Sanders envisioned during his 2020 presidential run, "Maybe, just maybe, instead of spending $1.8 trillion a year globally on weapons of destruction, maybe an American president . . . can lead the world and instead of spending money to kill each other, maybe we pool our resources and fight our common enemy, which is climate change."[80]

Such political and economic integration will not be easy, but working toward a global polity unified by the egalitarian ethos of our hunter-gatherer ancestors represents the highest measure of our success so far on the planet.

Downsizing the Military-Industrial Complex

In chapter 5, we note that the US military currently maintains more than 800 known bases in 80 countries. We argue that military personnel stationed abroad could be redirected into a civil defense force to provide lead monitoring and abatement, install filtration systems, and replace national lead-based infrastructure. Another benefit of drawing down this massive imperial infrastructure is that we would be reducing what is presently the nation's and the world's largest institutional carbon emitter.[81] Again, while our solutions must be internationalist in their scope, there can be no real solution to climate change unless we drastically reduce the carbon footprint caused by American empire. We must doggedly promote and support candidates who challenge American imperialism and perpetual war.

Retrenching our carbon-spewing war machine will not only allow us to redirect federal discretionary spending, redeploy skilled personnel, curtail emissions, and promote a more peaceful world with less armed combat, destruction, and death, it will also reduce other forms of environmental damage linked to our massive military presence. Indeed, in addition to being the largest carbon emitter in the world, the Department of Defense produces more hazardous waste than the five largest US chemical companies combined. A troubling but little-known fact is that nearly two-thirds of the United States' 1,200 Superfund sites are abandoned military facilities or sites that support military needs.[82] Throughout these bases and in other theaters of American-driven war across the last century, our armies have left their toxic vestiges via depleted uranium, oil, leaded jet fuel, pesticides, defoliants like Agent Orange, and lead, which wreak havoc on human brains. Leaders of the future must be elected with mandates to draw down US hegemony around the globe.

CONCLUSION

In 1942, Viktor Frankl, a Viennese psychiatrist and neurologist, was arrested and placed in a Nazi concentration camp. Four years later, after having suffered the horrors of the experience, in which much of his family—including his pregnant wife—were lost to the Nazi pogroms, Frankl published his seminal book, *Man's Search for Meaning*. In it, he developed a theory that sustaining meaning in one's life represented the most essential element of human existence: "Being human always points, and is directed, to something or someone, other than oneself—be it a meaning to fulfill or another human being to encounter. The more one forgets himself—by giving himself to a cause to serve or another person to love—the more human he is."

As we face down a future defined by crises—of inequality, economic collapse, pandemic viruses, and escalating environmental catastrophes—there is renewed wisdom in Frankl's insights. Climate change represents a looming existential calamity that calls on us to unify across normal lines of opposition and "give ourselves" to a larger cause: the survival of our society now and for our future ancestors. In doing so, we stand on the precipice of a moment that Frankl would say has the potential to make us more human.

Indeed, the world that we want—one that is ecologically sustainable and offers peace, inclusive prosperity, and basic dignity to all citizens—is within our grasp, and the GND is an initial policy expression of this vision that must continue growing internationally in scope. But our window for acting is relatively short, and in that time, we will need to rewire our brains, think beyond the derangements of capitalism, and initiate drastic changes in our society if we are to reverse environmental breakdown and its neurologic and other consequences. In doing so, we may discover a wellspring of deeper compassion and commitment to one another that will, in addition to reversing ecological catastrophe, quench our ever-present search for meaning.

Baby boomers across the political spectrum would seem poised to make climate change a part of their defining legacy.[83,84] Having contributed to bringing our species to the brink of disaster, boomers are positioned to return full circle to the more egalitarian, collectivist ideals of their youth and redeem the promise of the sixties by making one last generational push to secure a future for the species. As journalist and poet Caitlin Johnstone has written,

> What we need is not just our healthy impulse to collaborate, but to collaborate in a wise and intuitive way that is not manipulated

> by the propaganda narratives of the powerful. We need an *enlightened* collectivism in which we all collaborate toward the good of the whole, not because we've been manipulated into it, nor even just because we've been convinced to by compelling arguments, but because we've become wise and compassionate enough to understand that that's what's best for everyone.[85]

But we'll leave the last word to legendary conservationist Rachel Carson, who, in a graduation speech in June 1962 at Scripps College, conveyed a message that remains more relevant than ever:

> The stream of time moves forward and mankind moves with it. Your generation must come to terms with the environment. You must face realities instead of taking refuge in ignorance and evasion of truth. Yours is a grave and sobering responsibility, but it is also a shining opportunity. You go out into a world where mankind is challenged, as it has never been challenged before, to prove its maturity and its mastery—not of nature, but of itself. Therein lies our hope and our destiny.

8

Occupy the Nursing Home!

Breaking Down Walls and Breaking Out "Socialceuticals"

Sitting in the confines of an especially bleak nursing home in the western suburbs of Milwaukee, 30-year-old Anne Basting felt her frustration building. For weeks, she had been forcing herself to volunteer at the facility—a nondescript, pale beige building thick with the pungent smell of urine—where she struggled to engage residents on the dementia care unit in activities and games. On the floor's common room, the television boomed gameshow blather at terrific volumes, pierced only by the occasional alarm trilling down the unit's long corridor. It was chaos. Residents sat hunched in wheelchairs, depressed, drugged into oblivion, and largely unresponsive to Anne's efforts at engagement. Queries to spark reminiscence about holidays, families, children, pets, and sensory reactions mostly fell flat. Anne felt as if she were operating in an aboveground catacomb of lost souls who were irretrievably broken.

Still, she kept coming back. In her seventh week as a volunteer, Anne decided to take a page from a different book—literally. She found a magazine on a side table, thumbed through it, and tore out an advertisement of the Marlboro Man staring off into the distance, trademark cigarette dangling from his lip. Glossy image in hand, she walked into the common room with a few art supplies—a sketch pad and a magic marker—and held the picture up to four residents gathered around a table. Rather than asking them to conjure memories from their own past, which had been eliciting catatonic nonresponses, Anne instead asked them to *imagine.*

"Okay. Let's make a story up," she said, holding up the picture of the Marlboro Man. "Who can tell me about this man? What do we want to call him?"

Almost instantly, the residents sprang to life:

"The man is Fred Astaire!"

"And what's he doing here?"

"He fishes for food but is so sick of fish that he wouldn't eat another one if you fried it in gold!"

Freed from the burden of having to remember, not to mention the indignity of being subjected to monotonous games like bingo and balloon volleyball, the residents were now becoming animated and playful. Anne continued leading her charges deeper into the story, using the magic marker to stroke every spoken comment on the sketch pad. As the narrative unfolded line by line, becoming progressively more farcical, the residents who had previously sat idle in the chaotic common room, editing themselves into silence, were now effusively laughing, singing, gesturing, and firing off enthusiastic observations:

"Where does Fred live?"

"Oklahoma!"

"What is it like there?"

[singing] "Oklahoma where the wind comes sweeping down the plains! Where the waving wheat can sure smell sweet, when the wind comes right behind the rain! There are lots of skinny rivers. And skinny trees!"

"Is he married?"

"Yes, to Gina Autry. They work in the rodeo. He does calf roping and she does barrel riding. They have three dogs, Bozo, Sandy and ABCDEFG. They will have a big Christmas dinner on a white lace tablecloth with candles. They will eat goose!"

Forty-five minutes later, when the story about the Marlboro Man had run its natural course, Anne looked around at the lively eyes and lilting body language of the residents and felt the chaos of the common room melting away. Compared to the prior seven-week slog, this "felt like a miracle."[1,2] Indeed, in that moment, on an otherwise unassuming afternoon in the mid-nineties, TimeSlips, an improvisational creative storytelling activity, was born.

Over the decades, Anne has honed the technique and developed a standardized process that has now been taught to more than 3,000 people

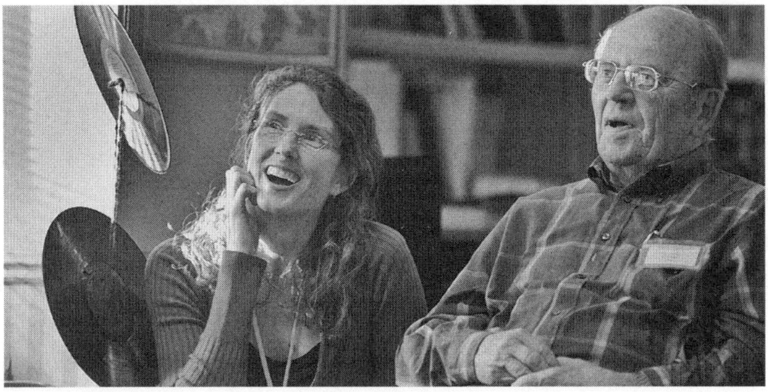

Figure 8.1. Anne Basting works on a creative community care project with an elder resident in Milwaukee, Wisconsin.
Source: Photograph courtesy of Anne Basting.

in 47 states and 18 countries, who are using the TimeSlips storytelling technique to unleash imaginative energies in nursing homes just as she did several decades ago. In 2016, Anne, now a full professor at the University of Wisconsin, Milwaukee, was honored with a prestigious MacArthur Foundation Genius Award for TimeSlips and for her work using creative methods in the care of elders (figure 8.1).

Certainly, fusillades of creativity, wit, and artistic performance are not what come to mind when we typically think about nursing homes—spaces that most people generally fear, loathe, and avoid. Mentioning a nursing home usually conjures imagery of dull fluorescent lights, overworked staff, bland food, and residents slouched in wheelchairs, bathed in the dull soporific glow of daytime TV. As the satirical newspaper the *Onion* darkly joked in one of its article headlines featuring a fictional 93-year-old woman named Janice Humphries, who lived in a nursing home: "Family Fears Grandmother Aware of Her Surroundings."[3]

But things are changing. Over the past several decades, there has been a revolution afoot to humanize long-term care homes and transform them into dynamic living spaces embedded in authentic communities rather than dark, foreboding warehouses of the elderly. Our friend Anne and many others have contributed to a larger movement to break down the walls of nursing homes and infuse them not only with the expressive arts but with rich community relationships, intergenerational activities, and opportunities for purposeful engagement, even for those with advanced memory loss. So how did we get here, and how might nursing homes continue to evolve in the future?

In this chapter, we begin turning our focus to look at how elders in our communities are faring in the era of American dementia. To do so, we first explore the history of long-term care in the United States, examining the role of the neoliberal order in shaping these relatively new institutions—many of which are still beholden to a powerful profit motive—and discovering the pockets of resistance that have helped transform care for the elderly in recent years. Not only will we meet some of the leaders of the movement to "occupy" and reinvent nursing homes and share examples of *socialceuticals* (relationship-based activities that are proving far more effective in supporting people living with dementia than any drug, device, or supplement), we will also explore strategies for how readers can bring creative talents and interests into age-segregated institutional spaces to unlock moments of genuine human connection. Nursing homes, you will come to see, are places of great ambiguity and contradiction; in them, we encounter the comingling of despair and hope, sadness and creativity, ruthless market forces and the generativity of the human spirit. Let's take a closer look.

HOW DID WE GET HERE?

Origins of Systems of Long-Term Care

As a species, human beings have tended to look after the sick and disabled within the familial or social unit. Archaeological remains are limited but show substantial evidence of our paleolithic hunter-gatherer ancestors caring for and even venerating senescent or injured relatives long after their "productive" years as members of itinerant bands. Even as we transitioned to sedentary agricultural civilizations, societies in the East and West generally maintained social mores and legal codes to ensure relational responsibility for aging parents as they grew older.

It wasn't until recent centuries that these relatively stable patterns of committed eldercare were disrupted. As rising industrialization and urbanization fragmented family units and frayed social ties, nation-states and religious organizations in Europe and North America increasingly stepped in to embrace a role in caring for indigent elders. Starting in the

1700s, new institutions called *poorhouses* (or *workhouses*) arose to care for those who were dependent, needy, widowed, or otherwise unable to provide for themselves, including the mentally ill. Effectively, these institutions segregated the disadvantaged as outcasts and exchanged basic food and shelter for often grueling work. Staff in poorhouses were untrained, and sanitary conditions were barely tolerable. Within these restrictive spaces, infectious diseases like tuberculosis ran rampant, and, as depicted by Charles Dickens, orphans were often warehoused alongside the elderly.

Such institutions predominated until roughly the early 20th century, when shifting demographics (because of increasing lifespans) and dramatic perturbations in the political economy of the era (such as the Great Depression) gradually overwhelmed poorhouses and made systemic reform necessary. New state- and religious-run facilities called *convalescent homes* emerged to provide long-term care and basic sustenance expressly for elders for a nominal fee. Given the general success of these institutions—at least relative to the squalid poorhouses of the past—the US government saw fit to invest in them at the federal and state level. In the sixties, Medicaid (government insurance for the poor) and Medicare (largely for those over 65) were introduced as part of the Social Security Act to establish a basic human right: ensuring that seniors could obtain the care needed to stay as healthy as possible.[4] These social democratic programs gave elders access to convalescent care no matter their economic situation. As the neoliberal turn commenced in the seventies, robust federal payment sources from Medicare and Medicaid quickly facilitated the growth of a new nursing home industry, and for-profit operators began developing chains of nursing homes, motivated by economies of scale.

From a nursing home design perspective, the demographics and market forces of the mid-20th century led to the creation of large, often architecturally uninspiring structures, built to resemble hospitals and maximize occupancy. Inside, these facilities often had long straight corridors and prominent nursing stations, and they were built with high occupancy in mind. Residents frequently shared bedrooms with others, as one would in an inpatient setting. Speaking of residents, men and women who were admitted were often medicalized as "patients," with staff often knowing little about those in their care, their accomplishments in life, or their personal, familial, and cultural preferences.

These poorly trained staff were forced to work long hours doing the physically, mentally, and emotionally strenuous labor of providing personal care to residents, increasing numbers of whom were living long enough to develop dementia. As patients with advanced cognitive challenges entered the institutional ranks during the seventies and eighties, sedating residents with psychotropic drugs became a common and overused practice, as did the use of physical restraints to control those with agitation. While certainly a step up from the grimy poorhouses of the 1800s, institutionalized residents were treated less like dignified elders and more like diminished human beings, who were simply being put out to pasture in age-segregated domiciles until they expired. The late Oliver Sacks, who trained and worked as a neurologist in the mid- to late 20th century, described the depressing nursing home ambience of the era in similar terms to what Anne Basting encountered in the facility in Wisconsin as late as the nineties: "There was now little left but sitting, zombie-like, in front of the now-never-turned-off TV."[5]

Attempts at Nursing Home Reform

These systemic shortcomings in institutional care elicited reform efforts that have unfolded over the past several decades. In 1987, a major effort to transform the industry occurred with the Nursing Home Reform Act. This legislation was based on work led by Sid Katz, a geriatrician who chaired an Institute of Medicine (now National Academy of Medicine) panel on improving the quality of care in nursing homes. The basic conception behind this effort was to optimize care and outcomes by moving from measurements of nursing home structure (for example, safety features and staffing) to more meaningful human outcomes (such as quality of care and quality of life).

This favorable shifting of the therapeutic goalposts helped spark architectural and programmatic innovations to late 20th-century institutions. For instance, starting in the eighties, special care units (SCUs) for people living with dementia emerged as a new design concept. Concentrating on innovations to provide more nuanced care for those challenged by memory loss, this movement improved and humanized environments through music therapy and other arts-based programs and physical space redesign. In such units, institutions increasingly tried to conceal the more medicalized vestiges of mid-20th-century convalescent homes (such as long corridors and visible nursing stations) and develop more welcoming design elements (for instance, individual rooms, circular paths inside and outside facilities to allow people to exercise and wander safely, and so forth). As a response to the depersonalization of past institutional care settings, incoming residents were encouraged to bring their own furniture and life mementos to furnish more personalized, homelike spaces. Underlying this shift was a new theory: that aberrant elder behaviors were a function not just of the *individual* but also of impoverished *environments* that did not stimulate individual minds, encourage social activities, or support the humanity of residents.

The Person-Centered Care Revolution

For the last three decades, attempts to reform, demedicalize, and ultimately humanize nursing homes have been bolstered by a global reform movement called person-centered care (PCC). This pioneering effort, undertaken by leaders across the world, aimed massive attention and resources specifically at the task of improving the relationship between staff and residents and delivering higher quality care to elders, who had previously been subjected to impersonalized and inhumane institutionalized care.

The PCC revolution is most often associated with the work of Tom Kitwood, a British medical doctor and psychologist who was a major intellectual force behind the movement. Kitwood, an ordained priest who was heavily influenced by Christian theological beliefs as well as the humanist psychology of Carl Rogers, Carl Jung, and the philosophical and spiritual work of writers such as Martin Buber, used the term PCC to bring together a set of ideas and practices—in his words a new "paradigm"—aimed at developing high quality interpersonal care that respected and honored those with dementia, affirming their selfhood rather than flattening it.

At the core of Kitwood's critique was the aforementioned belief that people living with dementia were more deeply affected by the external factors that surrounded them than was commonly recognized by a reductionistic medicalized model, which framed the condition as an isolated pathology in individual brains divorced from psychosocial needs. Ignorance of the rich personhood of people with dementia and disproportionate focus on brain pathology fostered by the medicalization of senility,

Kitwood believed, had led to impersonal, instrumental care practice. The PCC movement promoted the belief that cognitive changes occurred in living persons who could both be negatively affected by poor care environments and positively affected by a more supportive milieu.

The main accomplishment of the PCC model was to deepen institutional curiosity about the subjective experiences of residents. Increasingly, nursing homes made efforts to allow residents to bring artifacts of their lives into their new homes as well as collecting life-history narratives from each resident so that staff could incorporate biographical knowledge into PCC planning and practice. Such an adaptation (pioneered in part by one of our friends and colleagues, Jim Gruber in Cincinnati, Ohio) enabled caregivers to see residents as people with meaningful histories rather than patients who were facelessly fading away in hospital beds and recliners. By sensitizing staff to individual stories, PCC advocates believed that the workforce would be more acutely aware of the idiosyncratic environmental triggers that could impede or promote quality of life for individual residents, as well as becoming more highly attuned to verbal and nonverbal forms of communication. So too could nursing homes more effectively provide living spaces, programs, and activities to help elders preserve worthy, valued social identities. Kitwood flatly rejected the fatalistic but paradigmatically dominant notion borne of the "politics of anguish" that dementia was an inexorable decline. He wrote:

> Far more can be done to sustain personhood than was formerly believed[6]. . . It has become clear, also, that the view of dementia which accompanied the old culture of care was "paradigmatically wrong" . . . In the paradigm that we are rejecting the unit of analysis was usually to be an isolated human being with a failing brain. Here, then, is an extreme version of the methodological individualism that has dominated both clinical psychology and psychiatry.[7]

For Kitwood and PCC advocates, a new and more egalitarian philosophy would infuse institutional care. The patient was not merely an atomized individual; rather, the *self* was relational and interdependent, and a reduction in personhood was a natural consequence of a reduction in opportunities for reaffirming social interaction and solidarity. Kitwood famously condemned what he termed the "malignant social psychology" prevalent in a medicalized Western society—in essence, the provocative and dehumanizing cultural scripts deployed as part of the *shock politics* we examine in chapter 3—that strategically positioned people living with dementia as defective and diseased. These mischaracterizations, while perhaps rhetorically useful for advocates and fundraisers seeking scarce public resources in the American dementia era, engineered a host of dysfunctional relationships that reduced life-affirming interactions and precipitated cognitive decline. Chiefly, they justified a physical separation of "dementia victims" from "normal, nondemented people" and rationalized forms of ritualized, routinized, inflexible care with minimal regard for peoples' subjective wishes, desires, needs, and fears. A reduction in social network and meaningful relationships—a "loss of place," as it were—would invariably manifest in a reduction in personhood and quality of life. Dementia thus came to be seen not as an irreversible trajectory of decline, but rather as a process that could be modulated through proper societal and institutional care and engagement.

Practically speaking, a PCC philosophy slowly transformed nursing care around new practices and standards. Institutions sought out the voice of residents and families in shaping care approaches and empowered them through appointments to internal advisory councils. Staff training around better communication skills and relationship building became standardized and widely implemented. Increasingly, institutions paid more attention to individualizing the dying process and providing comfort and pain management in end-of-life care.

As the structure, culture, and mission of many eldercare organizations changed in accordance with the permeating values of the PCC movement, so too did the provision of care. Specifically, the focus on individual well-being ushered in a new era of highly evolved arts-based approaches, which could be tailored to an individual's needs, to provide biopsychosocial stimulation in support of quality of life, preserve a social role with value, and embrace the strengths and capacities of residents with dementia. A wide variety of nonpharmacological and behavioral interventions emerged, including bright light therapy, massage and touch therapy, music therapy, physical activity, memory training, homeopathy, validation therapy, reminiscence therapy, aroma therapy, stimulated presence therapy, acupuncture therapy, Montessori training, and other such biopsychosocial activities. It was, of course, also in this culture-shifting context that TimeSlips was invented, with Anne Basting using creative improvisational storytelling to cut through the stagnation of the dementia unit in Milwaukee and stoke the imaginations and creativity of residents in her care to draw out their personhood.

Validation Approaches

The PCC movement also spawned other worldwide innovations in institutional care. One approach, called *validation*, developed by social worker and actress Naomi Feil in Cleveland, Ohio, sought to affirm the lived experiences of people with dementia by finding relevance and meaning in their day-to-day perceptions rather than "correcting" or redirecting them. Prior to the PCC movement, the dominant mode of relating to people in nursing care was *reality orientation*. In this medicalized paradigm, residents were constantly reminded of the "facts" of their existence (for example, the date, time, location, identity of others)—essentially being bent to the normative reality of the staff. In contrast, validation therapy oriented the caregiver toward understanding and *validating* the world as seen by residents and thus providing comfort by making them feel that others understood and affirmed their worldview. Naomi developed methods to retrain and reskill nursing home providers to bring greater empathy to bear in understanding elders. Like Anne Basting, her methods incorporated the use of narrative, music, arts, and touch to reach into the minds and spirits of those who might even have lost the power of speech.[8] Naomi's approach proved particularly useful for people with severe dementia and is now taught to care teams around the world.

Culture Change and the Death of the Nursing Home

While modern reform efforts have focused predominantly on providing more humane care for residents, other visionaries within the movement have pushed for deeper culture change throughout the institutional structure of nursing homes.

Bill Thomas is one such figure.

Bill, a geriatrician, guitar player, thespian, playwright, and entrepreneur among other pursuits, is a major mover and shaker in the culture change movement. While training in medicine at the University of Rochester, he and his wife and professional partner, Jude, helped found the first culture change organization, the Pioneer Network, in 1997 with the goal of continuing to push nursing homes toward more humane and holistic models of care. Shortly after, Bill and Jude founded the Eden Alternative, an international nonprofit devoted to improving quality of life for elders in institutional care. Building on the philosophy and ethos of the PCC movement, this group of advocates pushed for nursing homes to further elevate their standard of care and become even more homelike, with residents and staff empowered to develop their own ideas for improving (and deinstitutionalizing) the community from the ground up. Integration of pets and plants, as well as children and other community members, was also used to break down institutional barriers and revitalize formerly sterile, isolated, and institutionalized environments. For Bill, a free spirit known for wearing a black T-shirt emblazoned with the word LOVE in block letters, the focus of culture change at nursing homes was as much the care of the human spirit as the body and mind.

In 2001, Bill and Jude moved on from transforming large facilities to creating a model based on smaller-scale homes called Green Houses. Supported in 2005 with a $10 million grant from the Robert Wood Johnson Foundation, the project had by 2011 built more than 100 homes designed for 10-12 residents, transforming physical environments, philosophy, culture of the setting, and organization and training of the staff to enhance the quality of care for people living with dementia, as well as maximizing remaining personhood. Features of Green Houses often included open kitchens, central rooms for social interaction, easy access to the outdoors, and private rooms and bathrooms with a focus on creating a powerful sense of homeyness and a balance of openness with privacy that was mindful of staff engagement and relationships. Now reinvigorated as the Green House Project 2.0, the initiative continues to pursue innovative architectural forms and program practices, like Best Life[9] for people with memory challenges. Best Life focuses on validating positive accomplishments of people with dementia, and its training programs for staff use new technologies like virtual reality to help carers become better educated about dementia and develop deeper empathy for residents.

Nonetheless, even a disruptive and successful innovator like Bill, who has been committed to challenging the very notion of what a nursing home can be, has grown weary of the arduous task of trying to fundamentally transform procrustean long-term care environments. As Bill told us, "Institutions are institutions because they're good at replicating themselves. They are built on purpose to deflect, diminish, and redirect change." In recent years, he has come to terms with the limitations of institutional change and turned his imagination beyond nursing homes altogether and to *community*-centered care—which he views as the next major paradigm shift in eldercare. As he told us, "I learned that in order to really create something new and different it's not worth my time and energy fixing an existing theory. It's incumbent on me to develop a new theory. We need new tools and new language, and humans themselves can create the communities they need."

Bill's new vision involves looking beyond the horizons of long-term care institutions and taking on the weightier challenge of helping extant communities evolve to become friendlier for people living with dementia. In contrast to the change-averse nature of nursing homes, Bill's philosophy regards communities as organic, constantly in flux, adaptable, and able to nimbly adjust to changing circumstances to care for elders in situ rather than institutionally. Next chapter, we focus on emerging age- and dementia-friendly communities and delve into Bill's fascinating new high-tech vision for a post-nursing home, community-based care model in greater detail.

ROLE OF THE MARKET: NEOLIBERALISM AND PROFIT IN THE LONG-TERM CARE MARKETPLACE

There is, of course, a darker side to the evolution of nursing homes in the American dementia era. Given that the modern long-term care system emerged just as hyper-capitalist forces were being unleashed in the late 20th century, the market-driven political economy of the last several decades has invariably shaped the way we as a society institutionally care for the elderly—not always for the better.

The influx of state and federal dollars for institutional care in the sixties motivated a new generation of entrepreneurs who saw nursing home care as a potentially lucrative and untapped market. As the industry grew, so too did the variation in quality care and innovation across facilities. Even so, many for-profits appropriated the language of reform to capture market share without actually making material or cultural improvements in the provision of more humane care. Organizations commonly embraced

PCC and culture change as a branding strategy and committed to only superficial changes without actually operationalizing direct care practices in line with PCC principles. The divide between organizational word and deed ultimately is part of what pushed people like Bill Thomas to seek solutions outside the long-term care system altogether. As Bill told us when we asked about his take on the industry over the last several decades, "We have paid a heavy price for neoliberalism."

Today, approximately 70% to 80% of the long-term care industry (housing 1.3 million elders) is composed of for-profit institutions, and large multistate conglomerates own a large share of the infrastructure.[10] International research shows that quality of care tends to be lower in private homes as a result of cost cutting around the margins to increase profits.[11,12,13] Studies in Ontario, Canada, where I (Peter) work part time, have shown that during the COVID-19 outbreak, for-profit facilities had significantly higher death rates compared to nonprofits.[14]

These shifts represent a particularly troubling harbinger for the middle class. The outsize presence of for-profit institutions in the long-term care industry has gradually shifted the housing market for seniors toward private higher-end facilities. While those at the lower end of the income distribution remain reliant on state and local programs such as Medicaid (Medicare does not currently cover senior housing or long-term care services), postretirement elders who have too much income to qualify for government-subsidized housing and too little to live in higher-end luxury housing developments (over $100,000 in annual costs) or pay for home health aides (over $50,000 annually) have been placed in an increasingly precarious position. Many have found themselves in a Kafkaesque predicament where it is simply most expedient to deplete their life savings to qualify for Medicaid.[15] A team of researchers led by Caroline Pearson at the University of Chicago have studied the class divisions in senior care, which have been exacerbated by the market forces unleashed during decades of neoliberal restructuring. In a 2019 study, they projected that by 2029, there will be 14.4 million such "middle-income seniors." As the researchers concluded: "While many of these seniors will likely need the level of care provided in seniors housing . . . 54% of seniors will not have sufficient financial resources to pay for it."[16]

The disproportionate presence of the private industry in long-term care has other social consequences. As long-term care organizations have grown in size, they have also acquired major political power and developed strategies to flex their muscles at both federal and state levels to ensure that regulation (such as Centers for Medicare and Medicaid Services [CMS] oversight) does not impede profit. Wealthy nursing home operators frequently donate to politicians or are themselves politicians with undue influence on state regulatory and reimbursement legislation. As regulation of facilities has waned in the neoliberal era, driven by these politically influential factions with skin in the game, there has been a troubling trend toward diminished care, safety, and neglect (as well as poor treatment of frontline workers who make, on average, $24,000 annually[17]) that harkens back to the poorhouse era. So too have there been instances of outright theft. For instance, during the COVID-19 lockdown in 2020, a Federal Trade Commission investigation revealed that some nursing homes were coercing their patients into signing over pandemic stimulus checks, falsely arguing that the facility had a claim to the payment if the patient was on Medicaid.[18,19] Moreover, in the midst of the pandemic, the *New York Times* reported, horrifically, that for-profit nursing homes were taking advantage of a lack of regulatory oversight to evict vulnerable residents, since housing discharged COVID-19 patients could bring in at least $600 more a day in Medicare dollars than people with relatively mild health issues.[20]

Irresponsible management of for-profit facilities has, in recent years, led to high-profile collapses of whole chains, resulting in the displacement of residents and necessitating government intervention (the "socialism for the rich" that Martin Luther King assailed) to bail out failed private ventures (corporate welfare).[21,22] Like the financial collapse of 2007–2008 and New Orleans after Katrina before it, the eldercare industry has become yet another cautionary tale about what can happen when zombie market forces and profit motive run amok in a highly deregulated environment. For instance, one major scandal recently uncovered by the Center for Investigative Reporting[23] involved the proliferation of unscrupulous "care" organizations. These assisted living facilities—refurbished residential spaces often embedded in neighborhoods where a small number of elder residents live and are cared for by live-in staff—have been marketed as a cheaper alternative to larger nursing homes. The pop-up industry, which has become the darling of the get-rich-quick business world, is largely devoid of regulation. Consequently, entrepreneurs have seized the opportunity to flip and renovate cheap properties (such as foreclosed homes) and generate cash flow by drawing monthly rents from elder residents ($4,800 per month and up to $6,500 if dementia care is required, according to the National Investment Center).[24]

Because owners are operating in a largely unregulated milieu, where there is little oversight and no medical expertise requirement for staff or directors, many have found it maximally profitable to staff their facilities with undocumented immigrants. Recent investigative reports have established hundreds of cases of labor law and minimum wage violations, with workers commonly being paid as low as $2 to $3.50 per hour (approximately $800 per month). So too are workers often expected to provide 24-hour care to residents and are charged a fee for their "housing" within the facility, which often entails sleeping in living rooms, hallways, or garages. Although subjected to miserable working conditions, exploited staff are often kept in check by the looming threats of owners reporting their undocumented status. Investigative reporting has uncovered instances of owners withholding passports as well as surveilling and physically abusing workers. As journalist Jennifer Gollan, who first broke the scandal, has argued, because the current regulatory oversight regime is "complaint driven," with state and federal regulators responding only to grievances from workers or advocates, and because workers lack an organized labor body to protect their interests, regulators are often blind to massive systemic abuses. Meanwhile, this "demented" business arrangement has proved highly lucrative for owners of home care properties, who are able to earn upward of $250,000 a year per property.[25]

Day Care Services

Although we have emphasized institutional long-term care, where much of the energy for reform has been focused, for the past century, efforts to provide services in community have also been evolving. In an effort to keep older people living in their own homes or those of relatives, services can be provided in the home or in nonresidential day care settings. For example, the current National Adult Day Care Services Association was itself created in 1996 but dates its origins to the 1970s as part of the National Council on Aging, further claiming that the first adult day care programs were created in the 1940s and 1950s. Some day care programs have included people with different levels of cognitive impairment, whereas some have been dementia specific. Some were nursing models, and others more socially oriented or integrative of art, music, or intergenerational interaction.

Most day and home care services are private pay and for-profit. These types of programs are relatively expensive and therefore typically exclude people in socially or economically disadvantaged situations, who are probably at most need for services. Such community-based initiatives are trying to position themselves with new business models and create collaborative networks to play a role in emerging integrated health care systems. All the involved organizations are trying to position themselves as essential components of such collaborative networks. Over time, federal programs like Medicare and Medicaid have paid for an increasing number and range of community services. Some private long-term care insurance also pays for respite services, as well as institutional long-term care.

In general, as we explore in greater detail in the next chapter, there has been more emphasis in recent years on locating the heart of programs in communities rather than institutions—a shift made even more important during the COVID-19 pandemic, when institutional clustering of vulnerable elders facilitated massive loss of life (over 40% of the overall death toll in the United States as of spring 2020). As with long-term care, however, reimbursement models and political influence have tended to support the status quo: inefficient, expensive, acute-care-focused enterprises that do not provide good value (or really even basic good care) for the money. In this "system" the neoliberal model largely prevails, and those with money acquire access to superior care.

SOCIALCEUTICALS, PSYCHEDELICS, SIMULATIONS, AND ROBOTS: RECENT (AND FUTURE) INNOVATIONS IN LONG-TERM CARE

Market forces and their "deranged" consequences for our elders aside, some positive shifts are also happening in long-term care that continue to carry forth the torch of the PCC and culture change movements and humanize our approaches to caring for the physically and cognitively frail. Below, we examine a few notable trends.

Socialceuticals Today

The momentum that PCC and culture change have generated for therapeutically integrating the expressive arts into care environments as a means of supporting sensory enrichment and interpersonal relationships has continued peaking in recent years. Our late friend Richard Taylor, a loquacious Texan diagnosed with young-onset dementia in his early fifties, who went on to become a strong and vocal advocate for PCC and culture change, helped popularize a concept for this new generation of interventions that he called "socialceuticals." This playful construct, which combined the *social* emphasis of the PCC movement with the *-ceutical* suffix connoting a healing process, reflected a range of activities in the arts—music, painting, gardening, dance, storytelling, and so on—that all seem to have therapeutic value exceeding traditional pharmaceutical approaches and none of the side effects. When we asked Richard to define what, to him, a *socialceutical* meant, he poured forth with an elaborate but illuminating definition: "Nonpharmacological, relationship- and community-based, psychosocial-spiritual interventions that foster purpose, improve QOL, and end the segregation of the cognitively frail."[26]

That's admittedly a mouthful. But today, socialceuticals launched by the PCC movement are taking on rich and diverse forms, even beyond TimeSlips, with all using the arts to tap into something quintessentially human. Let's consider some examples of socialceuticals that we can safely prescribe for individuals and society:

- *Meet Me at MoMA*[27]: In 2019, researchers discovered a painting in an Indonesian island cave that was the oldest pictorial record of storytelling in the world. In the image, which was dated at 43,900 years old, hunters that were half-man and half-animals engaged in a game drive to round up and ambush small pigs and buffalo indigenous to the island. This remarkable finding underscored the power of story and image for human beings across tens of thousands of years.

  This intrinsic proclivity to image and story has informed a program called Meet Me, first launched in the Museum of Modern Art (MoMA) in New York in 2006. Meet Me was developed within the museum's galleries as a pilot project to provide an immersive visual arts experience for people with dementia and their caregivers. On the museum's off days, the organization opened its doors specifically to nursing home residents to observe works of art under the guidance of a trained museum guide. Groups of up to six people with dementia go from painting to painting in different wings of the museum, with trained guides facilitating wide-ranging conversation about the art relating to color, design, impact, and interpretations of the "story" being told. As with TimeSlips, the activity creates a failure-free context in which there are no right or wrong answers. As might be expected of a human activity so deeply inscribed in our species, the emotional quality of artwork often unlocks expressiveness and poignant feelings in viewers who may be otherwise challenged by advanced memory loss.

As word about MoMA's initiative has spread, its leaders have developed training manuals, and the program has begun to appear at other art museums across the world. Research has shown that such gallery-based programs support quality of life, enjoyment, and relaxation, as well as promoting a sense of identity and social inclusion for people living with dementia,[28,29] while also reducing cortisol levels.[30] Researcher Mary Mittelman of New York University has also found that the program often has positive effects on the museum staff and leadership. Other, more economically oriented research has shown that for every $1 invested in arts programs like Meet Me at MoMA, there is a return-of-investment between $3.20 and $6.62.[31] But ultimately, the effectiveness of this socialceutical exists in its ability to reconnect people with dementia to the primal power of image, story, and social bonds.

- *Alive Inside*[32]: Similarly, ethnomusicologist John Blacking has written that music is so intrinsic to the human experience that it is "there in the body, waiting to be brought out and developed, like the basic principles of language."[33] Indeed, this dynamic is especially powerful for people with memory loss, as the ancient cognitive systems that predispose us to music (which are thought to be significantly older than language) can be activated and engaged in highly stimulating ways. As depicted in the 2014 film *Alive Inside* (featuring Oliver Sacks), there has been a recent focus within long-term care organizations on developing individually tailored music playlists for people with dementia. Organizations that commit to the PCC principle of knowing residents in their biographical totality can carefully select music that reflects peoples' past musical tastes and connects with their emotional lives in ways that improve mood and quality of life.

Often, older music from a person's formative years proves more appealing, as people's long-term memories are better preserved. In *Alive Inside,* a particularly moving scene depicts a nursing home resident—hunched, detached, and nonverbal like the residents Anne Basting encountered in Milwaukee—sparked into wide-eyed amazement and voluble interaction with carers as he listens to old hits from his youth by the musician Cab Calloway. The documentary won a Sundance Film Festival Award in 2014, and the *Alive Inside* approach has quickly spread worldwide, including at Penn State College of Medicine, where students have used small grants to purchase iPods and customize playlists for residents of area nursing homes.

Building on the success of individual-focused listening, there has been a push to make the *Alive Inside* experience more social and intergenerational. Currently, over 500 schools have helped train children and youth to engage with elders in this way, with over 30,000 uses of the Alive Inside app. At Penn State, students have recently developed projects to include family members and caregivers in a shared listening experience.[34] There are ample opportunities for musicians to contribute their talents and passions to the care of elders, which we examine later in the book.

- *Community choruses*: Another innovative socialceutical involving interpersonal relationships forged around our innate predilection for music has been the recent formation of nursing home choruses. Research has shown that participatory singing in a choir can have positive health benefits for regular community-dwelling older adults, and recent efforts have introduced this concept for people living with dementia in various community settings (for example, community centers, senior centers, faith-based organizations). Under the direction of a chorus director, elders—and sometimes their caregivers and family members—will train to perform choral repertoire in public. Not only is participation in a choir cognitively stimulating, it can also foster social interaction and bonding, camaraderie, mutual support, and a sense of joyousness and belonging.

Researchers from the University of California, San Francisco, have evaluated 6-month-long participation in community choirs across 12 senior centers, showing that elder singers experienced reduced feelings of loneliness and increased interest in life.[35] The group has developed a manual that describes how the study and program were designed, the formation of community partnerships, and program delivery and maintenance. It also includes practical details (such as how to do vocal and physical warm-ups, recommended qualifications and training of choir directors).[36] The Alzheimer's Association, to their credit, has also supported local efforts to replicate the success of the community choir concept. The Minnesota-based group Giving Voice keeps a current repository of community chorus efforts around the world.[37]

- *Opening Minds through Art*: Beyond static image and music, expressive visual art is also a potent socialceutical. Opening Minds through Art (OMA), developed by artist and gerontologist Elizabeth Lokon at Miami University, in Ohio, is an intergenerational art-making program tailored for people with dementia. Using structured art-making processes that emphasize the remaining strengths of people challenged by memory loss, OMA allows participants to express their creativity, again in a failure-free setting akin to TimeSlips. In OMA, nursing home residents are paired with volunteers—generally undergraduate students at universities across the United States who are trained to support the elders' creative expression—and meet regularly in a small group setting to cocreate expressive art. The partnership has proved mutually beneficial, with students significantly improving their attitudes toward nursing home residents affected by dementia,[38] and residents in turn experiencing improvements in their well-being (for instance, social interest, engagement, and pleasure).[39]

  More recent efforts have sought to involve medical students in the OMA process, with the hope of bettering attitudes toward older

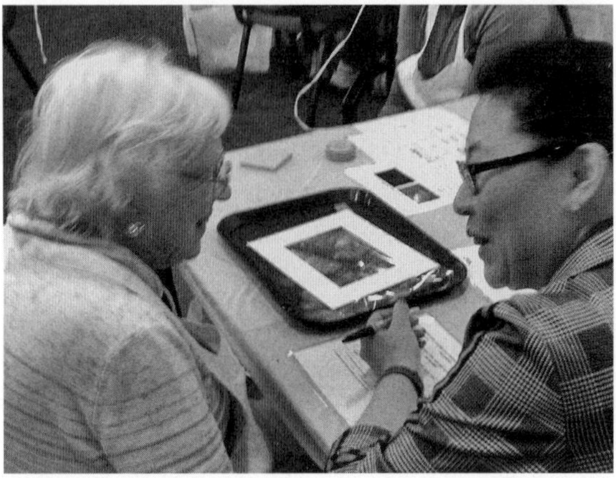

Figure 8.2. Students like Sage Gee at Penn State College of Medicine make weekly visits to Country Meadows retirement community in Hershey, Pennsylvania, to facilitate Opening Minds through Art sessions.
Source: Photograph by Daniel George.

patients with memory loss and potentially nudging more young doctors toward careers in geriatric care (figure 8.2). Medical students at Penn State have recently developed a new wrinkle in OMA that involves family members collaborating with residents in the cocreation of art.[40] Pulling those closest to the artists into the socialceutical activity enables family members to observe their loved one in moments of creative generativity. Such powerful interactions, which, like TimeSlips and Meet Me, use art and expression to engage imagination and to center the remaining strengths, capacities, and dignity of elders with memory loss, help unseat the fatalism, sadness, and dread that can so often color the perceptions of family members toward their aging relatives.

- *Alzheimer's Poetry Project*: Another injection of the arts and sociality into nursing home care has involved the use of poetry. Trained facilitators use written verse to inspire creative self-expression in people living with dementia, reduce their social isolation, and provide social and intellectual stimulation. Gary Glazner (Alzheimer's Poetry Project)[41] in the United States and John Killick (Dementia Positive)[42] in the UK launched similar projects in the nineties and have become the international "poet laureates" of Alzheimer's. Both visit nursing homes, where they model how to engage residents one-on-one or in large-groups to read classic poems people learned in their youth and cocreate poetry based on the words, thoughts, and feelings of those affected by cognitive impairment.

Similar to the TimeSlips improvisational storytelling approach, both use a form of call-and-response in groups around particular themes (such as seasons or old films) to engage the collective imaginations of residents around the spoken word. Frequently, both approaches prompt the group with songs and movement. When residents are freed from the task of having to remember (or guided back to more intact long-term memories by the evocation of canonical poetry) and are unleashed into the realm of imagination and humor, spoken insights can be remarkably expressive and imagistic, leading to the creation of surreal, nuanced, and at times hilarious poetic forms.

As of 2020, Glazner's program was annually providing upward of 500 sessions that serve over 10,000 people with dementia. More than 30 states and seven countries have implemented the Alzheimer's Poetry Project in various languages, from English to Polish to Japanese.[43] Research suggests participation in poetry sessions results in improved participant attention, engagement, communication, and mood.[44] So too have studies suggested a transformational effect on the attitudes and perceptions of those who attend the sessions, including high school and medical students and care staff.[45]

- *Dance*: As Anne Basting witnessed during her first immersion into TimeSlips at the Wisconsin nursing home, it is not uncommon to see residents, once invited into a more imaginative realm, become so possessed by the creative flow that they begin singing and dancing. Indeed, dance has also proved to be an effective socialceutical in itself—a multifactorial brain health intervention that includes elements of aerobic exercise, balance, music, social interaction, and often even storytelling. As an embodied artform with deep evolutionary roots for our species, it taps into both the ancient cognitive systems predisposing us to music and proprioceptive stimuli (embodied memories like riding a bicycle) that are often preserved

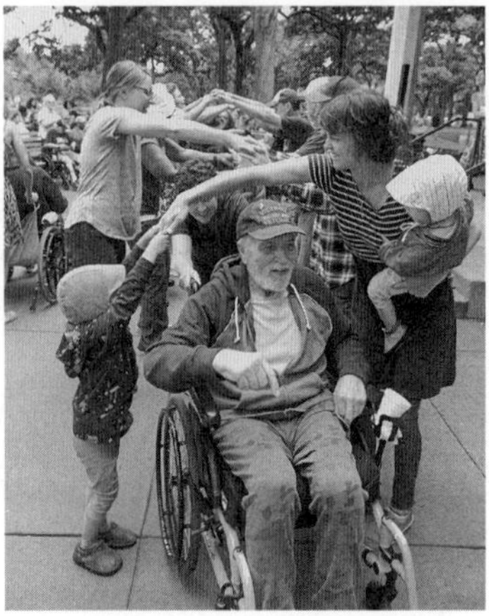

Figure 8.3. An intergenerational improvisational dance unfolds during a Kairos Alive! event.
Source: Rich Ryan for Kairos Alive!

deep into the dementia trajectory. Research has found neural and other benefits in elders who have participated in extended dance programs.[46]

Several national programs—Dance for Parkinson's, Kairos Alive!, and Dance Exchange—have emerged in recent decades to promote the artform in nursing home settings, and all are centered on the elderly, often those with cognitive impairment. Dance for Parkinson's was developed by the Mark Morris Dance Company in New York and is now led by David Levinthal.[47] The theory underlying it is that physical motion inspired by positive emotions elicited through music is a particularly salutary intervention for people with a condition that can cause slowing and freezing of body motions.

Kairos Alive! is based in Minneapolis and Dance Exchange in Washington, DC, with both incorporating elements of intergenerational dance for people living with dementia.[48] Kairos Alive! uses modern improvisational dance forms in various community and institutional settings, including museums, community centers, hospitals, and nursing homes (figure 8.3). Facilitators get people moving and relating to one another by having fun and leaning into disinhibition. Research has demonstrated improved physical and emotional health, as well as overall quality of life.

Similarly, Dance Exchange, which was founded by Liz Lerman, a MacArthur Fellowship–winning choreographer and dancer, uses dynamic group methods to facilitate dance in community settings. The group's toolbox, available on their website, can be used to guide people in appreciating the value of physical movement and the power of embodied narrative. Some of their most creative work challenges participants not just to move but to think more deeply about the role of science in society and their relationships to nature.

- *Elder clowning*: We often think of clowns as figures of the absurd relegated to circuses or children's birthday parties. And yet, for generations, clowns have played a unique archetypal role for human communities. In recent years, there have been attempts to leverage the unique role of the *trickster* in the human subconscious as a therapeutic intervention in nursing homes. Consequently, *elder clowning* has become an internationally recognized trend in long-term care.

  When working with persons affected by dementia, trained elder clowns thrive by using some of the same principles that have informed PCC and culture change efforts. For instance, therapists use touch, eye contact, nonverbal communication, validation, and emotional mirroring, as well as humor, music, movement, magic, and jokes to connect with those with cognitive challenges on their terms.[49] The red nose of the clown is a powerful and disarming symbol that serves as a tacit invitation to step out of normal institutional boundaries and into a more playful, absurd, and joyful realm—one that can elicit reciprocal playfulness and mutual laughter in an often serious, tightly managed setting, where those cathartic emotions can be hard to come by. Our Canadian colleague Pia Kontos has found that elder clowning has reduced moderate to severe behavioral and psychological symptoms of dementia of nursing home residents.[50] At present, therapeutic clowning networks are growing around the world, and assisted living homes are also hiring stand-up comedians to work with residents.[51]

- *Nature interventions*: The therapeutic effects of green spaces have long been established,[52] with studies finding, for instance, that exposure to nature is strongly correlated with well-being, vitality, and life satisfaction,[53,54] as well as reducing pain, stress, and anxiety in hospitalized patients.[55,56,57,58,59,60] More recent studies in long-term care have explored how different types of garden settings—including outdoor and indoor community gardens, wander gardens, Japanese gardens, gardens for birdwatching, and so forth—can reduce depression, agitation, anxiety, verbal and physical aggression, inappropriate or disruptive behaviors, number of falls, pacing, and exit seeking.[61,62,63,64,65,66,67]

Additionally, evidence indicates that interacting with a garden can help restore aspects of life that dementia can disrupt—for instance, improvements in sleep, mood, affect, psychological well-being, social relationships, level of engagement, and sense of community.[68,69,70,71,72,73,74,75,76,77] As with dance, the simple proprioceptive act of gardening can help people with dementia recover a sense of who they were before their diagnosis by providing a setting in which to enact a sense of identity, agency, and independence, as well as spontaneous evocation of past memories.[78,79,80,81] Building in purposeful, altruistic dimensions to gardening—for instance, by having residents grow food for donation to local charities or mentor younger gardeners—may further enhance the socialceutical benefit of cultivating produce.

No less than the aforementioned Oliver Sacks noted the profound effects of gardening on his patients with dementia. The late neurologist argued that in four decades practicing medicine, he had come to rely on two forms of nonpharmaceutical therapies that were vital for those with memory loss, namely music and gardening. Sacks, who was himself deeply enamored with green spaces during his life and sought out botanical gardens as part of his self-care, wrote:

> As a physician, I take my patients to gardens whenever possible. All of us have had the experience of wandering through a lush garden or a timeless desert, walking by a river or an ocean, or climbing a mountain and finding ourselves simultaneously calmed and reinvigorated, engaged in mind, refreshed in body and spirit. The importance of these physiological states on individual and community health is fundamental and wide-ranging. I cannot say exactly how nature exerts its calming and organizing effects on our brains, but I have seen in my patients the restorative and healing powers of nature and gardens, even for those who are deeply disabled

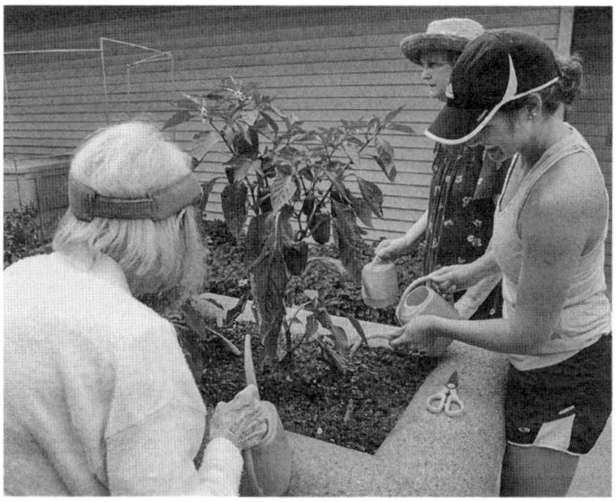

Figure 8.4. Penn State medical student Abby Styck gardens with nursing home residents in Michigan, who donated all grown produce to local charities. *Source:* Photograph courtesy of Abby Styck.

> neurologically. In many cases, gardens and nature are more powerful than any medication.[82]

Sacks wrote specifically about his patients with advanced dementia, people "who may have very little sense of orientation to their surroundings" and expressed frank amazement that the physical and sensorial act of gardening could—like song, story, dance, expressive art, and other activities deeply embedded in the human condition—awaken "embodied memory" in a way that caused a metamorphosis in those with severe memory loss. For Sacks, these patients may have "forgotten, or cannot access, how to tie their shoes or handle cooking implements. But put them in front of a flower bed with some seedlings, and they will know exactly what to do—I have never seen such a patient plant something upside down."[83]

Gardening is low cost and can be done in various care settings—even in windowsills, in greenhouses, or on the rooftops of buildings in areas where space may be limited. As such, it is a powerful socialceutical, or perhaps more appropriately *eco-socialceutical*, with great potential for improving the quality of life of people with dementia. At Penn State, medical students have begun evaluating the effects of gardening for nursing home residents who have also donated grown produce to food-insecure neighbors, focusing on how this added element may influence sense of purpose (figure 8.4).

Psychedelics in Long-Term Care?

Speaking of the healing power of plants, the failure of pharmaceuticals (and antipsychotics) in dementia care has not only sparked a new generation of socialceuticals, it has also prompted thinking about other compounds derived from the natural world that might offer a somewhat unorthodox therapeutic value for nursing home residents. Some in the field are catching the resurgent wave of psychedelics, which have reentered mainstream allopathic medicine after being internationally banned in the seventies.[84] A small but growing evidence base suggests that compounds like psilocybin (magic mushrooms), MDMA, LSD, ketamine, and dimethyltryptamine may be effective in controlled medical settings,[85] with researchers observing preliminary benefits for psychedelics in treatment of depression, anxiety, substance addiction (tobacco/alcohol), PTSD, obsessive-compulsive disorder, migraine and cluster headaches, eating disorders, and in palliative care for patients facing terminal cancer.[86,87]

The mechanisms underlying these benefits remain biopsychosocially complex, but—in a clinical sense—the compounds are believed to engender greater cognitive and emotional flexibility and increase communication across brain regions while fostering a broader and more sacred perspective, which potentially helps users extricate themselves from loops of negative affect and harmful thought patterns. Naturally, some have started to ask whether these compounds—especially if used at lower doses—could provide benefit for people with dementia, as well as their caregivers. In 2020, our colleagues at Johns Hopkins University, one of the international leaders in the resurgent era of psychedelics, launched an exciting preliminary study focused on participants diagnosed with mild dementia that one of us (Danny) is collaborating on.

Despite psychedelics being criminalized since the culture wars of the sixties, their use in Western medicine has been quietly building for decades. In fact, as a medical student in the seventies, I (Peter) undertook a psychiatric rotation that included work at Spring Grove Hospital, a state hospital for those who were chronically mentally ill with conditions like schizophrenia, and was also exposed to the world-class Maryland Psychiatric Research Center program on psychedelic therapies. There, staff administered LSD and music therapy guidance not merely to terminally ill patients and persons suffering from alcohol addiction, but also to mental health professionals—a personal experience that reinforced for me the powerfully and potentially life-changing effects of this class of drugs.

Even with psychedelics reemerging into mainstream biomedicine today, it is unclear whether they will have a role in caring for the elderly, and the idea should be treated with warranted skepticism until more scientifically rigorous research bears out clear benefit and safety. Given the recent ascendance of the socialceutical movement, however, one intriguing potential application of psychedelics in long-term care would identify strategies in which the compounds could, as Peter witnessed during his training in Maryland, enhance the effectiveness of arts-based therapies that guide people with dementia in creating meaning and forging relationships around shared aesthetic experiences (for example, music therapy, painting, dance, gardening, and so on).[88] With their capacity to deepen the spiritual significance of artwork and other sensorial experiences and imbue users with a sense of unity and mystical awe, psychedelics could theoretically augment feelings of relatedness to institutional or naturalistic settings (for example, gardens, green spaces, art galleries, music rooms, and so on), enhance imagination and creative expression, and intensify bonds with fellow residents, caregivers, and family members.

Moreover, one of the emerging key mechanisms of psychedelics is their ability to foster equanimity in some users by reducing the ego's dominion over consciousness. Given the psychological benefits observed in patients with terminal cancer—in which about 80% of participants showed clinically significant decreases in depressed mood and anxiety after treatment, and some lost their fear of death altogether—some believe that the ego-attenuating properties of psychedelics could potentially offer benefits in nursing home care, although research must bear this out and address myriad scientific and ethical questions. Whereas antipsychotics have proved largely ineffective (and dangerous) in treating agitation, antisocial behaviors, and delirium, psychedelic treatments that disrupt the ego's hold on moment-to-moment consciousness and potentially allow unbinding from acute physical and mental suffering, as well as inflexible, habitual patterns of cognitive activity and negative affect, could, if borne out by research, represent a safer and more effective alternative.

We might also imagine the potential therapeutic application of psychedelics for use with caregivers and family members. It is well-established that those closest to people living with memory loss can suffer disproportionately as a result of observing their loved one's decline—thanks largely to the overwhelmingly negative cultural scripts born of the seventies that have defined dementia as a tragic "loss of self." Some believe that, if psychedelics are used carefully in a clinically controlled setting, there may be comfort in guiding caregivers and family members through a psychedelic experience—one that could yield greater insight into what it feels like to "lose oneself" and thus foster deeper empathy for the cognitive changes their loved one is undergoing. Specifically, the revelation that one can "lose one's mind" and yet still experience moments of clarity, transcendence, beauty, joy, and numinous connection to others and the natural world could help prime caregivers to view their loved one's "decline" in less monolithic terms and affirm the "okayness" of having dementia (what researchers refer to as the *noetic* effect of psychedelics that leads one to greater wisdom and insight). Psychedelics may also guide caregivers in exploring other creative, expressive, and sensorial means of connecting with their loved ones (that is, socialceuticals).

Of course, as we have written elsewhere,[89] in addition to establishing effective dosing regimens, researchers will also need to holistically consider the set and setting in which therapies are administered, as well as the intention and expectations participants bring to the intervention, all of which have been found to be vital to the success of psychedelic therapies. Investigators will need to rigorously establish clinical standards, safety protocols, and guidelines that minimize risk of adverse events and maximize quality of life while also addressing ethical concerns (such as consent/assent). Presumably, adoption of psychedelic therapies would require extensive institutional caregiver reskilling beyond PCC to facilitate positive outcomes and avoid dangerous or improperly supervised usage (for instance, emotionally unpleasant triggers in institutional environments). It will take time to evaluate the types of arts interventions (such as tailored music playlists) and settings (gardens, private rooms) that best support beneficial outcomes, as well as the profile of people with dementia who may stand to benefit (psychedelic approaches will not work for everyone).

Certainly, the path to using psychedelics as therapeutic adjuncts in dementia care is daunting and may ultimately prove to be of little help to patients or society. After all, if there's one thing we've learned in our consideration of drug development for Alzheimer's during the neoliberal era, the graveyard of failed compounds is quite crowded. The question of whether there are potential benefits to be had in psychedelics for dementia care, however, seems worth consideration when drug development is so fraught with challenges and inconvenient truths. Ultimately, we are living at a time when we are facing down major existential issues—including a deadly global pandemic affecting our most vulnerable and the basic survival of civilization in the face of catastrophic climate change. Like COVID-19 and global warming, caring for an unprecedentedly large elderly population is a unique and urgent human challenge, which will demand of us new ideas, thoughts, feelings, connections, and bonds to break through current stagnation and forge new schemas of meaning to inspire, organize, and sustain existentially necessary actions. Psychedelics, if used responsibly and with the right intention, may be a tool to help us face down, adapt to, and overcome some of the major challenges of our era.

That said, should psychedelics prove effective and gain FDA approval, we must also be vigilant of how the hyper-capitalist forces of the American dementia era will commodify these complex therapies[90] (which have been used carefully, ritualistically, and with sacred purpose by human communities for tens of thousands of years) and exaggerate the relative benefits vis-à-vis risks for shareholder benefit. Some argue that because of the nature of psychedelic therapy—which isn't merely a matter of popping a daily pill but rather involves a therapeutic guide, careful idiosyncratic attention to set and setting, and emotionally complex reintegration—it is a modality less commodifiable by market forces. Even so, investors are already sinking money into the promise of psychedelic therapies, and we well know the totalizing tendencies of the deregulated capitalist marketplace.

As a final word: while we, as skeptics of pharmaceutical approaches, remain ambivalent about psychedelics, we also believe drugs can have powerful effects on the brain, sometimes for good and sometimes for ill. It is important to keep open minds about different approaches as well as maintaining a healthy critical stance. In a broad cultural sense, contemporary society seems to be adjusting its views about psychoactive drugs like marijuana and other compounds. It thus seems important that people living with dementia and their caregivers not be excluded from such conversations about both their potential harms and benefits.

Dementiavilles: The Recent (Controversial) Emergence of Simulated Environments

On the topic of altered states, some organizations and entrepreneurs have taken the PCC/culture change concept of making people "feel at home" within institutions to its logical extreme, building simulated environments for elders that support a realistic illusion (or perhaps more appropriately, "delusion") that people are reliving earlier life stages. Such environments are predicated on a principle of *therapeutic deception*—the notion that illusory environments that evoke a sense of normalcy and comfort for people living with dementia can be beneficial to their quality of life.

In 2013, an institution called Hogeweyk in the Netherlands gained international media attention—particularly after a visit by CNN health reporter Sanjay Gupta—and has become colloquially known as Dementiaville. In 2014, Peter visited the 150-resident facility with Vicki de Klerk, the daughter of Naomi Feil, founder of the international validation therapy movement we learned about above. Validation, of course, asks us to try to see the world (past and current experiences) through the eyes of the elder with dementia, and Hogeweyk is engineered in extreme fashion around this concept. Its designers have developed spaces decorated in the manner of traditional Dutch homes to validate residents' beliefs that they are inhabiting an earlier time and place. So complete is the commitment to the verisimilitude of an authentic Dutch village that the designers built a nonfunctional but authentic bus stop, where residents wait to catch a bus to "head home." Individual rooms are designed to match various forms of Dutch social life, with several even mimicking colonial Indonesia for those who had immigrated to Holland from the former imperial outpost. The elder community-at-large is invited to shop at functional grocery stores, attend the theater, and eat in simulated restaurants.

The project has been frequently compared to the movie *The Truman Show*, a dark comedy featuring Jim Carrey playing an adult who had been raised from birth by a corporation to live in a simulated television gameshow village. Truthfully, Hogeweyk had for me (Peter) a similar sense of unease to it, and it was impossible not to notice that its developers are operating with a bullish business mentality. The fact that we were charged 300 Euros for a one-hour conversation as part of the tour seemed excessively entrepreneurial.

Other community-based programs are being developed based on using the physical environment as an all-encompassing pneumonic device. In San Diego, the Glenner Center (on whose advisory board Peter sits)—a day care for people with mild to moderate dementia—built a replica municipal town square inside an old industrial building. This simulated space recapitulates an urban environment from 50 years ago, including a clothing store, city offices, a gas station, museums, a diner, movie theater, schools, and other places one might find in or near a town square. The project integrates standard activities like meals, music, exercise, and art for people living with dementia and occasionally also their families. Glenner is currently developing similar programs in California and elsewhere. So too are other "dementiavilles" opening in Western countries (such as France and Canada).[91] With dementia representing a $400 billion industry,[92] we may see an increase of such facilities, and potentially the franchising of particularly successful and popular organizations.[93] As a society, we will doubtlessly need to wrestle with the ethical ambiguities of these spaces, and specifically the question of whether any therapeutic benefits realized through such deceptions outweigh the potential indignity of subjecting nonconsenting elders to an immersive illusion at the end of their lives (and removing them from "normal" communities without their consent).

Long-Term Care and the Digital Revolution

The use of computers, social media, monitoring systems, personal lifestyle measurement devices, virtual and augmented reality, and various forms of digital entertainment are increasingly influencing programming and practices in long-term care. Such "robot" carers can monitor for falls, provide simple conversation, and even perform rudimentary physical caregiving tasks. Part of the larger trends toward automation, these digital approaches claim to be able to enhance quality of care (such as improved safety) while diminishing the need for human staff.

Japan is leading the way in robotic technology, as the country has a particularly acute shortage of human long-term care workers given their low birth rate and rapidly aging populations, not to mention low use of immigrant care workers compared with other countries. As we bolster our caregiving workforce to care for increasing elder populations, we might best view robots, not as a "replacement" for embodied caregivers, but as assistive devices that can free staff to truly do the humanizing work of PCC and culture change.

HOW WE CAN RESIST

Nursing homes are spaces of ambiguity and contradiction, where we see a convergence of sometimes dark colonizing market forces but also the inspiring humanity and creative wellspring of people like Anne Basting, Bill Thomas, Oliver Sacks, and others. Given that these institutions are so morally complex, it is worth thinking about how we might "occupy" nursing homes in our own backyards to continue doing the work of infusing eldercare environments with the life-affirming values of the PCC and culture change movements.

Humanizing Long-Term Care Spaces

As Naomi Klein has argued, as we face down climate change, we desperately need to build an economy based around love and mutual caring rather than profit and destruction. The act of locally ensuring the well-being of our elderly is inherently low carbon, low tech, and renewable. The question is, how can we bring creative talents and interests into aging spaces to unlock moments of genuine human connection? Every reader will have a different answer to this. Perhaps you can personally volunteer at a nursing home, donating your artistic or practical talents to enriching the environment. Maybe your role will be to mobilize other groups you're involved in—co-workers, religious congregations, book clubs, Boy/Girl Scouts, and so on—to break down the age-segregated walls of nursing homes, deliver socialceuticals (such as TimeSlips), or set up valued infrastructure (community gardens, for example). Such acts are aggressively unprofitable and noncommodifiable. They generate not revenue but moments of enjoyment, purpose, fulfillment, and human bonds, building community solidarity and bridging between generations. A healthier society needs more of this.

Increasingly, people are exploring innovative ways to break down age-segregated walls and make long-term care facilities into *shared sites* for people of different generations. One particularly life-affirming partnership is the practice of colocating preschools within nursing homes, a trend that started in Japan in the seventies and has spread throughout the world. As we explore further in chapter 10, blending the generations in a school setting produces myriad reciprocal benefits. Most obviously, the presence of young children helps long-term care residents fend off the loneliness, physical and cognitive stagnation, and depletion of purpose that can be endemic to institutional settings. So too are children generally indifferent to the signs and symptoms of dementia and meet elderly residents nonjudgmentally in the moment. In turn, children gain access to caring elders (who may not be present or proximate in their nuclear families) and form deep bonds as they learn, play, and grow with older friends. Although logistically challenging, forging these sorts of shared-site partnerships in our communities can go a long way in breaking down arbitrary age barriers and humanizing institutional care spaces.

Policy

Finding the balance in the regulatory environment for long-term care to foster innovation for the future while protecting current clients and residents is challenging. Ideally, programs should be started as demonstrations that can be systematically evaluated and then, if found to provide an adequate cost-benefit ratio, more fully implemented in the system as a whole. Such is the case with the programs of all-inclusive care (PACE) supported through both Medicare and Medicaid. Concerned citizens can watch for state and federal legislative efforts to implement such innovations.

With regard to senior housing, researcher Caroline Pearson and her colleagues have projected that the average annual cost of assisted living and medical needs will be around $62,000. They suggest that the housing sector could accept lower profit margins, offer less luxurious housing, take advantage of technology, and subsidize middle-income residents with higher-paying ones. The government could create tax incentives, expand subsidies and Medicare coverage of nonmedical services, and create a long-term care benefit.[94]

We could also follow Japan's lead in reducing the market and creating a national long-term-care insurance system.[95] As journalist Meagan Day has written, a national single-payer social insurance policy, which could potentially be passed as part of healthcare reform, would provide comprehensive coverage for home- or community-based care for anyone (regardless of income) who is experiencing difficulty performing daily tasks. Such a policy, the potential benefits of which were illustrated quite dramatically during the brutal spread of the COVID-19 virus through clustered residential care facilities, may be rendered even more necessary in the next decade, when 10,000 baby boomers will turn 65 each day. Of a single-payer program, Day writes:

> This would have three major benefits. First, everyone would have access to the care they need, not just those who are fortunate enough to have a willing and available family member nearby. Second, informal carers would receive necessary relief, allowing them to live their own lives with the knowledge that their loved ones are getting the care they need. (This has strong feminist implications, since adult women bear the brunt of informal care work.) And third, formalizing long-term care would create millions of new jobs, easing unemployment and stimulating the economy overall.[96]

Including Many Voices in Reform

As we approach health care reform more generally, whatever form it takes, we need to be vigilant that geriatric services, programs for those with chronic conditions, primary care, and public health are not neglected as the hospitals and specialists continue to vie for their already excessively large piece of the health care pie. So too should we ensure representation of people living with dementia at the local, national, and international levels so that we are not talking at them or about them but *with* them as active participants with a voice.

We must try to hear all voices and seek to call forth those often not heard. But even as we celebrate the ascendancy of the speech of those with a diagnosis of dementia and other labels like MCI (mild cognitive impairment), regardless of source, we must maintain a critical stance, as no voice is immune from having a political agenda. Whereas we feel the pain of caregivers, we will challenge even that source of authenticity and authority when it appears distorted by false expectations and promises. Lived experience is individualized, and some advocates speak for all people with dementia in ways that can also be self-serving and potentially exclusionary (for example, of those with dementia who cannot speak anymore). Some in this conversation space have unusual dementias (for example, little progression), which necessitates skepticism for their ability to speak for all. In reclaiming their humanity, these proponents can be celebrated for their courage but not excused from the critical stance we should take to all human voices.

CONCLUSION

After Anne Basting had established TimeSlips in the midnineties, her next question was what to do with the wellspring of rich, imaginative narratives she had collected from nursing home residents. A playwright at heart, Anne's initial answer to this question was to take aspects of those stories and weave them into a larger dramatic work, which could be enjoyed by the broader public. She synthesized the stories she had collected—the creative oeuvre of dozens of people with "dementia" who had participated in TimeSlips—into a successful off-Broadway theatrical production that ran in the late nineties.

Anne's instincts to bridge from age-segregated nursing homes into community spaces reflects a larger pattern in the field over the last several decades. Next chapter, we hone in on this trend, which has engendered community-based approaches to care, looking specifically at national and international movements that envision a future where we do not segregate the cognitively frail in institutional settings but rather care for them in well-integrated age- and dementia-friendly communities.

9

A Bridge beyond Loneliness

The Gathering Momentum of Age- and Dementia-Friendly Communities

"I'm going to the hospital, son. You probably won't see me again," said the old man through the screen door of his trailer park home.

As I (Danny) had done many times before, I showed up at the gentleman's doorstep in Hershey, Pennsylvania, to drop off his daily Meals on Wheels delivery—a tray of hot food and a bagged lunch bundled with milk, an apple, and a sandwich. Although he'd always received each meal with the same gruff gratitude, I knew little about my white-haired neighbor, except that he lived alone and had no family in the area. While our list of meal recipients from the local Agency on Aging almost always noted emergency contact information for each person—usually friends or kin—his simply listed the trailer park landlord.

Although I never asked, I presumed the man was dealing with fairly serious complications from diabetes. Each time I saw him, his legs were heavily bandaged, with swollen ruddy toes sticking out of orthotic slippers. When I would knock on the door, he would rise from his chair with a grimace and saunter over, oxygen tank in tow. Today, he remained in his recliner, calling out at me through the screen door in a faltering voice, as he delivered his fatalistic prediction that would, unfortunately, prove prophetic.

Delivering for Meals on Wheels is one of the more intimate ways one can gain an on-the-ground sense of just how much our community-dwelling elders struggle in their later years, as well as the insufficiency of our efforts to mitigate their loneliness and loss of meaningful place in society. On my route, I've commonly seen elderly neighbors living with open wounds, subsisting in abject squalor, coping with severe and untreated memory loss, and enduring arduous medical treatments like chemotherapy without the aid of family or friends (and with virtually empty refrigerators). Over time, the experiences of delivering hundreds of door-to-door meals flow together into a single stream that carves out a basic truth: *we need a healthier society that is more embracing of our elders.*

How did we reach this point of such deep disconnection from our graying neighbors, not to mention our aging family members? And how does this predicament reflect the political-economic forces of the unhealthy society we examine in previous chapters? In this chapter, we explore these questions, considering the costs of elder loneliness and imagining strategies for remedying this symptom of our American dementia. In doing so, we describe national and international movements advocating for age- and dementia-friendly communities, which are currently gathering momentum, and establish ways in which we can render our own neighborhoods more humane and age friendly. This will require us to think about elder loneliness not merely as a lamentable cultural phenomenon but as a political-economic problem with potential structural solutions.

"HELLO IN THERE": CAPITALISM, ALIENATION, AND LONELINESS

As we've seen throughout the book, neoliberal restructuring has not been kind to our most vulnerable citizens—and that includes the elderly. Just how, and why, has the situation deteriorated for the aged in our society as we've progressed into the American dementia era?

For starters, as our lives have gradually become subsumed in the free market over the last four decades, we have found ourselves captive to an economic system that defines our value almost exclusively in terms of our productivity. To be fully human within this social order is to be a functioning economic actor within markets who produces value and also participates in society as a vigorous consumer. When people, whether because of old age, injury, infirmity, or other misfortune, are unable to do so, they effectively become diminished—perceived as detracting from economic growth rather than contributing to it. As Bill Thomas, the gerontologist we met last chapter, told us: "Old people especially pay a price for neoliberalism, because if your worth is mediated entirely through the market, and you become less economically productive as you age, then your worth in society is devalued by aging." This tension would surface in the culture quite starkly during the 2020 COVID-19 pandemic, when the extended lockdown necessary to protect elders and others more susceptible to the deadly virus clashed with imperatives to maintain economic business as usual (especially in the absence of robust extended relief from the federal government). The implication of hyper-capitalist logic: the health of the economy trumps the health of our elders, the latter of whom are de facto regarded as a market inefficiency and thus disposable. In a healthier society, balancing risks during acute emergencies like epidemics would draw on collective wisdom. But when the profit motive so distorts and dements our thinking, it makes rational, value-rich deliberation nearly impossible.

Overall, the subaltern social positioning of the elderly during the hyper-capitalist drift of the last forty years has inverted the more traditional social arrangement we touched on last chapter wherein, for human societies throughout history, an aging person's status within the community actually *increased* with age. While post–New Deal American society at least enshrined some semblance of collective moral commitment to the elderly by instituting safety net programs like social security, Medicare, and Meals on Wheels, which provide material protections for those no longer fully participating in the labor force, the neoliberal order—with its systematic efforts to reduce the role of the state in favor of markets and doctrinal promotion of individual responsibility—has gradually weakened our collective support for the aged, who are, in a cold economic calculus, regarded as a burdensome "surplus" who drain from society.[1] Recall from chapter 3 how this dynamic is often expressed through the crass language of "demographic tidal waves" and "silver tsunamis," or analogized to natural disasters (such as Hurricane Katrina)[2] that dramatize the growing economic "burden" of the elderly. In contemporary neoliberal shock politics, characterizations like this are commonly weaponized to argue for "urgent and necessary" cuts to elder-focused safety net programs, which live under constant threat of being dismantled by both major political parties in an age of grinding austerity and deficit hawking.

Our tendency to regard noneconomically productive elders, especially those with dementia, as a demographic "problem" has been one contributor to weakening their standing in society. Other political-economic and sociological factors have contributed to this fragmentation as well. Over the past several decades, the climbing average life expectancy has led to more adults—like the ailing gentleman on my Meals on Wheels route—living later in the lifespan than past elders did. Meanwhile, family sizes have shrunk, and in an era of globalization, financialization, free labor flow, and sprawling suburbanization (and exurbanization), working-age adults have increasingly relocated their families over wider and wider distances. As a result, children and grandchildren are more geographically scattered from older relatives than at any other time in human history. And even when families *are* able to live near their older relatives, the financial precarity that defines our era has made it a near-necessity to have two-earner families. This shift has gradually transitioned eldercare responsibility away from familial and social support systems and largely into the private assisted-living sector—yet another displacement into the market of our commitment to one another.

Outsourcing the care of our aging family members to a long-term care industry dominated by corporate interests (and thus the profit motive) has not only expedited the physical separation of elders from nuclear families, it has also further eroded our day-to-day interactions with our frail and aging neighbors. Of course, not everyone can afford to buy into the private long-term care market. As we've learned, the United States, unlike many industrialized countries, lacks a broad public program covering long-term care, which means that many who are aging but have insufficient savings to opt in to the independent / assisted living housing markets (but are not poor enough to qualify for Medicaid) must figure out a way to age in place, often without direct help from family members.[3] As a society, we simply choose not to pay for the cost of humanely caring for all aging citizens—to organize our economy around profit and market forces rather than collectively addressing universal human needs across the lifespan.[4]

At the community level, austerity policies implemented in the wake of the 2007-2008 Wall Street financial crash have further reduced services for older people, resulting in the closure of senior centers, adult education provision, libraries, leisure facilities, and the tightening of eligibility for home- and residential-based care.[5,6,7,8] Growing inequality has deepened economic insecurity across all age groups and subjected elders to financial distress.[9] Indeed, 34% of older adult individuals and 22% of couples are not poor enough to qualify for social programs and services but do not have enough money to make ends meet.[10]

Altogether, this inauspicious confluence of factors in the era of American dementia—devaluing of the elderly; disconnection from family; fewer intergenerational households; ever-eroding social protections, services, and safety nets; and insecurity around housing and living expenses later in life—has led a disturbing trend toward disconnection, loneliness, isolation, and precariousness for our aging neighbors and increased vulnerability to neglect, violence, and abuse, from the trailer parks in the Appalachian foothills of central Pennsylvania to overcrowded midwestern nursing homes and throughout the rest of the country.[11,12] Nearly one-third of Americans older than 65 currently live alone, and half of those over 85 do.[13] Research has consistently shown that, while self-reported loneliness tends to peak at several points across the lifespan (the twenties and fifties), its highest crest occurs in elderhood (the eighties and beyond).[14]

In 1971, the late American folk singer John Prine sang that "Old people just grow lonesome, waiting for someone to say, 'Hello in there . . . hello.'" Five decades later, market fundamentalism, the retreat of the state from its commitments to citizens, and a more atomized, alienated, disconnected, and overworked society has made the situation arguably bleaker, and the "hellos" even harder to come by. In continuing to think about brain health in an unhealthy society, it is critical to examine the material effects these deteriorating social conditions are imposing on the bodies and brains of our aging neighbors every day.

Applying an Ecopsychosocial Lens: Toxic Effects of Loneliness

Loneliness has become *the* watchword of the neoliberal era, and not just in the United States. In the United Kingdom, a country that has been similarly transformed by hyper-capitalist logic, loneliness is considered such a pervasive social ill that a new cabinet position, Minister for Loneliness, has been created to measure the problem and develop a societal response. In 2017, the commission appointed to study the loneliness epidemic discovered that more than 200,000 elders in the UK had not had a conversation with a friend or relative in more than a month (*a month*).[15] In evaluating the health consequences of such pervasive disconnection, the commission concluded that feeling distress from lack of social contact was as physically harmful as smoking 15 cigarettes a day.[16]

In Japan, the world's oldest country, where over a quarter of the population is 65 or above, the crisis of loneliness is manifesting in unforeseen—and rather Kafkaesque—ways. Between 1985 and 2015, as neoliberalism reordered Japanese society just as it has the United States and UK, the number of seniors living alone increased by 600%, and state pensions have failed to keep up with cost of living.[17] Over roughly that same period, the country has witnessed a dramatic rise in deaths of isolated elders whose decayed bodies sit unnoticed in their houses for weeks or months before being found by police or landlords—a gruesome epiphenomenon of the zombie era that the Japanese refer to as "lonely deaths."[18] So too has Japan observed a concurrent spike in elder crimes like shoplifting and weapon possession.[19] Since these petty crimes are strictly sentenced in Japan, an astounding *one in five* current inmates in the Japanese carceral system is a senior citizen. What is driving this bizarre trend in elder crime?

In a word, loneliness.

According to a 2017 government report, half the Japanese seniors caught shoplifting live alone, and 40% say they rarely speak to or lack family. Jail, on the other hand, not only offers safety and stability, warmth, caring supervision, and three nutritious meals a day, it also removes a financial burden from the lives of elders and their families and guarantees a sense of community through daily social interactions. So, in essence, neoliberalism has helped engineer a grim societal reality whereby seniors in one of the world's most economically powerful countries are willfully trading their personal liberty for respite from loneliness, financial precarity, and the prospect of dying in isolation.

While solitude can certainly have its benefits, chronic loneliness is inescapably toxic for social animals. Ample evidence suggests that loneliness and its attendant depression, isolation, diminution of social networks and social activity have varied deleterious effects throughout the body and brain, which can accelerate physiological decline.[20] As former US surgeon general Vivek Murthy—who on leaving his post authored a book about the urgency of the loneliness epidemic and the healing power of human connection[21]—has bluntly warned, loneliness upregulates the stress response and is inexorably associated "with a greater risk of cardiovascular disease, dementia, depression, and anxiety."[22]

Given what we know about the intimate relationship between the health of the heart and that of the brain, the link between loneliness and deteriorating cardiovascular health is particularly concerning. A recent systematic review and meta-analysis found that loneliness and social isolation take such a long-term toll on the vascular system (via higher blood pressure and increased hypothalamic-pituitary-adrenocortical activity[23,24,25,26]) that they increase risk of coronary heart disease by 29% and stroke by 32%.[27] Other studies have linked greater perceived social isolation with an increased risk of death for patients with heart failure.[28] So too has social isolation been associated with insomnia—another major risk factor for dementia.[29] Lack of sleep stresses the vascular system and impairs the brain's metabolic self-cleaning capacity. Beyond these effects, researchers have shown that insomnia born of loneliness puts people at twice greater risk for premature death than those with robust social interactions.[30]

Unsurprisingly, loneliness has been found to predict greater cognitive decline[31] and double risk of dementia.[32] Researchers from Harvard and Peking Universities analyzed 12 years of data from men and women aged 65 years or older and found that loneliness and depressive symptoms were related to risk factors of worsening cognition. Loneliness has also been associated with higher inflammation, greater amyloid burden, and lower brain-derived neurotrophic factor, which contributes to new neuron growth and synapses formation, as well as reducing risk of dementia and stroke. People who are lonelier have also rather unsurprisingly been observed to be at higher risk of mental health problems.[33]

Taken together, this body of growing literature illustrates how the alienation, loneliness, and atomization sown within an unhealthy society organized around individualism, consumerism, profit motive, and markets is *quite literally* proving to be a threat to the brain health and general well-being of our isolated elders, not to mention the rest of us who are aging.

The Protective Effects of Social Bonds

On the flip side, ample evidence shows that social engagement, the preservation of social networks, and perceptions of usefulness, purpose, belonging, and connection to community can be positive forces for the brain health of the elderly. Echoing our evolution as a species that developed over thousands of generations in small, tight-knit bands of hunter-gatherers (not to mention the more recent trade-offs inherent in the community-seeking behavior of Japanese elder "criminals" over the last several decades), researchers have specifically linked social engagement to lower risk for dementia[34] and age-related cognitive impairment.[35] Even beyond brain health, studies spanning the past three decades and across multiple continents have established strong associations between social integration and survival.[36,37,38,39]

Other studies have linked social activity with greater feelings of usefulness, suggesting that improved self-perceptions and a more purposeful bearing might improve general health outcomes for elders. Multiple studies undertaken in several countries have supported an association between decreased feelings of usefulness/purposefulness and reductions in global functioning outcomes (that is, mobility, activities of daily living, and increased mortality).[40,41] For instance, a study of elderly Japanese adults aged 65 and older found that on measures of usefulness to society and to others, participants who felt "only a little" or "not at all" useful were twice as likely to die over a six-year follow-up period, in analyses that adjusted for a range of sociodemographic factors, comorbidity, depression, self-perceived health, and social network characteristics.[42]

In another study in Japan, a seven-year longitudinal measure of 43,000-plus adults found that individuals who believed that their life was worth living (in possession of what the Japanese call *ikigai*, or "that which makes life worth living") were (1) less likely to die than were their counterparts without this belief; (2) more likely to be married, educated, and employed; and (3) reported lower levels of stress and better self-rated health.[43] Results from these studies complimented the Helsinki Study, in which Finnish adults aged 75 years and older who felt themselves to be "more needed" were less likely to die over a 10-year follow-up and less likely to enter an institutional facility over a 5-year follow-up.[44] A four-year study of French citizens aged 60 years or older similarly showed that an increasing sense of uselessness predicted an increase in disability,[45] and researchers have confirmed similar findings in the United States.

Other studies have found that a sense of belonging consistently produces more favorable health outcomes across a range of ethnic groups.[46] Interestingly, *National Geographic* has conducted an international study called Blue Zones, looking at regions where the world's healthiest and longest-living people reside. They identified Blue Zones in wide-ranging locations—from Greece, Japan, and Sardinia to California—all of which shared a strong sense of community and a respectful integration of elders into the broader social fabric.[47]

In terms of strategies to assist elders in forging protective bonds, studies have consistently pointed to *volunteering* as being associated with improved health outcomes for aging persons. Perhaps this is not surprising since, in addition to bringing people into relationships and social networks where they can feel valued and purposeful (that is, a greater sense of ikigai), the act of volunteering increases physical, social, and cognitive activity, and in turn, those increases lead to improved health outcomes via a range of physiological and psychological mechanisms. Accordingly, recent studies have shown volunteering at any number of hours to be associated with higher levels of cognitive functioning[48] as well as better physical health and longevity.[49] Staying connected and purposeful, as well as avoiding the isolation and lassitude of advancing years, are powerful and underappreciated determinants of health for our aging neighbors.[50]

Given our expanding knowledge about the toxic effects of loneliness and the flipside benefits of social integration and volunteering, it is heartening that movements are afoot around the world to push back against the dreary loneliness engineered by the neoliberal reordering of society and to modify our communities to more meaningfully integrate elders.

EXAMINING THE AGE- AND DEMENTIA-FRIENDLY CITIES MOVEMENTS

Movements Born of Ageism

The very need for a concept of cities that endeavor to become more age and dementia friendly is in some sense an indictment of entrenched societal biases toward aging in the hyper-capitalist era, as it implies a default *un*friendliness toward those who are aged or affected by memory loss that requires societal remediation. People commonly refer to this tendency as *ageism*, a term coined in 1969 by the influential geriatrician Robert Butler. While the phrase connotes a cultural bias akin to racism or sexism that leads us to view our graying neighbors as "irrelevant," "burdensome," or otherwise diminished (see the OK Boomer meme referenced earlier), it is also true that ageism can be applied to people across the aging spectrum, including children.

The age- and dementia-friendly movements both interrogate ageism toward elders, but the former provides more latitude to challenge our neoliberal-inflected ageist tendencies to detract value from, or render irrelevant, *any* individuals who have diminished economic productivity. In a world where there will soon be more people over the age of 65 than under the age of 5, and where people over 65 are 50 times as wealthy as those under 35,[51] it will be critical to challenge ageism wherever it may occur along the aging spectrum. Ultimately, the goal should be to achieve sustainable societies built on social democratic principles that—instead of creating a stark market-based landscape of winners and losers—guarantee basic material and environmental security and dignity of human beings at every age. Can the age- and dementia-friendly movements assist us in pursuing this goal? Let's learn more about their respective visions.

The Age-Friendly Communities Movement

The World Health Organization launched the age-friendly movement in the early 2000s, at a time of relatively strong economic growth. While the storm of financial collapse was brewing in the deregulated finance and housing markets of the post-Clinton era, the movement's initial goals were to link urban design, architecture, and social policy in ways that ensured elders were actively involved, valued, and supported with infrastructure and services to meet their needs and help them age in place.[52] When the Great Recession hit in 2007-2008, the economic floor collapsed, and the resulting austerity policies that aggressively scaled back the welfare state and public investments also altered the goals of the age-friendly movement.[53] Consequently, while the essence of the WHO's age-friendly vision remains, it has evolved within an era of crisis defined by disparity, austerity, precarity, and climate change, integrating the goal of pursuing *equity* and addressing *social disadvantage*, while acknowledging the need for sustainability to be at the forefront of any planning.[54]

In the United States, the WHO's push to make communities more age friendly is being coordinated and promoted by the American Association of Retired Persons (AARP), which has rebranded the movement as *livable communities*. This initiative supports neighborhoods, towns, cities, and rural areas that wish to adapt in ways that improve the thriving of people of all ages—building walkable streets, age-friendly and intergenerational housing, more robust transportation options, access to social services, and opportunities for social and civic participation and inclusion. Beyond development, it aims to use education to foster an age-friendly ethos across various sectors, from the arts, businesses, community groups, emergency services, health and social services, to housing and transportation. Thus far, the AARP has focused its efforts disproportionately on assessing the adaptations of urban communities, delegating the responsibility of making transformational plans and acting to local communities. Toolkits for community adaptation have been developed to provide guidance.[55]

Generally speaking, the age-friendly movement is premised on the overwhelming evidence presented above, which has shown that—in a positive sense—elderly folks who remain active and maintain or create new social bonds and roles that stabilize selfhood and sense of purpose will generally experience better health outcomes than those who disengage from society and social commitments. Proponents believe that life events, aging, and environments interact materially with the biology of the body and brain to precipitate neurologic and behavioral transformations that are protective or pathological—a conceptual framework readers might recall from earlier chapters as *entanglement theory*.[56] While it is natural that life-course transitions faced by older adults (for example, retirement and loss of professional identity, loss of mobility, increases in disability and illness, loss of spouse, diminution of social networks) put elders at risk for social isolation and loneliness, age-friendly advocates believe some of these factors can be mitigated through coordinated planning, community education, and the buffering of protective social relationships through activities like volunteering.

Critics argue that, much like the person-centered care and culture change movements, the *age-friendly* concept must not merely serve as a "branding exercise" for cities,[57] and that proponents must truly commit to reaching out to socially excluded groups in low-income communities and more adroitly embrace social, class, and ethnic diversity in planning. They also argue that a better job must be done to integrate rural communities into the age-friendly developmental vision and challenge wider inequalities and injustices in a more consistent and coordinated way.[58,59] Elders from different socioeconomic strata—for instance, the gentleman on the

Meals on Wheels route in Hershey—should be *centered* in this movement and have a key role in the planning and reverse engineering of public spaces rather than planning being decided from the top down. That said, others critique that communities should be designed not merely for elders but rather as livable places for people of all ages, especially since children and youth are subject to ageism (unfair discrimination on the basis of chronological age), loneliness, and rising deaths of despair. Ultimately, having a sense of purpose is essential to being human at any age.

The Dementia-Friendly Communities Movement

Dementia-friendly communities are focused more specifically on improving inclusion and quality of life for people living with dementia. Whereas the age-friendly movement draws its vision from entanglement theory, the call for dementia-friendly communities takes its conceptual cue, largely, from disability studies, which has long challenged negative stereotypes of disabilities while promoting strategies for the inclusion and participation of people who are differently abled.[60] Although conceptual models for dementia-friendly cities vary across cultural contexts, most have been organized around some combination of the following attributes:

- increased community awareness about dementia and more humane attitudes toward those affected;
- provision of supportive resources, opportunities, and trainings for caregivers and families (dementia support, advance planning, and so on);
- dementia support training for citizens of all ages;
- promotion of opportunities for meaningful participation in community life through dementia-friendly services, activities, and supports;
- modifications in physical environments and infrastructure to ensure safety and inclusion (housing, transport, neighborhood design, and so forth);
- increased dementia-friendly business and financial practices and reduced opportunities for fraud and abuse;
- increased screening detection, diagnosis, and specialized services for memory loss;

- reduction of stigma and acknowledgment of the potential retained by persons with dementia;
- promotion of independent living; and
- emergency preparedness.

In the United States, the Dementia Friendly America initiative[61] aspires to foster cities equipped to support people with dementia and their family and friend caregivers. The organization has far exceeded its initial goal of establishing 16 model cities by 2016, and new communities are becoming certified each month. Often associated with these programs are Dementia Friends initiatives to educate younger individuals on how to interact with people with cognitive challenges. As with the age-friendly movement, the dementia-friendly initiative has developed its own toolkit.[62]

One focus of the dementia-friendly movement that remains somewhat controversial is its advocacy for early diagnosis of memory challenges. While this may sound like a positive goal on paper, it also potentially extends stigmatizing *predisease* illness labels to more of the population. As our British colleague Carol Brayne has told us, because of the complicated ways labels like AD and MCI are experienced by human beings, and because of the hyper-capitalist imperative to create new "consumers" in drug markets, "We can't just allow people to sleepwalk into screenings and diagnoses." Thinking back to chapter 3 and the marketplace of memory, the question is how early and reliably clinicians can make an early diagnosis of dementia or MCI and how it actually helps people with cognitive challenges. Much evidence suggests that having an early label does not actually benefit people with symptoms and their families (it more clearly helps experts and companies who want to enroll people into trials, use more biomarkers, and sell more drugs). But the promise that we can pharmacologically "fix" brain aging better at an early stage has proved false.

Additionally, the dementia-friendly movement has focused much attention on the physical built environment with minimal acknowledgment of larger environmental concerns (that is, climate change and natural disasters, which disproportionately affect the vulnerable, including the elderly).[63] And finally the dementia-focused initiatives largely ignore the idea that dementia itself and other forms of cognitive disability can affect children and other ages in addition to elders, and are thus not inclusive of these other groups earlier in the lifespan.

MOVING TOWARD AGE- AND DEMENTIA-FRIENDLY COMMUNITIES

While these dual movements can be a bit abstract, they have provided both an intellectual energy and a practical framework that have guided recent efforts to creatively address the challenges of aging populations and revalue all members of society, regardless of cognitive functioning or economic productivity. In this respect, both initiatives challenge aspects of neoliberalism and provide hope for creating greater social solidarity. Let's explore some particularly compelling on-the-ground projects that have recently emerged from these fledgling movements, which we've been fortunate enough to be a part of.

A Village of Hope: 3D Printing an Age-Friendly Community on a Rural Mountaintop

On a cold morning in March 2019, I (Danny) stood shivering in an old abandoned elementary school perched on a frozen mountaintop in Clearfield, Pennsylvania. The scene looked a bit like a postapocalyptic zombie film set in Appalachia: an old shuttered building in the rural coal country of central Pennsylvania with crumbling ceiling tiles, gutted classrooms with overturned desks and chairs, and handwritten lesson plans from a decade earlier etched on the blackboard, frozen in time. As I walked through the school, my breath visible in front of me, I listened as representatives from the Clearfield County Agency on Aging described their vision to transition this abandoned building and lonely mountaintop clearing into a thriving 23-acre intergenerational, age- and dementia-friendly community.

The agency has forged a public-private partnership with geriatrician Bill Thomas and a new company he has established called Minka (a Japanese word for "peoples' house"). After growing disenchanted with the institutional stagnation in the nursing home marketplace, Bill's latest big idea has been designing 3D-printed compact homes (or *minkas*, as they are referred to in shorthand) that can help integrate aging elders into communities of the future, with Clearfield serving as a prototype of this vision. On the mountaintop clearing, which was a former coal mining site, Bill and his team are working with the agency to build 60 state-of-the-art modular homes outfitted with smart technology (for example,

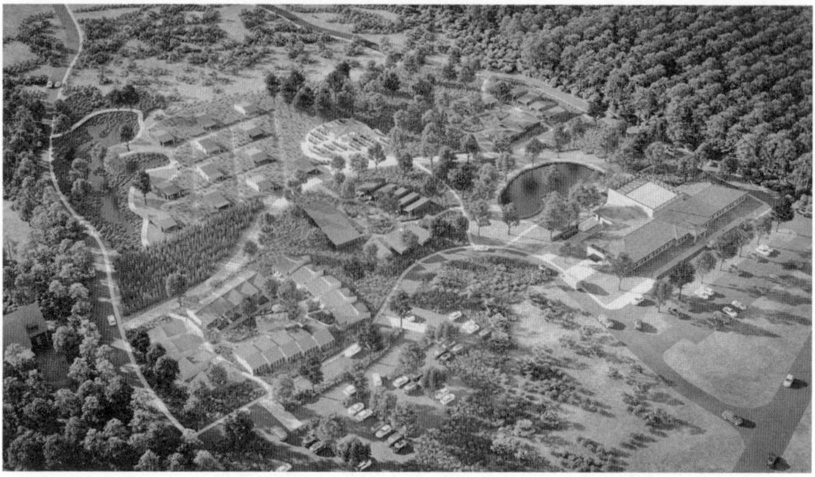

Figure 9.1. A digital rendering of the Village of Hope in Clearfield, Pennsylvania. *Source:* Photograph courtesy of Minka.

lights, GPS tracking, virtual family visits, and telehealth) and engineered to keep residents with physical and cognitive frailty safe without requiring hospitalization or institutional care. To make the village accessible, homes will be priced on a sliding scale based on residents' income (figure 9.1).

Thomas, who originally designed the 3D model home prototype for his daughter Haleigh Jane, who lives with a developmental conditional called Otahara syndrome,[64] is not merely interested in using the latest robotic gadgets to build a mountaintop geriatric techno-utopia. His vision is for the houses to serve as the material foundation of a broader "multi-ability, multi-generational inclusive community," which Thomas refers to by the acronym MAGIC. This means that, unlike traditional age-segregated nursing homes, people of all ages and physical and cognitive abilities will be neighbors in the village, with the decommissioned school repurposed into a mixed-use community center refitted with a health clinic, grocery store, café, and arts and theater space that binds the village.

All design elements of the mountain clearing—the landscaping, walking paths, common areas, parks, ponds, urban gardens, and wooded surroundings—will be aimed at fostering social connection, relationship building, and neighborly support to mitigate the toxic effects of loneliness and encourage protective engagement and social bonding. Indeed, for Thomas and his collaborators, building a village that weaves people into a textured living community based on the MAGIC ethos is the primary goal, taking precedence over a narrower, more reductive focus on "enhancing cognitive stimulation" or "increasing cognitive capacity," which we saw to be the guiding principles of the marketplace of memory in chapter 3. To Thomas, community's role ought to be helping people thrive and flourish no matter their age or level of cognitive function. This not only serves as a direct challenge to our societal tendency to segregate the cognitively frail in institutional settings, it also is a way of intentionally structuring a village to eliminate ageism and resist the neoliberal ascription of social value based on one's productive and consumptive capacity.[65]

If Thomas has his way, the project in Clearfield will merely be the first domino to fall. In a country that is facing down the impossibility of housing growing numbers of aging people in long-term care facilities and that has, during the COVID-19 pandemic, witnessed firsthand the deadly consequences of clustering vulnerable elders under a single institutional roof, modular homes offer a potentially radical challenge to the status quo of institutionalized housing and displacement, isolation, and endangerment of aging citizens. Compact homes can not only be arranged into cluster communities and small rural villages, as Thomas and the Agency on Aging are doing on the Appalachian mountaintop; they can also potentially be placed in spaces adjacent to urban neighborhoods and developments, or even in backyards in ways that safely embed elders in community settings, affording independence as well as organic connection to others and to beautiful landscapes and architecture. Having moved beyond long-term care institutions, Thomas predicts the rise of such *pocket neighborhoods*, where homecare providers support clusters of elders living in a common area. Increasingly, he believes that providers will focus not only on housing stock but also on developing community centers and other commons that can anchor people who are living in place, thicken social bonds, and add quality to their lives.[66]

By reimagining societal aging outside the limited purview of age-segregated long-term care facilities, Thomas and his colleagues see their purpose as developing new tools and concepts that allow people to create the intergenerational communities they need by dint of their own agency. As Thomas's collaborative partner Kavan Peterson has said, "If we can design communities to meet needs and not control symptoms, we can see better outcomes. For decades, the only story we've heard about aging is one of loss, decline and despair. But there is a new story. It is a story of connection, expression, joy and growth . . . told by people living with dementia, by those who love them, and by people of all ages who want to live in diverse and welcoming communities."[67]

Whether this age-friendly vision and ambitious social-engineering effort in coal country will succeed is unclear, but the work of Thomas and his colleagues represents a profound conceptual challenge to orthodoxies about caring for the cognitively frail, which have largely defined our approaches for the last hundred years and led to dire straits for elders in economically developed countries.

Intergenerational Cohousing Partnerships

Last chapter, we saw how hybrid nursing home-preschools have begun emerging to meet needs at both ends of the age spectrum. Such shared-site partnerships are manifesting in other forms as well, spawning highly innovative approaches to multigenerational cohousing.

For instance, in the Dutch city of Deventer, a retirement facility has partnered with a local college to offer students a chance to live with elders. In essence, students room and board for free in the community and, in exchange, provide ongoing volunteering with residents, including teaching them how to send emails, use social media, and Skype with family members.[68] This model has caught on in multiple countries, including in our backyard in Cleveland. At Judson retirement community, a long-term care facility we've been privileged to work with over the years, students from the Cleveland Institute of Music are offered free housing in exchange for weekly musical performances at each of the retirement community's campuses, as well as serving on musical arts committees, assisting staff therapists, and volunteering at community events.

Other emerging age-friendly housing models are being driven by universities that are building new living units on campuses for retirees. While this trend has been appropriately criticized by some as cynical, since institutions are effectively creating new revenue streams with deep-pocketed boomers seeking to "reexperience their youth," elder housing on university campuses does potentially engender new opportunities for reciprocal benefit (such as mentoring, lifelong learning, social support, and so on).[69]

Since housing is a basic human need for people of all ages, there are rich possibilities in all our communities for bringing generations together in such intuitive, mutually supportive, and reciprocally beneficial living arrangements. At Penn State, we are developing a program that will allow medical students to live in an assisted living home located right on the outskirts of campus. Essentially, students in their preclinical years will be given residence in a rent-free apartment in exchange for volunteering in the dementia-care unit, hosting socialceutical programs like TimeSlips and Opening Minds through Art. One can imagine how opportunities like this could be designed to involve students in the arts and humanities as well as other health trainee programs in ways that are professionally formative for students and protective and enriching for elders susceptible to the dangers of isolation.

Yet another trend has been the recent creation of hundreds of self-governed shared housing communities. As reported by the *New York Times* in 2019,[70] this "village movement" matches people who have unused housing with those who need housing—usually around shared experiences or values. Members of these communities, many of which are multigenerational and nested in housing complexes or converted apartments, often negotiate for lower rents in exchange for taking on community responsibilities (such as transportation, security, landscaping, maintenance, and so on). Others pay dues to hire coordinators to oversee services. Shared communities effectively become *microcommunes* that operate in a community setting outside an institutional framework. Such are the ways people are adapting locally to address the rising crisis of affordable long-term housing for elders in a country that does not (yet) provide a universal safety net for retirees.

Infusing Community Organizations with an Age-Friendly Ethos

Age-friendly principles can also stimulate inventive thinking about sharing resources and infrastructure as well as fostering unique partnerships. For instance, libraries and schools have begun connecting struggling young readers with mentors in residential care homes who find joy and purpose in teaching this skill to children.[71] As we explored last chapter in the Meet Me at MoMA program, museums are increasingly opening their doors to groups of people from long-term care homes and their caregivers, enabling elders normally excluded from such public spaces to enjoy social interaction and share in powerful aesthetic experiences in quintessentially human ways. Community spaces such as farmers' markets, community gardens, nature centers, and parks also have great potential to support intergenerational exchanges in urban environments. In each instance, an age- and dementia-friendly community vision and ethos can provide a theoretical base to challenge the invisible ageist stereotypes and open new avenues to use existing social infrastructure to increase social solidarity.

Reinventing Senior Centers

In this age-friendly spirit, significant attention has been paid to senior centers. Not only do proponents of age- and dementia-friendly communities view it as critical that these spaces remain solvent anchor institutions for elders in our communities in an age of austerity, there is also momentum behind the concept of reinventing senior centers as "intergenerational community centers."[72] Rather than arbitrarily segregating elderly cohorts in social activities, advocates are imagining ways modernized organizations could provide space for dynamic programming (exercise classes, book clubs, health screenings, health care services, and so on) while facilitating people from different generations coming together to nurture trust, empathy, and support through mutually affirming interactions. Japan, for instance, has proactively responded to its tragic problem of senior loneliness by investing public funds in the creation, staffing, and maintenance of senior centers, offering an array of age-diverse recreational activities, services, and social supports.[73]

At Penn State, we have worked with a senior center near our hospital campus to reimagine the facility as a shared site for medical school classes. Since 2016, we have staged a Culinary Medicine course for fourth-year students in the senior center's teaching kitchen (figure 9.2). There, elders join students to work collaboratively in the kitchen, where they practice cooking healthy meals and discuss interpersonal and socioeconomic aspects of meal planning and eating on budget. Infusing a medical school course with elder involvement at the senior center has enabled rich and unexpected learning opportunities. For instance, elders frequently bring their life experiences to bear in offering poignant personal stories (for example, being affected by eating disorders, not being able to afford produce, and so on) and exhortations (such as to be aware of nutritional limitations low-income individuals face) that help put the curriculum's nutritional science in a human context for developing health trainees.[74,75]

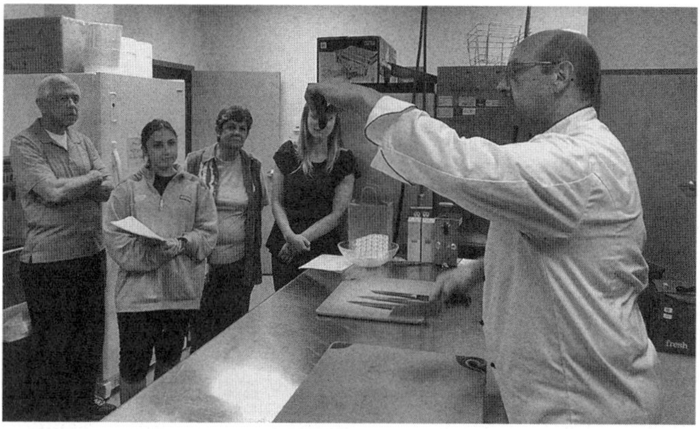

Figure 9.2. Medical students work alongside elders in a Culinary Medicine course under the guidance of chef Dave Gurdis and nutritionist educator Tomi Dreibelbis.
Source: Photograph courtesy of Tomi Dreibelbis.

Students have uniformly felt that this intergenerational dimension improved their nutritional-counseling skills and ultimately influenced elders' lifestyle choices. They have, for instance, commonly reflected that elder partners "had lots to offer as teachers," and that "their life experiences were an asset in discussing diet changes." Elders have been galvanized by the interaction with students. Frequently, senior center members express how pleased they were to successfully impart their own personal teachings to the students. For instance, one participant who had strongly urged students to be mindful of the needs of underserved patients wrote, "I feel it is important for doctors to be more aware of nutrition when working with patients. I suggested to the [students] that they be aware of nutritional limitations faced by poor individuals who don't have easy access to healthful ingredients." Such opportunities provide elders in Hershey—neighbors of the isolated gentleman who lived in the trailer park on my route—the type of social engagement and opportunity to feel a sense of purpose, contribution, and social bonding through volunteering that research has found to be so protective.[76]

In Cleveland, we have both worked with another innovative intergenerational community campus, Fairhill Partners, under the inspired leadership of our friend and colleague Stephanie Fallcreek.[77] Both the Alzheimer Center that Peter directed years ago and the Intergenerational School he co-founded with his wife, Cathy, Stephanie, and others in 2000 found their first real homes at Fairhill. The organization is exemplary for providing a diversity of services to meet the needs of elders and others in the community, for collaborative partnerships, and for a strong commitment to caring for the socially disadvantaged. Although concerned with the ongoing challenges of obtaining funding and managing resources effectively for their innovative programming, Fairhill is a place where humane values, rather than the bottom line, drive the mission.

As there are an estimated 15,000 senior centers across the United States, the prospect of using these organizations as transformative intergenerational community centers for age- and dementia-friendly partnerships surpassing the work we've done in Hershey and Cleveland is ripe with potential. It will be essential to aim public resources at any initiative to improve senior centers, which invariably means using progressive taxation—particularly of the ultra-wealthy. As journalist Meagan Day has written in arguing for investments in senior center infrastructure, "Jeff Bezos and Bill Gates don't deserve their billions nearly as much as every senior deserves to feel connected, cared for, and loved."[78]

Organizing across the Generations around Climate Change

As earth's ecosystems are increasingly disrupted by planetary warming, the effects will reverberate across all age cohorts, disproportionately affecting the most vulnerable at either end of the age spectrum. Given the rising precariousness caused by climate change and the need to build resilient, mutually supportive communities in response, cross-generational solidarity is powerfully consummated in efforts to protect the environment.

When this intergenerational dynamic comes together organically, it can be rather moving to witness. In mid-October 2017, I (Danny) joined several dozen demonstrators—including several of my medical students—in protesting the Atlantic Sunrise pipeline, a natural gas pipeline whose construction would tear through a tract of farmland owned by an order of Roman Catholic nuns living in Lancaster, Pennsylvania, just 20 miles from our medical school. We gathered in a harvested cornfield, buffeted by harsh crosswinds on the cold autumn morning, staying warm by huddling in close quarters and singing protest songs that rose above the industrial hum of machines idling in the background. The pipeline company (Transco/Williams) had been granted the legal authority to seize the convent's land against their will with the backing of US Marshals. As a bulldozer slipped into gear and approached the construction site ready to break ground on the convent's farmland, the protestors locked arms, giving themselves up for arrest in an act of civil disobedience against the corporate exploitation of the local community and the natural environment.

Many of the folks blocking the bulldozer could be described as pensioners, sporting white hair and silver beards. One of them was a woman named Rachel, who was shivering in the cold crosswinds as the bulldozer approached. I offered her my hooded sweatshirt and struck up a conversation to learn why she was willing to be arrested for this cause. She told me, "I'm doing this for my 6-year-old niece and 3-year-old nephew. The way things are going is so discouraging. I'm not afraid to be arrested—I was hauled off in the paddy wagon for protesting the Keystone pipeline, so I've been there, done that. We've all got to do what we've got to do."

When the bulldozer finally reached the work site, the phalanx of protestors encircled it, forcing the driver to cut the engine. Soon thereafter, the police closed in and arrested Rachel and the 24 others braver than I who were willing to be taken into custody. Those who left in handcuffs ranged in age from 16 to 86 and included three pastors and a high school student.

When it comes to fighting for our environment, corporate power is particularly formidable and has largely co-opted our government institutions at all levels in an era of neoliberal dominance. But the public health and ecosystem risks posed by fracking are too dangerous to ignore. The only way we can guarantee truly age-friendly cities of the future is to forge solidarity across generations and resist environmental degradation, especially where our poorest and most politically marginalized citizens are irreparably harmed by corporate power and environmental racism. Like my neighbor Rachel, we must be emboldened by an intergenerational ethic to block fracking wells and pipelines and selflessly engage in forms of civil disobedience in defense of current and future human beings.

In addition to finding local pockets of resistance in your communities, there are organizations that can connect you with opportunities to protect our ecosystem. For instance, the group Gray is Green is an online gathering place for older Americans who aspire to create a green legacy for the future by fighting for ecological sustainability as well as social and economic justice. The organization has a website that serves as a central clearinghouse of ideas and communications for adults interested in "greening their lives, learning about sustainability, advocating for sound public policy, being creative stewards or grandparents, emerging as elders, and mentoring young people."[79] Another group, Elders Climate Action, has a more policy-oriented focus.[80]

A Role for Technology? Self-Driving Cars as Age- and Dementia-Friendly Infrastructure

As a NASA engineer, Jaime Waydo helped land the first rover on Mars. Years later, she headed up Google's systems engineering team to launch the company's fleet of autonomous vehicles in the United States. Despite these lofty accomplishments, Waydo, who has since taken a leadership role with Apple's self-driving car project, has often found herself contemplating the implications of self-driving cars with respect to her aging mother. "My mom's getting older and having those hard conversations about you're not able to safely drive any more. We need to take your keys away," she told the *Guardian* in 2017. "A technology like this can really give a lot of people mobility for a very long time."[81]

Indeed, while a main lesson of the book is that no form of technology produced in capital markets is likely to be lowered in like a deus ex machina to "solve" complicated human problems, from the changing climate to the aging brain, people like Waydo and Bill Thomas animate the possibility that some market-based innovations *can* have a functional role to play in fostering communities that are more age and dementia friendly and mitigating alienation and loneliness for our elders. So what is the particular promise of self-driving cars as an assistive technology within age- and dementia-friendly communities?

As with Thomas's modular homes outfitted with smart and energy-efficient technology, autonomous electric cars could serve as a powerful and environmentally friendly infrastructure that helps people age in place, embedded in community rather than age-segregated nursing institutions. Cars equipped with self-driving functionality could not only extend independent mobility for people like Waydo's mother, who might not otherwise be able to safely drive, they could also remove some of the transportation responsibility from busy or geographically distant family members (for instance, travel to and from healthcare appointments) and quell anxiety about a loved one getting lost or being involved in accidents.

One can even imagine smart cars monitoring the well-being of riders (is there agitation or confusion?), communicating with family members via phone or video screen in a pinch, and perhaps offering ameliorative and pneumonic assistance (for example, calming music, verbal reassurance, and reminders). Ironically, self-driving cars offer the promise of preserving independence in elder drivers like Waydo's mother by taking a degree of it away.

Of course, by potentially extending independence in this paradoxical manner, autonomous cars also represent a means of keeping elders integrated into communities. Cars that could safely transport aging persons over long distances in rural America and navigate congested urban or sprawling suburban areas open up a wide array of social engagements beyond one's home. Given the toxic effects of loneliness and the benefits of active engagement (especially volunteering), one could imagine autonomous vehicles helping to facilitate social opportunities—for instance, by transporting elders to museums, libraries, parks, schools, gardens, soup kitchens, and other vibrant public spaces, where they could stay engaged and meaningfully involved in society.

Integrating elders in these ways would not only benefit their own biopsychosocial well-being, but also potentially strengthen the social fabric of communities. Age- and dementia-friendly cities that find ways to increase the presence of elders in shared social spaces can create more moments of intergenerational solidarity as well as refitting the remaining talents and strengths of aging persons into extant community needs. Such presence of those with memory challenges can perhaps help reduce the stigma associated with dementia and assist communities in developing greater compassion toward the cognitively and physically frail. So too can a broader presence of elders in community spaces offer opportunities for organizations and businesses that may be able to develop experiences and products for a clientele who have historically been excluded.

While we tend to think about the self-driving car revolution as a market-based initiative, it is intriguing to consider how the state might help scale the technology and aim it at meeting collective social needs. For instance, one wonders what a program like Meals on Wheels might look like if reorganized around a technology like autonomous vehicles? Rather than having meals delivered to discrete homes by volunteers, fleets of self-driving vehicles could instead pick up willing elders, like the gentleman in the Hershey trailer park, and transport them to central community venues for hot meals (or even collaborative meal preparation) and social interaction with other elders as well as community volunteers. After all, while receiving nutritious foods is certainly important, we have seen in this chapter how human companionship and thick social bonds are even more existentially nourishing. Ultimately, there are many practical and moral questions surrounding the self-driving car phenomenon, but it is an emerging technology worth keeping at the forefront of our imaginations as we pursue more age- and dementia-friendly communities.

HOW WE CAN RESIST

Become a Dementia Friend

As part of the larger dementia-friendly movement, countries have begun training citizens to serve as Dementia Friends. The organization Dementia-Friendly America defines a Dementia Friend as "someone who, through viewing a series of online videos or attending an in-person session, learns about what it's like to live with dementia and then turns that understanding into action." Trainees emerge with the ability to offer people with dementia and their caregivers a helping volunteer hand at community events, in caregiving groups, or in assisted living environments.

Other countries have aggressively implemented Dementia Friends programs. For instance, Japan has created over 8 million Dementia Friends (6% of its population), and millions more have been certified across the world. In the United States, training programs are offered across the country and take a relatively short amount of time to complete.[82]

Occupy Public Spaces to Make Them More Dementia-Friendly

In the late nineties, as Tom Kitwood's PCC movement was transforming the way we thought about caring for persons with dementia, a Dutch psychiatrist named Bere Miesen began developing a concept he called a *memory café*. Staged in community settings, in full public view, memory cafés were initially gatherings of people with dementia, their caregivers, and health professionals, but they quickly grew to involve others as well. The café is a place—sometimes an actual café, other times churches, community centers, or other local venues—where those who are concerned about aging can gather in a safe, engaging, and mutually supportive environment, and share stories, ideas, and resources. At present, there are memory cafés all around the world, and in all 50 states in the United States. If you are interested in learning more about starting a memory café, you can visit the memory café online directory.[83] Free training and assistance are also available through the Alzheimer's Association.

The memory café concept has continued evolving in recent years under the aegis of dementia-friendly communities, as people with dementia and their caregivers have begun "occupying" the types of cultural spaces mentioned above—schools, libraries, museums, zoos, food banks, markets, gardens, and so on—both to assert the presence of people with memory challenges in increasingly public settings but also to find ways to give back to the community through volunteer and cultural enrichment opportunities. This grassroots movement, called Momentia, emerged in Seattle, Washington, in 2013, on the heels of Occupy Wall Street, and is gradually spreading throughout the United States. Like Occupy, Momentia is largely leaderless and seeks to empower persons living with dementia as community organizers who set their own agenda at the local level. Organizationally, Momentia tells a different story about what it means to be a person living with memory loss—one that casts off the normal shock politics tropes of despair, decline, and isolation and emphasizes connection, growth, purpose, hope, and finding joy in the moment.[84]

Deliver for Meals on Wheels

To return full circle to the story at the outset of this chapter, one way to contribute to an age- and dementia-friendlier community would be volunteering for Meals on Wheels in your community.[85] Thanks to a federally funded infrastructure fueled by millions of employees and volunteers across 5,000-plus community-based programs in the United States, Meals on Wheels provides more than 225 million meals to 2.4 million older Americans annually, half of whom are malnourished or at risk of being malnourished.[86,87] While the benefits of the program are abundantly obvious, research has shown that the delivery of meals to peoples' homes improves diet quality, increases nutrient intakes, and reduces food insecurity and nutritional risk while fostering socialization opportunities, improvement in dietary adherence, and higher quality of life for elders.[88,89] So too does the program provide regular informal check-ins on the well-being of elder neighbors and allow people to live independently without institutional care.[90] Nearly 60% of recipients who live alone say the volunteer delivering the meal is the only person they will see that day, and nine out of ten recipients say Meals on Wheels helps them feel more secure and improves their health.[91]

Nonetheless, Meals on Wheels is the very type of social service program that often ends up on the neoliberal chopping block of Washington, DC, in our era of American dementia. Even with our ever-aging population, the organization is serving 16 million fewer meals than it did in 2005 because, while funding has remained stagnant during the age of austerity, food, transportation, and other costs have continued to increase with inflation.[92] In 2017, former President Trump's proposed budget included a plan to cut a community development block grant that contributed millions of dollars to Meals on Wheels funding. Mick Mulvaney, president Trump's director in the Office of Management and Budget, was quoted as saying, "Meals on Wheels sounds great [but is] . . . just not showing any results."[93] As the program draws a major percentage (35%) of its funding from the Older Americans Act, any future cuts to the Department of Health and Human Services could also potentially affect Meals on Wheels.

As citizens, we clearly need to stay vigilant of our political process and organize when "demented" cuts to programs of social uplift like Meals on Wheels are proposed by either party as part of austerity pushes. In fact, given that 6.9 million seniors live in poverty, with 9 million suffering from food insecurity, we should be lobbying our representatives to significantly *increase* funding for the Older Americans Act, which provides meals and other critical services.[94] We can also help imagine new opportunities in our politics. For instance, what if a federal jobs program actually created *full-time work* for people to not only deliver Meals on Wheels to elderly neighbors but also be trained as dementia supporters who could provide more thorough social care and companionship and facilitate meaningful community inclusion? As automation and globalization further reduce jobs in the US labor market, we can respond by investing in (low-carbon) caring economy jobs (such as eldercare) that "treat populations" by mitigating the loneliness, isolation, and fragmentation of our culture and restoring social bonds and dignity in our own neighborhoods.

CONCLUSION

I still make deliveries to the trailer park where the older gentleman with advanced diabetes used to reside. His home is now inhabited by another elder whom I've yet to meet, and passing the trailer on my route always makes me think back to our last meeting and how far we have to go in building communities that are more holistically embracing of isolated elders like him. Yet, thanks to broader movements to counteract the ageism, alienation, atomization, and loneliness of our era, there is at least the possibility of momentum toward a better future. Whether cohousing initiatives, intergenerational villages, environmental actions, and efforts to integrate elders into our community organizations are anomalies or part of a larger wave that can transform societal care of the elderly and help us move beyond the American dementia era is yet to be seen.

Nonetheless, the age- and dementia-friendly community initiatives appear to provide an ideological superstructure that can guide us toward greater cross-generational solidarity in the pursuit of a more humane, dignified, cohesive society, based around an advanced moral and egalitarian commitment to one another and to a sustainable earth. So too can they help us interrogate the political-economic structures that drive inequality, austerity, and precarity that affect us all. In the next chapter, we explore a place that has been strategically built with an age- and dementia-friendly spirit—the Intergenerational School in Cleveland, Ohio. Near and dear to our hearts, the school represents our most personal vision for the types of institutions that might help guide us toward a more healthy and humane society.

10

The Intergenerational Schools

Desegregating and Revaluing the Cognitively Frail

In John Keats's poem "To Autumn," the 19th-century poet describes his impressions while walking the outskirts of a small English village on a crisp September day. As he wanders the autumnal landscape, soaking in its sights, sounds, and scents, Keats makes note of the wistful decay of the maturing season but also its ripening, abundance, and fulfillment. To his poet's eye, autumn is a "Season of mists and mellow fruitfulness." Cast around this guiding image, the poem becomes a larger meditation on the oppositional nature of aging—a process that gives even as it takes away.[1]

When it comes to dementia, our ageist culture dwells mostly on the "mists" of aging—the mental fogginess, drifting memories, and gathering deficits of old age—while largely ignoring the fruits advanced years can bear. The deficit-oriented shock politics story of Alzheimer's, culturally dominant since the field's neoliberal turn in the seventies, has generated such deep fear and stigma that receiving a dementia diagnosis often initiates a *social death*, isolating those with memory loss from the broader culture and its protective social bonds.[2] Ours is a market-dominated society built around normative expectations of economic productivity and consumption that largely segregates its cognitively frail members, who no longer contribute economic value. Rather than celebrating the oppositional give and take of the "maturing season," our tendency during the American dementia era has been to place the focus almost solely on the latter connotation.

To resist this deeply immoral tendency, I (Peter) and my wife, Cathy, a child psychologist, along with many others created The Intergenerational School (TIS) in Cleveland, Ohio—an elementary school that embraces people of all ages (including persons living with dementia) and positions them within a learning organization that values the strengths, talents, and gifts they can bring to the education of children. All volunteers, even those most affected by the deficits of advanced brain aging, are granted special status within the school as *mentors*, who coach, motivate, and serve as learning partners alongside schoolchildren. Such inclusivity unlocks a situation all too rare in our culture, when people with otherwise stigmatizing dementia diagnoses can once again enjoy purposeful connection, as they rediscover valued social roles and forge intergenerational bonds.

In this chapter, we share the story of this special school and show how its uplifting mission to not merely *desegregate* but to *revalue* local elders, including the cognitively frail, is a potent strategy for resisting both the biological processes of brain aging and the social dislocation that is part of a dementia diagnosis in the neoliberal era. While TIS started as only one organization in one midwestern city, the underlying ideas, principles, and values that have made it an internationally recognized[3] age- and dementia-friendly learning environment can be infused into schools, libraries, religious institutions, and other public places in all our communities to bring generations together. In the spirit of Keats's poem, such spaces can manifest a more "fruitful" social role for cognitively frail neighbors, who, like the poor, are too often relegated to the margins of a hyper-capitalist society obsessed with economic productivity and youth.

Allow us to invite you inside TIS.

WELCOME TO THE INTERGENERATIONAL SCHOOL!

Initially located in a New Deal–era merchant marine hospital, TIS was founded in 2000—the first public intergenerational elementary school in the world (figure 10.1). The organization was the brainchild of me (Peter) and my wife, who came to a joint realization in the late nineties that learning models for both children and older adults were not fundamentally different in terms of process and environment, and that relationships, stories, and shared community experiences could deepen learning across the age spectrum. We reached out to Stephanie Fallcreek, president of Fairhill Partners, the innovative campus of services for elders and other community members mentioned in chapter 9, and she generously committed

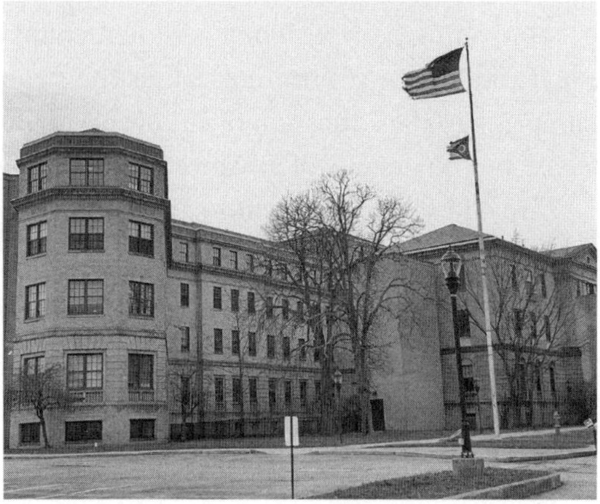

Figure 10.1. The Intergenerational School launched in 2000 in an old merchant marine hospital, which also formerly housed a Memory and Aging Clinic and an Alzheimer's Center.
Source: Photograph by Peter Whitehouse.

space in the building in which to realize the vision of the school. From this collaboration, TIS became a reality—a school based on the ideology that people of all ages and abilities could colearn alongside one another in developmentally appropriate ways, and that elders (even people with clinical dementia) could be valued members of a learning community. Organizationally, the school abandoned arbitrary age-based grade levels, instead creating multiage classes, where children of different ages but at similar developmental stages could learn with and from one another, as well as with elder volunteers.

When the school first opened its doors, it featured a staff of two teachers, an enrollment of 30 students in grades K–2, and several older volunteers, who were affectionately and appropriately called mentors. As TIS grew during its first several years, we reached out to Cleveland's aging community, developing collaborative relationships with elder organizations, assisted living facilities, and nursing homes that—thanks to the rise of the person-centered care movement in the nineties—encouraged aging residents to make visits to the school and young students to take field trips to residential homes. Through word of mouth, the volunteer pool of elders and the number of involved community organizations rapidly expanded.

Partnerships were also forged with the NIH-funded Alzheimer's Center that I (Peter) directed, as my ElderHealth clinic and research space were located on the third floor of the old merchant marine hospital (the school occupied the first two floors and basement). Patients in this clinic were sometimes offered an opportunity to volunteer in the school. By merely traveling down one story of the anchor-shaped building, elders diagnosed with dementia in the third-floor clinic would find their formal diagnosis rendered almost immediately irrelevant when they entered TIS on the lower floors, as mentors to children who were unaware of their disease labels and—having been educated about aging and its challenges as part of the school's curriculum—could nimbly adjust to memory lapses. In contrast to the age-segregated nature of modern schools, an observer walking the halls at TIS would see children sitting on couches and sharing books with various adult volunteers, including elders diagnosed with conditions such as early and late-onset Alzheimer's, frontal lobe dementia, and other severely stigmatizing clinical conditions.

Initially, the school's most "fruitful" strategy to integrate elders into the education of students was its Reading Mentor program, which paired each older volunteer with a cadre of younger students who were learning to read. While dementia can certainly cause a range of debilities, the intrinsic capacity to engage with the world through narrative often remains deep into the advanced stages of memory loss. Thus, even the TIS mentors with significant cognitive challenges retained the ability to read with a child (especially elementary-school-age books) and imaginatively engage around a story. Books in the school's reading collection were full of pictures and simpler words than adult books, and spontaneous stories would frequently blossom out of the preserved long-term memories of volunteers' own lives as they listened to children read stories aloud. As a mentor's memory condition progressed, family members or caregivers would often join them in their visits to TIS and assist in the reading sessions. Such commitment to preserving a loved one's volunteer role within the school led to a situation where mentors with otherwise disabling memory loss were able to continue contributing to children's growth and thereby resist their own "social death."

In 2009, an 84-year-old Reading Mentor named Barbara Kelsey, who had been diagnosed with Alzheimer's since her midseventies, was named the school's Volunteer of the Year in recognition of the hundreds of hours she spent mentoring students at the school each semester. Like clockwork, Barbara volunteered multiple mornings a week, visiting with her caregiver

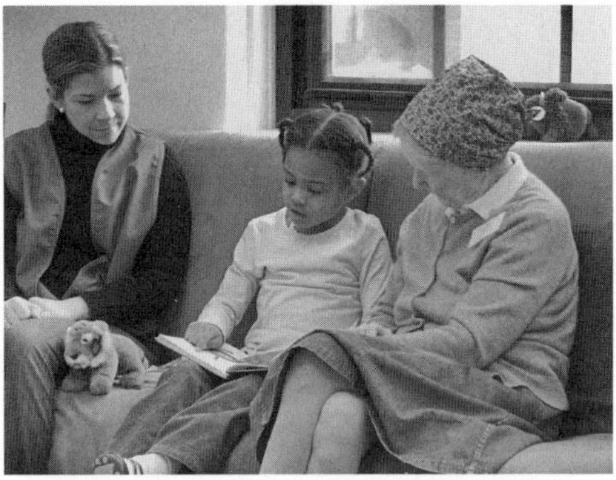

Figure 10.2. Barbara Kelsey (*right*) reads with an Intergenerational School student in the Reading Mentor program as her caregiver looks on.
Source: Photograph by Daniel George.

and working with the same group of students each visit. As she read with youngsters on couches in the TIS hallways, she formed close bonds with some of the students in greatest need of love and attention, and she had a special talent for meeting her charges in the moment, listening intently, and providing warm maternal encouragement (figure 10.2).

At the school's Volunteer Appreciation ceremony, Barbara heard her name announced and turned quizzically to her daughter Mary to ask why on earth she was receiving the award. Taking her mother's hand, Mary reminded her that she came to the school each week and was deeply appreciated for helping children learn to read and develop a love of books. Upon receiving this news, Barbara furrowed her brow. While her short-term memory loss was so severe that she could not remember her own ongoing visits to the school, the inclusive environment of TIS reinforced her remaining strengths, embraced her in nonjudgmental fashion, and helped her sustain a meaningful role in the Cleveland community.

Prior to her illness, Barbara Kelsey had been a library volunteer, teaching adults to read and delivering books to nursing homes and prisons. As her daughter Mary told us, "For my mother, helping other people in some way has always been part of how she defines herself. One of the great losses of aging in our culture is that people sort of fall out of the place they had for themselves—a place that had meaning." By offering a purposeful, community-based opportunity to share in the education of children and perform a meaningful social role, TIS provided Barbara

Kelsey an experience that far exceeded any pill, potion, or product in the marketplace of memory. Allowing elders like Barbara to be woven back into age- and dementia-friendly community environments in which they are able to flourish and contribute also powerfully rebuts the shock politics premise that illnesses like Alzheimer's vanquish one's identity to "zombie-like" depths—a misapprehension of the American dementia era that has helped justify the segregation of the cognitively frail.

Today, in response to community request, there are now three Intergenerational Schools in Cleveland, serving more than 700 students, with hundreds of individuals from numerous organizations—including multiple area nursing homes and clinics—participating as integral components of the schools. Each classroom works consistently with residents in long-term care settings, where, as with in-school volunteers like Barbara Kelsey, relationships can be built around common colearning experiences.

An Intergenerational Curriculum

Beyond the Reading Mentor program, TIS volunteers are integrated into the schools as active contributors to the curriculum. Teachers draw on the rich long-term memories many elders retain and weave oral history into lesson plans for students. For instance, after Barack Obama was elected president in 2008, a group of elders from a local assisted living home visited the school for an intergenerational discussion of the historic event. Students prepared interview questions for their older guests that explored memories of the earliest presidential election they had voted in and delved into the theme of race relations in the mid-20th century. During Black History Month, area elders (like Bill Leatherberry, a lawyer who worked for Ohio Congressman Louis Stokes on civil rights, and his wife, Diane, a patient of mine (Peter's) who marched in Selma and also mentored students in math and reading) are often recruited to the schools to provide personal stories that bring the African American experience in the United States to life (figure 10.3).

In fulfilling a mentoring role, elders often have a unique capacity to connect with younger generations, who are primed to soak up their stories. Last decade, Cleveland celebrated the 75-year anniversary of Cleveland native Jesse Owens's illustrious performance in the 1936 Berlin Olympics, where he won four gold medals, with Adolf Hitler and other high-ranking members of the Third Reich watching from above

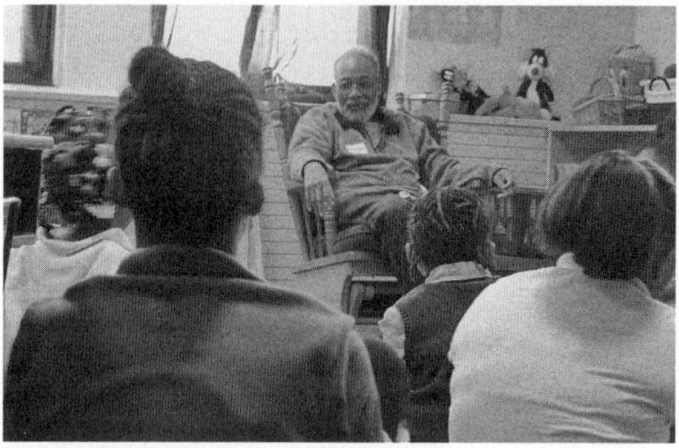

Figure 10.3. An elder participates in a Black History Month storytelling event at the Intergenerational School. *Source:* Photograph by Daniel George.

the Reichsportsfeld stadium. Hitler had famously declined to shake Owens's hand in public and urged that those of African descent be excluded from future games because of their more "primitive" physiques.[4] Gertrude O'Neal, a resident at a Cleveland assisted living home and TIS mentor had been born the same year as Owens (1913) and had befriended his wife, Minnie Ruth, before Owens (literally) catapulted to international stardom. Though in 2011 she was 97 years old, widowed, and a resident on a skilled care unit, Gertrude O'Neal participated in a Black History Month celebration at TIS and afterward chose to remain an active volunteer at the school. The subject of Jesse Owens, who passed away in 1980 but remains a folk hero in Cleveland, commonly surfaced in her exchanges with children, especially during the 75th anniversary celebration.

Several of the older students at TIS took a special interest in gathering an oral history about the legendary local athlete from Gertrude. For several weeks, they conducted research on Owens, learning of his humble upbringing in Cleveland, memorizing his accomplishments as an athlete at Ohio State and in the Olympics, and streaming grainy YouTube videos of his historic victories in Berlin with Hitler's steely gaze from above. Once prepared, they visited Gertrude at her assisted living home to interview her as she sat serenely in her wheelchair (figure 10.4). The students first asked what it was like to have known a celebrity who has been memorialized in movies, postage stamps, statues, street names, and even an asteroid discovered in Klet, Germany, the year of Owens's death. "Well," said Gertrude, "It was nothing big to me, 'cause I just knew him, you know? He was just a nice person, and rarely talked about it." With skillful prompting

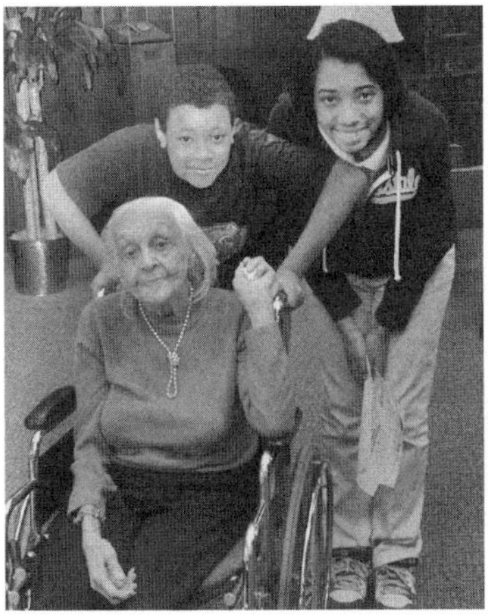

Figure 10.4. Gertrude O'Neal with two Intergenerational School students who interviewed her about Jesse Owens.
Source: Photograph by Daniel George.

from the students, she went on to discuss the apprehensiveness she and her friends had felt about Owens traveling into Nazi Germany, which promoted the odious doctrine of Aryan racial supremacy: "[We] didn't want him to go because of Hitler—he was an evil man," she said. The students then asked about the legend of Hitler refusing to shake Owens's hand. "Well, when we brought it up, Jesse just laughed," said Gertrude. "It didn't bother him. We got a lot of that here in the states; didn't have to go over there. That was the problem: he was used to it in a way. But not now . . . the world has changed all the way around."[5]

Intergenerational Activism

The school's hope is that this type of deep, narrative-based intergenerational learning can foster a spirited citizenship that will equip younger generations of students to push back against social and political-economic forces (such as racism, neoliberalism, militarism, environmental crises) that threaten the public good. Indeed, many of the school's children are from economically disadvantaged Cleveland homes and—like the children in Flint—have had lives shaped by the structural traumas caused by the income and wealth inequity, austerity politics, and public health failures of the neoliberal era. Frequently, we have observed moments wherein the wisdom of elders, including those with dementia, is instrumental in sparking a spirit of resistance in students.

Take Kay Fuller, a woman in her midnineties who volunteered at TIS despite her formal diagnosis of moderate dementia. In the sixties, Kay was living a comfortable life in a wealthy suburb a few miles from TIS,

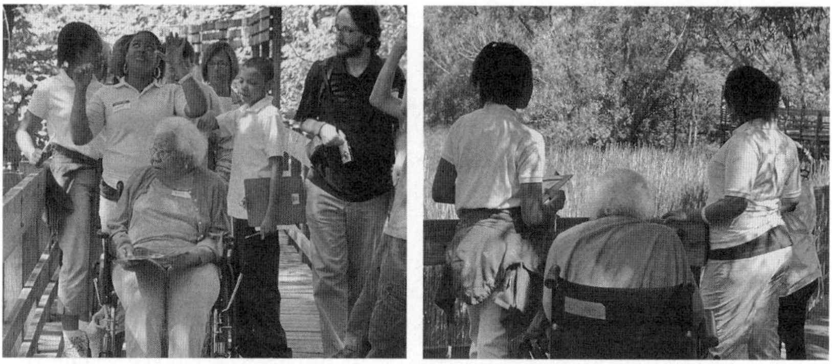

Figure 10.5A and 10.5B. TIS students accompany elders from a local assisted living home on a visit to a nature center on the Doan Brook, which was saved in the mid-20th century by Intergenerational School volunteer Kay Fuller and the Freeway Fighters.
Source: Photographs by Daniel George and Peter Whitehouse.

where she raised her three young children. It was the height of the post-Eisenhower freeway boom, and a corrupt county administrator was attempting to build a highway in her neighborhood that would tear through 200 acres of undisturbed marsh. In doing so, the development would despoil a stream called the Doan Brook, which ran by the then merchant marine hospital and emptied into Lake Erie, with leaded gasoline and other roadside pollutants. Upset by this turn of events, Kay joined an activist group informally called the Freeway Fighters and soon became a leader in waging a seven-year grassroots struggle against the superhighway, even testifying before Congress in Washington, DC. Finally, after nearly a decade of dogged advocacy by the Freeway Fighters, who rallied around the cry of "Ducks not Trucks!," the plan was scrapped. In the five decades since, over 300,000 children—including students at TIS—have taken classes at the nature center now located on the Doan Brook, whose relatively clean waters now flow into Lake Erie (figure 10.5).

A few years ago, TIS students visited Kay Fuller and some of her fellow Freeway Fighters (who, in their "maturing" years, had moved to a Cleveland assisted living home coincidentally located further downstream the Doan Brook) to gather oral histories about their advocacy (figure 10.6). During their visits, Kay energetically described to her young partners how the fight against the superhighway had thrust her into the unexpected position as a movement leader: "I just couldn't believe that they would put a freeway through there . . . but I never fought anything in my life! I

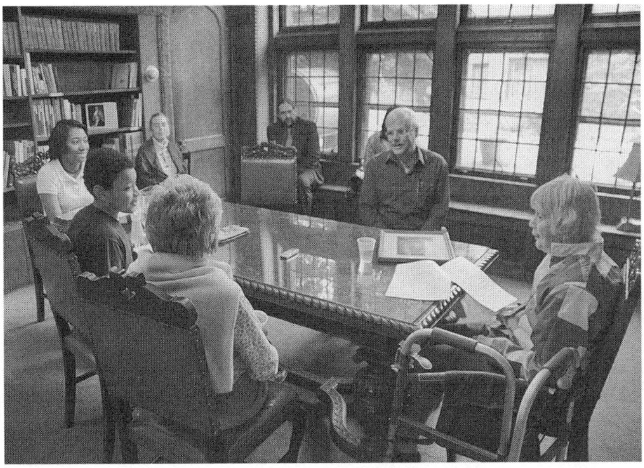

Figure 10.6. Intergenerational School students (*far left*) interview Kay Fuller (*right*) and her fellow Freeway Fighters at her residential care home to learn more about their grassroots struggle against a corrupt county official's freeway plans.
Source: Photograph by Peter Whitehouse.

had always been shy and afraid of my own voice, so I really had to work on it." When students asked what practical advice she would give their generation, she paused to reflect before saying, "I think you should take the lesson that if there is something that is worthwhile, you should be aware of it and fight for it!"

In students' reflective writing after the interviews, they expressed admiration for how Kay Fuller and the Freeway Fighters had mobilized to protect the local neighborhood. One wrote, "There are some things that you really need to stand up and fight for when you think they're wrong. You can't just sit there and let people run over you because that highway would've destroyed a beautiful part of this city that now is very integrated. It would have become neglected and empty."

This spirit of intergenerational activism takes on many forms within TIS. Consider the case of Mac Davis, a man in his eighties who came from a self-avowed "radical family" in Cleveland and often referred to himself as a "rabble-rouser" and "defender of the vulnerable." As a child in the thirties, he had campaigned for Franklin Delano Roosevelt, and now as a mentor in the school, he would often tell the TIS students with whom he volunteered the same story about distributing leaflets for FDR as a boy in Cleveland.

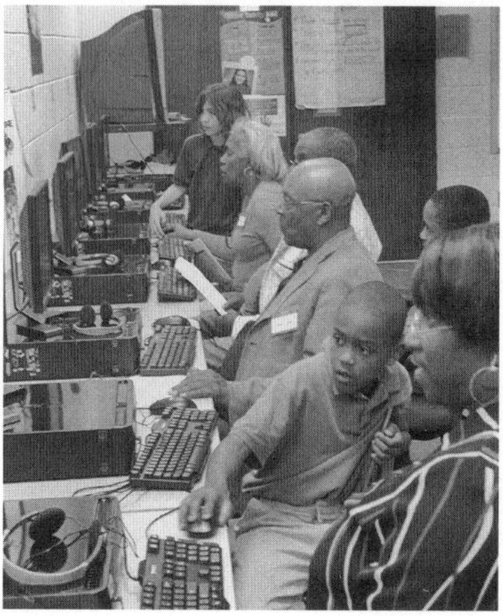

Figure 10.7. During the 2007–2008 Great Recession, Intergenerational School students taught elders how to create resumes and use PowerPoint. *Source:* Photograph by Daniel George.

Although professionally he had been a successful dentist, Mac was most proud of telling TIS students that, because of his passionate belief that healthcare was a "right for all rather than a privilege for the few," he had joined with other physicians in Cleveland to develop a progressive health management company. Their mission: to provide quality healthcare coverage for indigent Clevelanders and blind participating doctors to the income status of their patients so that service might be more equitable. In the midst of this active professional life, the students learned, Mac had also consistently volunteered abroad, providing pro bono dental work in developing countries.

The school's life-history curriculum with older students created a space that allowed the "mists" of Mac's short-term memory loss to clear and his stories about spirited citizenship to emerge and reanimate the principled foundations of his identity. He viewed the intergenerational classroom as providing him a special and all-too-rare platform to instill egalitarian values in a future generation. As he once told us, "I love children and enjoy seeing them expand their horizons and expose them to things they couldn't normally be exposed to. The older kids ask especially solemn and serious questions, and I try to help give them what I know that will help them live a better life and fight for a better life for everyone."

Over time, students grew quite close to Mac Davis, and it was impossible not to notice that his storytelling—while repetitive at times—was having an impact. One student wrote in a reflective essay, "Dr. Davis would

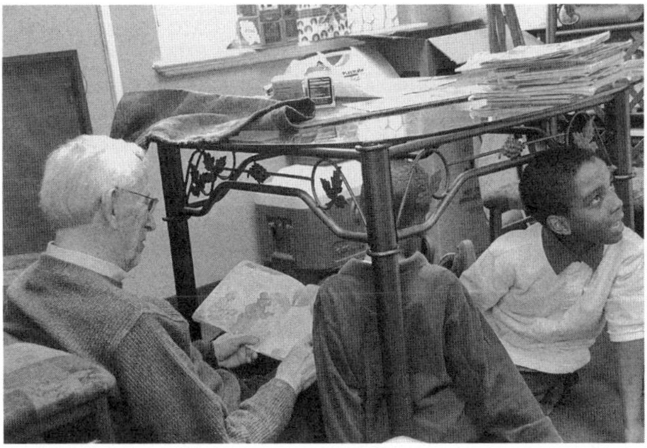

Figure 10.8. As a Reading Mentor, Mac Davis was expressive and engaging, often playfully breaking into character while reading stories with students. On occasion, he would propose that his group move under the reading table into their "clubhouse," which the students clamored for each time he visited.
Source: Photograph by Daniel George.

always make me aware for the future. I love to listen to him tell me about his past. His stories would kind of flow or sound as if they came out of a book with colorful pictures." During the 2007–2008 Great Recession, this particular student played a lead role in helping develop an intergenerational computer-based training workshop for elder African American community members seeking to learn new skills in the contracting job market (figure 10.7).

Of course, as is often the case in intergenerational programs, the benefits of Mac Davis's activism flowed both ways (figure 10.8). He had originally joined TIS as a volunteer at the urgings of his wife, who was concerned about how withdrawn and despondent her husband had become in the wake of receiving a diagnosis of "probable Alzheimer's" in 2000. Initially, he had withheld the diagnosis from friends, terrified of what he referred to as the "moral judgment" that could follow. Once he "came out" with his dementia, the social death Mac had so feared became a self-fulfilling prophecy, leading the once active and engaged Clevelander to increasingly brood around his room in the assisted living facility, many days refusing to get out of bed. The deepening depression and loneliness exacerbated his cognitive symptoms, creating a toxic feedback loop that his wife felt compelled to disrupt. Ultimately, she viewed the school as representing the best possible "treatment" for the slow mental and physical decline Mac was experiencing in the wake of becoming an "Alzheimer's victim." She frequently compared her husband's time at TIS to an uplifting drug: "It is definitely an upper for him. He comes back in a better mood, feeling high. Beforehand, he'll be tired and not want to go, and I'll say 'Well, you promised and it's time!' and he'll go and come back high as a kite."

As with Barbara Kelsey, volunteering at TIS presented Mac Davis with social space in which his career, life experiences, and long-standing activism could be reimbued with value. Breaking through his damning dementia diagnosis renewed a degree of quality of life that had been slipping away during his self-imposed exile at the assisted living home. Within TIS, there were ample opportunities for Mac to contribute to the lives of people from unprivileged backgrounds, as he had done since his formative, politically active youth. Such moments fostered the reassertion of his lifelong principles and the rediscovery of a sense of purposeful "fit" within the greater Cleveland community.

Applying an Ecopsychosocial Lens: Measuring the Benefits of Intergenerational Relationships

Given the anecdotal benefits for elders like Mac Davis, Gertrude O'Neal, and Kay Fuller, it is perhaps unsurprising that research has shown that long-term volunteering at TIS improves the quality of life of mentors. In 2011, we published findings[6,7] from a randomized controlled trial and longitudinal qualitative study establishing that elders—specifically persons with dementia—who volunteered at TIS over a 6-month period experienced significantly reduced stress, as well as overall improvements in quality of life, greater cognitive stimulation, and an elevated sense of purpose and usefulness. The reduction in stress was especially salient to the dementia caregiving field because of the multiple mechanisms that have been found linking elevated stress with increased risk of dementia and an exacerbation of cognitive decline (figure 10.9).

Beyond our study, a small but growing base of research has established that older adults who participate in intergenerational programs experience a range of biopsychosocial benefits, including gains in executive function and in the activity of prefrontal cortical regions;[8] increased engagement and interactions;[9] improvements in health status and

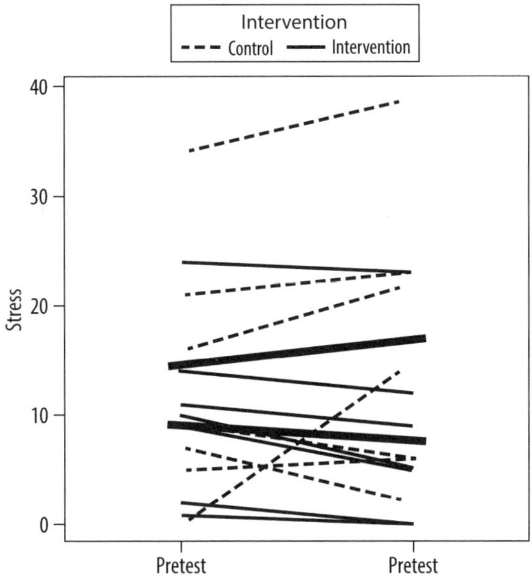

Figure 10.9. Each of the 15 lines represents a participant in the study over a 6-month period. Participants in the control group (*n*=7), who participated in an intervention at the assisted living home, are represented by a dotted line, while participants in the Intergenerational School intervention group (*n*=8) are represented by a continuous line. The thick bold lines represent averages for each group. The Beck Anxiety Inventory, a self-assessment instrument, was used to measure stress on a 40-point scale, with 40 representing high levels of stress/anxiety and 0 representing low levels. *Source:* Created by Daniel George.

well-being;[10] generational closeness, comfort, and empathy;[11] increased activity, strength, and cognitive ability;[12] mutually supportive interactions and the creation of meaningful relationships;[13] positive affect, confidence, and enhanced self-esteem supporting personhood;[14] lower levels of negative forms of engagement;[15,16] increased sense of social capital;[17] better psychological functioning and quality of life;[18,19] improvements in subjective health, social support, consciousness of loving community, and some aspects of physical performance;[20,21] improved immediate recall;[22] increased mobility;[23] and reduced stress[24] and agitation.[25,26,27,28]

There is also evidence that children who participate in intergenerational programs benefit through skill development (for example, reading, communication, and vocabulary), character building (sensitivity, patience, compassion, willingness to help, and so forth), and improved mood, enjoyment, and behavior.[29,30,31,32] They are also more likely to rate

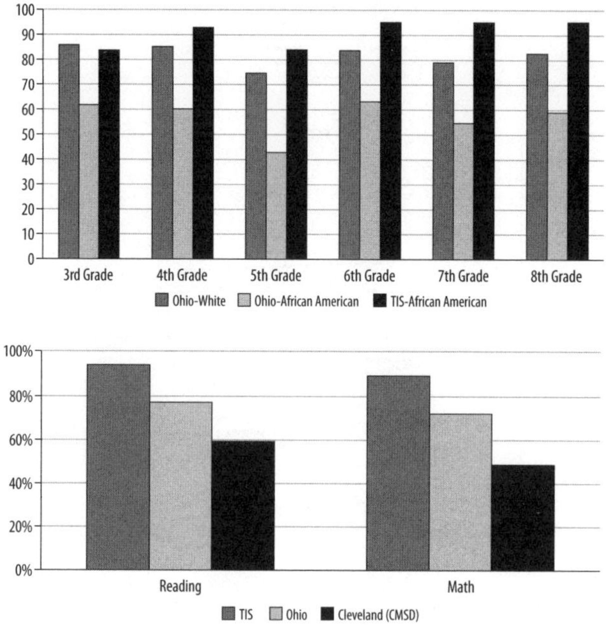

Figure 10.10. The Intergenerational School students consistently outperform students throughout the state on standardized tests (*top*); TIS students outperform their peers at the city (Cleveland Municipal School District) and state level in both reading and math (*bottom*).
Source: Courtesy of the Intergenerational School.

their health as "good" and demonstrate gains in the knowledge of dementia and more positive perceptions of older persons.[33,34] Programs that have brought undergraduates[35,36] and medical students[37] together with persons affected by dementia have reported positive attitudinal changes and enhancements in academic learning for younger persons.

We have also observed measurable scholastic benefits for TIS students—children who are predominately from minority backgrounds and living in poverty. In the school's vibrant learning environment, supported by daily interactions with caring older adults, students consistently post some of the highest achievement score results of any charter school in Ohio (figure 10.10).

INTERGENERATIVITY FOR THE COGNITIVELY FRAIL

Of course, these results demand we question *why* intergenerational relationships seem to be so mutually beneficial. Based on our research over the last several decades, we have developed a theoretical framework to try to explain this complex phenomenon, which we refer to as *intergenerativity*. A compound word combining *inter-* (between) and *generative* (producing life force), *intergenerativity* describes the meaningful fusion of ideas, emotions, and actions that can emerge in relationships when the arbitrary boundaries between generations, organizations, social groups, and individuals are dissolved. We intuitively recognize this dynamic in our cultural proclivities for things like *interpersonal* skills, *interdisciplinary* collaboration, and *international* partnerships, all of which convey emergent properties that occur when the arbitrary boundaries between isolated units are collapsed. Such concepts illustrate the power of intergenerativity to, as it were, go between to go beyond.

As a concept in developmental psychology, *generativity* even more specifically refers to the distinctly human need to *nurture things that will outlast us.* In Erik Erikson's theory of psychosocial development, the humanist psychologist famously identified a "seventh stage" ascendant during late adulthood that pitted "generativity" against "stagnation."[38] If adults were successful in this phase of life, an overriding sense of generativity could feed a sustaining sense of purpose and growth, even in the face of physical and mental decline. In the event stagnation prevailed, a biopsychosocial malaise could define one's later years and exacerbate the Keatsian "mists" of old age rather than yielding its "mellow fruitfulness."

When we think about the importance of generativity in the context of an ageist, atomized, and individualistic culture distorted and fractured by four decades of neoliberal restructuring and austerity policies, not to mention one organized in ways that segregate its economically unproductive elders, it is disturbing to think how many elders in the communities that exist in our American dementia era are actively struggling with stagnation. As seen in cases like Mac Davis's, the problem becomes even more pronounced for those diagnosed with a dementia, since the stigmatizing label not only marginalizes and segregates such people but the arbitrary (and ageist) boundary can also preclude opportunities to create, nurture, or self-actualize. For those who have spent their lives pursuing personal and professional goals only to find themselves marooned in assisted living institutions, being bereft of purpose and denied a meaningful place in the larger community fabric can be overwhelmingly saddening. As stagnation sets in, there is little opportunity to feel reciprocity, share personal stories, realize mutual goals, or affirm a meaningful social identity.

Put simply, our cultural positioning of the cognitively frail too often stifles their opportunities for generativity, and the effects of social dislocation, stress, and loneliness can be downright toxic. But by creating *intergenerational contact zones* like TIS, we can actively mitigate the deranged societal circumstances that sow stagnation among our aging and cognitively challenged neighbors.

While all the mentors described above embody aspects of intergenerativity, several volunteers we've come to know at TIS over the years are particularly illustrative of the concept. One was a woman in her late eighties named Jane Brooke, who volunteered at the school last decade. Jane was a former Cleveland schoolteacher, whose fun-loving spirit belied a failing body. In her early eighties, she had buried her husband, son, and sister, and the grief from those losses had hastened her decline and resulted in her placement in a locked unit at an assisted living home in the city.

She did not respond well to this transition.

Most days, chronic pain kept her in bed, and she was frequently agitated with care staff, finding comfort only in visits by therapy pets and children. Erikson might have termed her nursing home existence as a textbook case of *stagnation*—a deep-seated feeling of being disconnected and unable to meaningfully contribute—which gradually precipitated a physical, mental, and emotional decline. Yet, whereas Jane Brooke, like Mac Davis, was mired in obsolescence as a *patient* on the locked dementia unit, at TIS she flourished within a newfound generative identity as a *mentor*. Classroom activities were structured to foster this role: with kindergarteners, she became a Reading Mentor and participant in arts and music classes; with older students, she participated in history lessons that drew on her long-term memories and still robust capacity for storytelling.

Due to her chronic pain, Jane was bound to a wheelchair, but she was exhilarated by trips from the residential home to TIS. During each visit, she was instantly drawn to the children, particularly the younger students who greeted her arrival each week with a group song. When the children sang, they would act out the song, bobbing their knees in rhythm and wildly mimicking the movements of those around them, as they assumed the persona of the characters in the tune. Their youthful frenzy galvanized Jane, who would clap her hands (not always in rhythm), nod her head, and even hum or sing recognizable melodies as the students performed. When they finished, she would applaud while emphatically yelling "Bravo!"

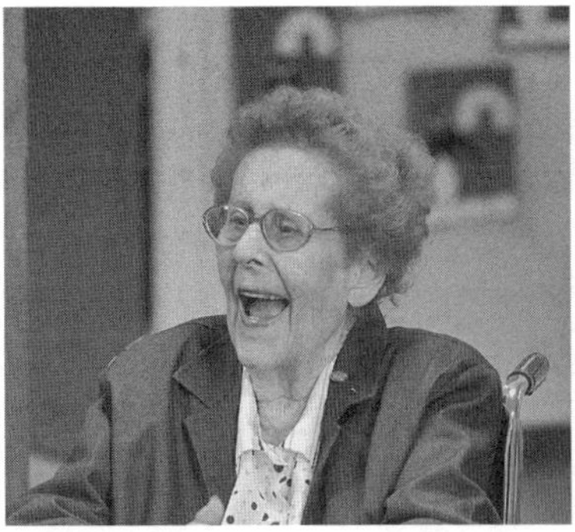

Figure 10.11. Jane Brooke smiles and dances as children sing a song for her and other nursing home residents at the Intergenerational School.
Source: Photograph by Daniel George.

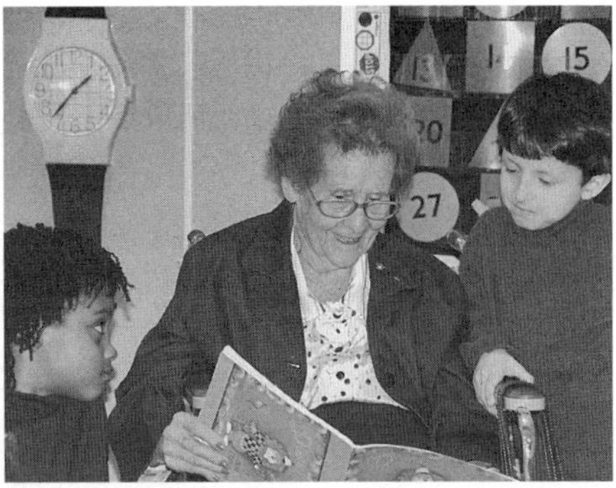

Figure 10.12. Jane Brooke reads with younger students at the Intergenerational School.
Source: Photograph by Daniel George.

Several weeks after she began volunteering, she was wheeled into the kindergarten classroom and, on entering, asked us, "Are they gonna sing for us?" which demonstrated an uncanny recognition of context and surprised everyone within earshot (figure 10.11).

The *intergenerative* nature of Jane Brooke's volunteering at TIS not only improved her quality of life, it also allowed her to reprise her role as a teacher. When she worked as a Reading Mentor, she would tell her younger partners, "You're going to be my friends today!" and emphatically insist that each child shake her hand with proper decorum before starting. She was an animated reader and would consistently praise the students she taught on the progress they were making (figure 10.12). At the end of each session, she would often remark that the children were "Bringing out old memories in me!" and invite students into her open arms, saying, "Come and give Old Jane a kiss!"

With the older TIS students, Jane spoke assertively—almost didactically—even as she so often failed to produce linear, logical sentences. Though a bit garbled, her effusive speech was often peppered with hearty adages, such as "When the going gets tough, the tough get going!" or "Never say never!" that were spoken flawlessly, with a practiced confidence, often accompanied by sweeping hand gestures. So too would she commonly refer to herself in the third person as "Old Jane" and boast of her indomitable spirit ("They try to bring the thing down, but *wham*, Old Jane comes right back at 'em!"). During life-history sessions with older

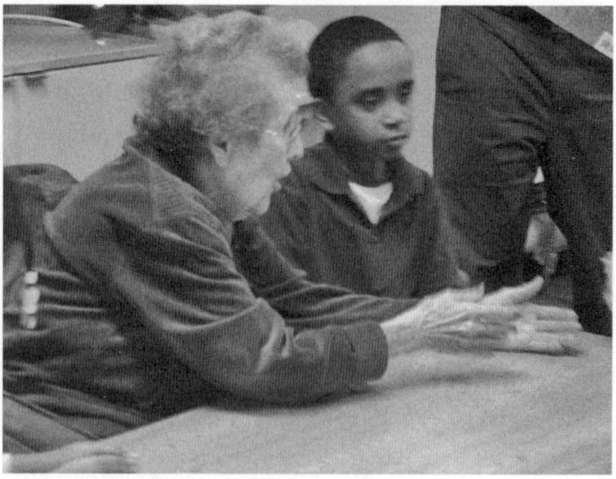

Figure 10.13. Jane Brooke works with older students at the Intergenerational School.
Source: Photograph by Daniel George.

students, she was sometimes able to recount long-term memories in a compelling narrative manner for long stretches of time. When she got into rhythm, the former teacher assumed a commanding mode of delivery, sweeping her hands, pounding the table, leaning confidently forward in her wheelchair in a way that stood in stark contrast to her comportment in the nursing home, which vacillated between cantankerous and meek (figure 10.13).

During one of her last visits to the school before she became too ill to make the trip, Jane reflected on her volunteering, giving voice to the intergenerative benefits enjoyed by elders and youngsters alike. She told us, "This is an education every time I come here—the kids really need people like us. For heaven sakes, we're trying to help children and we can still be doing this! It helps both sides of the picture!" At the time, we were hosting a reporter from NPR (Joe Shapiro), who was recording a story about the school for the program *Morning Edition*,[39] and when Jane spoke, everyone raised their eyebrows, startled by this insight.

As with Mac Davis, the noninstitutional environment of TIS selected for different aspects of Jane's personhood that harkened back to her younger days as a teacher and mother—social roles that had been largely rendered dormant in isolation at the assisted living home, where her primary identity was constrained to being a patient. The head nurses on her unit noticed dispositional changes in her before and after volunteering at TIS. Each used the words "exuberant" and "effervescent" to describe the manner in which she would return to the home, confirming that she would talk about the experience for days. One nurse told us, "She certainly enjoyed the interaction and just came back effervescent. She really just loved going. You couldn't always get her to do a lot of things, but, you know, as soon as you told her that's what she was doing, she would gladly get ready and go. Because she does deal with chronic pain, I mean, that is real." The second nurse similarly described the intergenerative transformation:

> She doesn't come out of her room a lot on her own. She'll go out with her [guardian] and her niece, but this is one thing she would actually go out to when we asked her—it seemed to have some purpose for her. She can actually remember going and is willing to get up and go out . . . and a lot of times she'll be in bed all day. So this is definitely good for her. We try a lot of times to get her to watercolor and ceramic class, and she'll go, "Oh I don't feel good, I'm not going." But this, after she'd been one or two times, then she would go and then go on about how much she likes the kids and what a great time she had.

However transformative those visits to TIS may have been, their effects tended to fade each week as the milieu of the locked unit returned Jane to ruts of dependency, helplessness, depression, and fixation on physical discomforts. This suffering seemed reinforced by the constant presence of care staff and the objects, sounds, smells, and signposts of a medical institution. In contrast, the energetic community-based setting of TIS was free of those elements, and their absence set the table for a greater sense of normalcy and self-efficacy for her, even as she advanced deeper into memory loss, chronic pain, and ill health. Perhaps this shouldn't come as a surprise. It again recalls Viktor Frankl's insight from *Man's Search for Meaning*: "Being human always points, and is directed, to something or someone, other than oneself—be it a meaning to fulfill or another human being to encounter. The more one forgets himself—by giving himself to a cause to serve or another person to love—the more human he is."

And yet, as was the case with Mac Davis, once people are branded with a dementia diagnosis, it is exceedingly rare to be asked to help another person. For those who have spent their lives pursuing meaningful goals in service of others, to find themselves gradually rendered superfluous in the eyes of their community due to the "mists" of brain aging is a painful reality to reconcile—one that can expedite feelings of stagnation. Breaking down ageist and ableist boundaries and serving as a volunteer with children can create a meaningful context for elders like Jane Brooke in which purposeful relationships can take root with children. When put in contact with a younger generation, "Old Jane" felt empowered as an educator, and it obliterated the patient-physician dyad that so often defined her interactions in residential care, placing emphasis on her remaining strengths while resurrecting well-worn generative roles as a teacher, mother, and grandmother. Such is the transformative force of intergenerativity to help cognitively frail elders resist the social death of dementia and preserve a sense of self and personal meaning within the protective structure of a community. There is a delightful (intergenerative) irony in the fact that "losing oneself" in service to children can be extraordinarily therapeutic for persons with advanced memory loss.

HOW WE CAN RESIST

Occupying Age-Segregated Spaces to Unleash Intergenerativity

Given what we've learned at TIS and in prior chapters, a natural question is how might those who live elsewhere similarly "occupy" other social spaces—schools, libraries, businesses, and so on—and infuse them with more intergenerational (and intergenerative) programs and activities? What might a healthier society that resists ageism and the "social death" of dementia look like in practice?

As a result of the success of the schools in Cleveland, in 2015 I (Peter) started an organization called Intergenerational Schools International (ISI), whose mission is to disseminate the power of intergenerational learning and intergenerativity in various other national and cultural settings.[40] Just as in the three schools in Cleveland, the pedagogical model is adapted to the community wishing to support such an organization. Hence it can be implemented in charter, public, or private schools as well as in other forms of learning organizations. ISI does not impose its model on others but works to include the elements of its learning philosophies and practices in other settings; however, the focus on learner-centered social construction of knowledge, built around cocreating collective wisdom, is promoted wherever the model is disseminated.

Currently, I (Peter) am working in Asia, North America, Africa, and Europe to build intergenerational knowledge centers that respond to different community needs, like private schools, afterschool programs, or career-training programs. Such knowledge centers are being located in schools, community centers, long-term care facilities, and other places of learning. The abovementioned concept of *intergenerational contact zones* has been proposed to signify that intergenerational relationships can be fostered in various locations with different purposes.[37] We are in the process of developing individual and organizational curricula that will allow people around the world to expand their knowledge about intergenerative learning.

We have also seen such intergenerative projects organically take root at local levels in the United States. For instance, last decade, I (Danny) gave a public lecture about TIS to an audience in Hershey, Pennsylvania, and was afterward approached by a 16-year-old girl named Grace Wagler, who wanted to launch an intergenerational reading program in her hometown that reflected the values and vision of the school. Partnering with leaders from the public library, a local retirement community, and our medical school, Grace and her team of Girl Scout volunteers successfully developed an Intergenerational Reading Club, which aimed at increasing reading and literacy skills in children while fostering social interaction, cognitive stimulation, and quality of life for residents in the assisted living community, some of whom had dementia diagnoses.

On Monday through Thursday evenings during the summer, elementary-aged children would meet for an hour in the retirement community living room to read library-borrowed books alongside residents (figure 10.14). While the program was technically a drop-in format so that families could participate as often as they liked, most children attended regularly. Eight of the twenty-seven overall participants were from families that had recently immigrated to the United States; therefore, the program was an opportunity for children from India, China, Korea, and Turkey to practice their English reading skills with an older mentor. When the children returned to school in the fall, many parents reported that their child had improved an entire grade level in reading over the course of the summer and asked that the program be extended into the fall. Not only

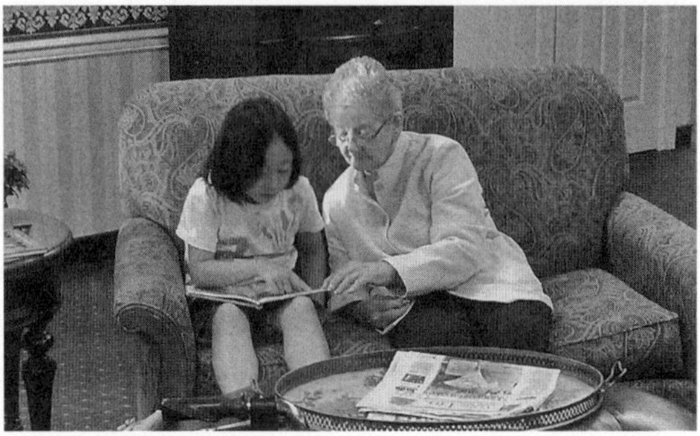

Figure 10.14. Reading mentors share books with children in Hershey, Pennsylvania, as part of the Intergenerational Reading Club.
Source: Photograph by Daniel George.

were children provided with reading practice during summer months, this personal growth presented intergenerative opportunities for elders to purposefully contribute to the education of a younger generation.[41]

Grace and her fellow volunteers continued innovating on the TIS model by creating a second program, called Intergenerational Storytime, for residents on the locked dementia unit. This program paired preschoolers (ages 3 to 5) with residents who were inclined to read, draw, and interact well with kids. Both children and elders would meet in an activity space within the unit to hear a story read by a children's librarian. After listening to the story, children and residents would sit together to draw pictures reflecting on story themes. Feedback from parents was universally positive, and many expressed that their children improved in the ability to sit quietly, listen, and follow simple instructions, while gaining valuable experience socializing outside their own family setting and showing compassion and respect to elders. Indeed, we have seen time and again that activities emerging from the arts (that is, socialceuticals like music, storytelling, and dance that have deep evolutionary roots and engage imagination, tap into emotions, elicit memories, allow for the creation of new meaning, and facilitate social bonds) provide the richest opportunities for meaningful intergenerative programming.

Best Practices for Starting Intergenerative Programs and Partnerships

It is vital for any successful intergenerational program or partnership that there be a *champion* who represents each of the different age groups involved, as well as genuine support from leadership. In a school–care facility partnership, there must be individuals from both organizations who believe in the power of intergenerational relationships and who are equally engaged in planning and implementing the programs to ensure benefits for all participants. School-based programming needs a designated coordinator who facilitates logistics and programmatic components while also monitoring the well-being of the older participants, especially those with cognitive challenges. This includes making sure elder interactions with students are appropriate and positive, and being in contact with any caregivers in the event a problem arises (for instance, an expected mentor not arriving at school). A well-designed program will avoid overburdening staff.

There are, however, existing barriers to program success. Chief among them would be the public's ageist misapprehensions, biases, and fears about dementia (and for that matter, aging in general), which we've found to be a limiting agent for intergenerational program participation. A prime way to address this issue is for organizations like libraries, museums, and schools to actively embrace elder involvement in communal activities and programs and promote a more humanizing narrative about persons living with memory loss, one that resists ageist rhetoric born of the anguished shock politics of the American dementia era.

CONCLUSION

As we discuss throughout the book, people are hungry for transformative change and primed to organize and act in local communities that have been degraded, materially and spiritually, by decades of hyper-capitalist restructuring. While our misguided cultural story about Alzheimer's—that dementia is a dread condition defined by cognitive "mists" that uniformly ravages selfhood and reduces individuals to undignified (and unproductive) zombie-like shells of themselves—has done much damage over the past several decades and coarsened the way we treat and relate to people challenged by memory loss, we can push back against this symptom of our American dementia and engage our aging neighbors with the empathy, inclusivity, and dignity they deserve. The Intergenerational Schools are but one example of how more humane ideas and principles can animate community institutions to *desegregate* and *revalue* the way we think of people diagnosed with dementia. Our experiences at TIS show that people living with memory loss—even quite advanced forms of dementia—can still make *major* contributions to their community in their "maturing season" and suggest that all of us can do more to foster meaningful, community-based relationships and social bonds for persons living with dementia that are intergenerative for communities. Ultimately, just as we argue with respect to resisting dementia, *our fight for brain health* must come to be viewed as *a fight for one another*—but especially the most vulnerable—as we move toward a healthier society.

Postscript

As we finalize our book, which was delayed in publication due to the COVID-19 pandemic, we want to provide a few relevant updates.

First, Biogen's drug aducanumab, the monoclonal antibody targeting beta amyloid protein, which we discuss in chapter 2, is, as of this writing, still being considered by the FDA despite the fact that the organization's own expert panel voted down the drug in November 2020 based on the low quality of evidence.

Main concerns about the drug remain its low-efficacy, its cost, and the possible long-term loss of public trust that may result from approving a massively expensive drug with such limitations. There are also concerns about the way Biogen, the FDA, and the Alzheimer's Association are "collaborating" and about the scientific integrity in this process. In our era of "American dementia"—in which the market incentives of the hyper-capitalist political economy are too often the driving force of societal change rather than truth, methodological rigor, and public health concerns—none of this is surprising. But as we continue to pursue an elusive "cure" for Alzheimer's, it is necessary to be clear-eyed about the forces that govern modern pharmaceutical development, the institutions of the neoliberal state, and the leaders of advocacy organizations. Mark Twain famously observed that "history doesn't repeat itself, but it often rhymes," and—in the Alzheimer's field—we see how the allure of fame and fortune distort the actions of people and organizations that have falsely promised an end to Alzheimer's across decades.

It is also worth reflecting on what the past year of the pandemic has exposed about our nation's long-term care system and the human rights disaster caused by market forces within. A staggering one-third of all US deaths from COVID-19 have occurred in nursing homes, and recent research has shown that significantly higher mortality risk accrued to residents of for-profit institutions as well as those with non-unionized staff. In the US, nearly 70 percent of nursing homes operate as for-profits, with many large chains and independent facilities being owned by private equity firms. In prioritizing investor profit, market forces appear to have engineered insufficient investment in staffing and personal protective equipment, inattention to safety protocols, and distorted data regarding quality of care, the combination of which allowed the deadly virus to run rampant in these homes, killing over 175,000 vulnerable elders.

Extended lockdown resulting from the virus's devastation in nursing homes has caused residents to suffer from long-term isolation from family, friends, and fellow residents, jarring interactions with masked care staff, and confusing phone and video calls with loved ones in the outside world. Emerging from the pandemic gives us a chance to reevaluate not only our societal approach to caring for the elderly but also how we can address the structural factors that allowed the pandemic to disproportionately disrupt the lives of other poor, vulnerable, and at-risk communities, including children. Perhaps COVID has also offered us a chance to behave in wiser ways toward future epidemics as well as the looming climate crisis. Ultimately, our book remains a charge to think critically about our "American dementia" and act in principled ways that bring about healthier brains and—even more importantly—a healthier society.

Daniel R. George and Peter J. Whitehouse
April 2021

Appendix

An Intergenerational Interview with the Authors

In this appendix, we hold an intergenerational conversation about what we have learned in writing the book and what ideas and practices related to the brain, aging, and societal health we see emerging in the near future. At the end, we use a dialogic process facilitated by Peter's friend and colleague Kristin Bodiford, an expert in social construction, relational research, intergenerational learning, restorative justice, and community development, around the central question surrounding our joint authorship: what have we learned about intergenerational collaboration by writing together? Speaking in spring 2020, during the onset of the COVID-19 pandemic, we also reflect on how the virus is reshaping society and what it means for dementia and brain health.

It has been ten years since you wrote The Myth of Alzheimer's *together. What has changed in the Alzheimer field, and what difference do you feel the book has made?*

PETER: Like society, the field is more polarized now than in 2008. Money, and hence political power, is aligned with biomedical science and lay organizations with limited moral scope that focus on cure and not adequately on prevention and care. Fundraising using unrealistic and sometimes demonstrably false premises and promises has become perfected as an artform. Using the shock politics strategy, the Alzheimer's field competes with other diseases, like cancer, to create more individual fear and social concern among its potential victims. On one hand, the experts and advocates generate angst and, on the other, hypocritically call for destigmatization. The faith in ultimate biomedical fixes is an example of how nonskeptical science and unbridled optimism constitutes scientism.

The perpetuation of the amyloid "hypothesis" is an example of such ability to push an idea in the face of contradictory data and misleading conceptions of biological processes. As we wrote about in the first chapters of this book, currently the field is trying to define Alzheimer's and *predementia* by using expensive and unproven biomarkers. like imaging, CSF, and blood tests. The boundaries between what is unknown and what is known and what is research and what is good clinical practice continue to be blurred in unethical ways. Clearly, the main beneficiaries of the research enterprise have been the researchers and their advocates and not patients and society. We have been offered (much false) hope at an enormous price and a huge opportunity cost. As we've written in this book, there are other ways to address the individual and social challenges of dementia and other societal priorities (social and environmental justice), but they are being ignored because of the almost psychotic-like focus of the field on simplistic but unrealistic solutions based on fundamental misconceptions, like the existence of a single condition called Alzheimer's that is clearly separable from aging.

In the preface to our first book, I was relatively gentle on my colleagues for their lack of attention to a bigger, more realistic picture of cognitive aging, but I am less inclined to be so today. We have learned too much (or should have) about the complexities of dementia, made so many false predictions, promised too much, and ignored the other existential challenges in society. Social injustice and environmental degradation have grown as problems since I started in the field and are not only important for addressing brain/cognitive health, but for the very survival of our civilization.

All that said, the neoliberal influence on the field is being challenged by lack of success in drug trials and some modest degree of skepticism about past and current exaggerated promises. The messages of *The Myth*—essentially that the "disease" was not a single entity, is related to aging, and likely not addressed through reductionistic biological approaches—have largely been proven to be true. The book was successful as a leading voice in the effort to realize that Alzheimer's is heterogeneous—a belief that has now become well-recognized. Still more problematic is how Alzheimer's disease(s) are related to aging. But even though billions of dollars have been spent on the quest, we still have no way to clearly diagnose Alzheimer's as separate from the continuum of cognitive aging, despite numerous claims to the contrary.

However, on a positive note and as reflected in this book, greater emphasis on public health, improvements in care, and the role of the arts and humanities in addressing the challenges of dementia is emerging. My own suspicion is that other societal priorities will rob Alzheimer's, as it is viewed today, of the limelight. The greatest threats to brain and general health are superstorms, heat waves, droughts, migration, air and water pollution, political unrest, economic disasters, and a list of more important issues than finding cure for Alzheimer's. What we need is a "cure" for neoliberalism—in other words, more effective treatments of the cultural American dementia. Such success would improve health for everyone alive today and in the future, including everyone facing age-associated cognitive challenges.

DANNY: Compared to a decade ago, there is now a palpable feeling of skepticism around the amyloid hypothesis—you can feel it. Articles that you see in mainstream publications like the *New York Times,* the *Washington Post,* or the *Atlantic,* which have largely echoed the establishment-industry-advocacy line about Alzheimer's drug development for decades and treated an amyloid-based cure as a fait accompli, are now openly questioning dominant theories and positing that the hypothesis may be wrong. Such reporting would have been seen as heretical a decade ago but—in the context of Alzheimer's research—the Overton window (the range of acceptable ideas in popular discourse) appears to have shifted in response to the wave of pharmaceutical failures. I think many in the field, at least in private, would concur with our observation that this book is being published in the midst of a major paradigm shift for Alzheimer's.

Obviously, Peter, myself, and others believe the population revelation studies showing falling risk for dementia have been a major finding since *The Myth of Alzheimer's* and were, as much as anything, the impetus for writing this book. We are utterly overwhelmed with information in our era, and these studies have sort of come and gone without much fanfare in the mainstream media. But if you had told someone a decade ago that dementia rates would be found to be *declining* in the US and other Western countries, but without a big leap in drug development or biotechnology, it would've been almost unfathomable. I think in this book we are saying to the reader: the historical, scientific, and political-economic lessons are there for us (healthier societies equal healthier brains), if we want them.

Sure, we can and should keep pursuing a cure (or cures) and effective (and cost-effective) treatments for this syndrome, but there is overall a much greater impetus to invest in prevention and care than there was a decade ago. Society is perhaps, on the whole, less enamored with innovation fantasies surrounding Alzheimer's than we were when *The Myth* came out. In a way, it seems similar to how the general public feels about fighting the so-called war on terror now versus [20 years ago], when there was, regrettably, a greater public appetite for armed conflict abroad and a belief we could fully eradicate terrorism at the barrel of a gun.

In terms of the difference our first book made, I think we somewhat aggressively planted a flag in the ground with our skepticism about Alzheimer's as a disease construct and a critique of amyloid-centric theories. While that meant taking a large brunt of criticism at the time, because of the shifting Overton window in the intervening decade, our views are now more-or-less mainstream in the field. I suppose it's less a matter of others following our lead than it is a function of the preponderance of contrary evidence simply overwhelming the old paradigm (in the manner Thomas Kuhn described), but I'll take it.

How have your own views changed most fundamentally, and how did that influence the writing of this new book?

PETER: Since writing the first book, I have become even less connected to the biomedical world and more involved in the world of public health, intergenerational education, and the arts and humanities. I have ramped up my critique of the shallow value considerations in medicine, often represented by narrowly focused bioethics. Writing the new book with Danny has allowed me to understand the concept of neoliberalism. What I used to call "the unholy alliance between unregulated capitalism and unskeptical scientism" now emerges as market fundamentalism.

I see collective political-economic actions to the challenges of dementia, like public health interventions, as more important than individual responses, like lifestyle changes. I have become even more convinced that changing peoples' minds about dementia and Alzheimer's can be a point of cultural leverage to shift our thinking and valuing away from simplistic linear thinking and unrealistic solutions to complex societal problems. I have invented and promoted the concept of *ecopsychosocial health*, which we describe in chapter 7, to draw attention to health as based on interdependence and connectivity. Much of modern biology is reductionistic, and it needs to attend to complex systems and broader conceptions of how life works. We need a dramatic shift in the nature of science as an interconnected and human activity and its relationships to the larger culture, including art. With that shift will come a necessary "spiritual" transformation in what we consider our humanity, both individually and collectively.

DANNY: I think there is probably a generational dynamic at play in how we react intellectually and emotionally to this question. For people my age (millennials), our twenties and thirties—the formative years of our adult lives—have been defined by things like the Enron scandal; 9/11; endless illegal wars in Iraq, Afghanistan, and elsewhere; the financial and foreclosure crisis; austerity regimes; the Flint catastrophe and widespread lead poisoning; serial mass shootings; the COVID-19 pandemic; and a litany of other spectacular societal failures.

Unlike boomers, who were more established and materially in a bit better position to weather these major events, people my age have largely been shaped by the all-around precarity we write about throughout the book. Things don't feel right in our society, especially much of the received wisdom about the glory and innovation of American capitalism. For many of us, nothing has really gotten better as adults, and each day seems to bring slightly worse and more destabilizing news about our society and world. As we touch on throughout the book, life expectancy has gradually declined in the US, with 150,000 people (36,000 millennials) dying from deaths of despair each year, and many more feeling perpetually lonely, anxious, alienated, and depressed at the declining state of things. Materially speaking, we earn 20% less than our parents, carry massive crippling debt, and—for many—the prospect of buying a house and securing all the other basic trappings of the decent life our parents' and grandparents' generations enjoyed feels frankly unobtainable. And in the background, we have a rapidly warming planet that may produce cataclysms threatening the existence of our species, or at very least creating immense widespread suffering. Our current political-economic organization seems incapable of doing anything to collectively change our fate in any of those areas.

That's heavy stuff, and I think the grimness of our era has largely informed my generational orientation in the world. Similar to David Foster Wallace's fish parable described in chapter 1, millennials are starting to ask: how can this political-economic system we were born into represent the "best of all possible worlds" when so many are living in poverty; when worldwide environmental disasters driven by industrial-capitalist economies are proving so deadly; when people are literally dying of loneliness and despair, rationing insulin, and suffering from random misfortunes; when we face a reality of being constantly at war for unspecified reasons? I know we can be insufferable at times (ha ha), but I also think millennials generally have a sense that things need to fundamentally change, that no sane society would be organized like this, and that capitalism (and American empire) are fading and need to be replaced with better, healthier, and more sustainable political-economic orders. We are a generation finely attuned to the mechanisms of power and the deep corruption in a political system where nothing really feels clean or fair, and the main question for us is whether we can meaningfully restructure the failing societal institutions of our fading empire as we become the dominant electoral force.

I feel that, in beginning to reject a mythos about America—a dying neoliberal consensus and imperial order that no longer feels viable, millennials have been much more open to new ideas, including democratic socialism. For many, a vision of a different, more humane and dignified world, where people don't have to suffer unnecessary and random cruelties, and where we could imagine political and economic systems actually contributing to human flourishing has crystallized over the last decade, starting with the Great Recession, building as a rogue, largely disorganized, but galvanizing movement via Occupy Wall Street, and gaining a brief institutional foothold during Bernie Sanders' unlikely presidential run in 2016 and 2020. Millennials could potentially reject the "theology" of free-market fundamentalism, since we know, generationally, that we increasingly possess a more favorable opinion towards socialism than capitalism. Without a doubt, these tectonic generational shifts within the culture over the last decade have shaped the thesis of our book.

Now, somewhat ironically, the revitalized society many millennials envision is not some far-off utopia but rather a harkening back to the social democratic order that prevailed after World War II, which allowed the boomers to by-and-large enjoy stable and prosperous lives. We are basically looking at the past, as well as at current social democracies like the Scandinavian countries that make economies cooperative, worker friendly, and redistribute excess wealth the market produces as social spending and asking, why can't we—in the wealthiest country ever to exist on earth—have things like equal, free access to quality healthcare, debt-free college education, and decent childcare and parental leave? Why can't we have a living wage, a jobs guarantee with secure pensions, a right to a home, and financial security? Why do we need to accept such vast inequalities in income and wealth and the looming precariousness working-class folks live under? Speaking personally as someone who studies brain aging, the fact that the population revelation studies from chapter 4, that identified declines in dementia for those who came of age in the postwar era of social democratic consensus, seem to gesture at the neurological benefits stemming from this type of increasingly desired political-economic organization is a really powerful confluence. The goal, it seems, is to complete the work of FDR and to make peoples' lives and basic dignity less dependent on the vicissitudes of markets.

Obviously, whether we're talking about Alzheimer's or any other social issue, our understanding is limited by the historical and cultural forms through which we interpret the reality in front of us, and we must humbly accept that our claims to truth are never fully "correct" and that the things we believe in could be wrong. Even so, in this cultural moment, the shared societal (and environmental) traumas sown by hyper-capitalism, set alongside our scientific data about dementia and the failures of science, technology, and open markets to make an impact, have coincided to produce a particular interpretation of the facts at hand. This book is very much a repository of the ideas, feelings, and generational yearnings in the zeitgeist. While I feel strongly about the argument we are making in this book and the moral principles we are basing it on, I'm also aware that things may change, and that science, with its mechanisms to course correct, can challenge the convictions we feel in the present moment. In other words, I'm aware that, as a millennial with leftist political leanings, I may have my own interpretive biases, but I still feel a strong sense of conviction in the message and mission of this book.

As a result, and as we say in the preface, it feels like there is a stirring in our species right now—a broader and necessary awakening—and I hope our book's message is one vibrating note in the growing chorus calling for necessary changes in a society on the brink of economic- and climate-driven hardship. It would be admittedly strange to feel a sense of optimism about where we are headed, but I would welcome it with open arms.

In your opinion, what is the single most important takeaway from this book for your readers?

PETER: Essentially, economics and politics are critical aspects of brain health when we consider it broadly, as we should. The scientific, clinical, and moral failure of narrow biomedical approaches are apparent. Community development and public health efforts are keys to a better future for maintaining brain health and health in general. I am increasingly using the word *decolonization* to capture what we need to do, particularly the baby boomers. Our minds have been occupied and our brains washed by ideas that no longer work in the world we have created using them. It is time to humbly admit ignorance and try learning some new ideas about and behaviors towards ourselves, each other, and nature.

DANNY: I agree with you, Peter. Science doesn't exist in a vacuum, and we need to consider political economy as a critical factor whenever we think about Alzheimer's or any other illness. How does the ordering of our society and the structures of power materially impact the distribution of risk and resiliency? How could it be different? Making our societies less "unhealthy" necessarily means thinking politically and in terms of working-class power rather than our current oligarchic rule by elites.

To that, I'd add that, in public health, we need to relearn how to "think the state." This means going beyond our usual tendencies to conceive of prevention at the individual or abstract level and instead imagine how the state, recaptured from the corporate and societal elite and subject to true democratic processes, can act to maximize a public good like brain health across the whole population, largely by universalizing access to material resources we know to be alimentary (for example, healthcare, living wage, higher education and vocational training). Again, this demands a moral imagination broader and deeper than the reducing valve of the ruling class and corporate media has typically allowed. It also demands that we see politics for what it is: a fierce competition over scarce resources that materially impacts our collective health down to the cellular/neuronal level. This is a fight we have to be tough about and win if we care about human health.

Hopefully our book shines a light on past brain health-supporting actions taken by "the state" after the New Deal (for instance, the GI Bill and subsidized higher education, antismoking campaigns, increased access to health care, efforts to remove lead from our products and environments) and helps readers imagine different political horizons in the future that could further improve the public's health more holistically and with respect to Alzheimer's diseases. That would be the most important takeaway—having the readers operationalize the argument we are making in their own civic lives.

What are the three most important policy actions that you feel will create a better future for people with dementia?

PETER: The great thing is that these suggestions will not only improve the quality of life of people with dementia, but all of us. One, raise taxes on the wealthy, especially the extremely rich, and at the same time realize that taxes are not bad but represent our social commitment to each other. As a part of this, we need to reimagine the nature of wealth as more than money and redefine its role in society.

Two, reform health care to minimize the neoliberal influences and to maximize prevention and community development. As we argue, this is connected to addressing climate change, the greatest threat today to people with dementia and in the near term to brain health and health in general for all of us.

Three, develop science policies that reward outcomes rather than perpetuating the celebration of unfulfilled and unrealistic promises of cure and other powerful biomedical interventions. As a part of this effort, constrain the political and economic influences of the pharmaceutical, device manufacture, and so-called health industries in general. Reframe and broaden our conceptions of what constitutes evidence for taking social action. Enhance education and learning in every aspect of life.

DANNY: Anything that improves the material conditions of the working class. From my view, single-payer healthcare, living wage, free education, and vocational training across the board are examples of policies critical to attaining a healthier society and healthier brains. Obviously, getting neurotoxic heavy metals like lead out of our homes, soil, and drinking water would also be close to the top of any list of policy actions.

Now, specific to a population of people with dementia, we write in chapter 9 about age- and dementia-friendly communities, and there are clear policies that can foster the development of towns, cities, and municipalities capable of better accommodating elders—for instance a universal long-term care insurance program. Given our belief in the power of socialceuticals within long-term care environments, investing in the arts is critically important. Trying to nudge medical students into geriatrics (we currently have 7,000 nationally but will need an estimated 33,000 by 2025)[1] and family medicine is another crucial societal adaptation that we probably won't make much headway on until we remove the excessive debt burden of medical school, which—thanks in part to the financialization of the economy during the neoliberal turn—has ballooned to over six figures for most students, creating a weighty financial incentive that pushes far too many good caring doctors into lucrative subspecialties. We've got a lot of work ahead of us.

What are the three biggest roadblocks to making the changes that you describe above and throughout the book?

PETER: The dominance of money in our politics is a key roadblock. For example, Supreme Court decisions like Citizens United that have sold our political system to the wealthy will be difficult to reverse. The politics of fear and mistrust undermine democracy. Citizens need to be better informed about their role in a democracy and the power of science but also its limitations—prioritizing such education has been difficult.

DANNY: I agree with Peter that special interest money saturating Congress is a main roadblock, since politicians are more or less middlemen for capital. The wealthy in our society—millionaires and billionaires, corporate interests, and the like—have leveraged the extreme wealth generated through free-market enterprise in the American dementia era to essentially capture the political process as well as the corporate media, think tanks, and other institutions that shape and manipulate public opinion. Despite former President Trump's pledge to "drain the swamp," there are presently over 12,000 lobbying firms and 4,000 PACs working the levers in DC. Truly, the foxes run the henhouse, and it is only through organizing nationally against our real enemies and building people power among the 99% that we can break their hold on the levers of structural power.

Second to that are imaginations that are arbitrarily limited by neoliberalism, largely due to the aforementioned corporate-owned media, which has a material interest in preserving our current sclerotic order that protects the interests of the ruling class, divides the working class with culture war distractions, and redirects popular anger away from the real sources of their suffering and deprivations. As the brilliant comedian George Carlin once observed, "The reason they call it the American Dream is because you have to be asleep to believe it."

There is so much corruption and false consciousness to peel away before we can actually start making necessary changes to pursue a healthier society (and healthier brains). With a political system so dysfunctional and beholden to capital and the ruling class, change will only come through mass mobilization that overwhelms our internally rotten political system. Again, this is why I think someone like Bernie Sanders, who galvanized democratic socialism and has shown a blueprint for reviving organized labor and rebuilding solidarity across the working class to pressure and win back concessions from the state (that is, capital), has served as such an important figure at this moment in history. Perhaps it's too early to say whether Sanders' "revolution"—or at very least the ideas and spirit of organized working-class resistance and solidarity he has unleashed—will succeed in living beyond him and whether our lives can become more dignified and less precarious in a fairer society. His loss was a major blow, and the decade ahead feels deeply fraught and uncertain.

How could the Alzheimer's Association and other major advocacy groups help create a sea change in the field to take us in the right direction?

PETER: Be more critical of scientism—unrealistic faith and promises of success; emphasize prevention through public and community health; see themselves as a better organization by advocating for a less self-serving agenda. They really have distorted the public policy space by making false and unrealistic claims about the value of always-promised, but not-realized, simplistic scientific fixes. If they really want to benefit people at risk for dementia (all of us) and society at large, then focus not just on individual lifestyle but also community health. Could we imagine the Alzheimer's Association leading efforts on lead abatement and eliminating other neurotoxins in our environment as a truly moral enterprise as well as an effective intervention? Could they stop competing with other diseases based on fear mongering?

DANNY: Show leadership on some of the issues we've identified above. Don't play it politically safe; stand on principle. This doesn't mean launching some radical and quixotic advocacy agenda; it simply means being evidence based and willing to stand up to power. As Peter said, if you know the neurological costs of lead poisoning, why not be a leading voice pushing the state on large-scale lead abatement, especially in our poorest areas? If you know the dangerous effects of global heating on the elderly and on brain health, why not champion the fight against climate change? If you know the profound benefits of education on cognitive reserve, why not lobby for free education for all from kindergarten forward? If you know the effects of head injuries on risk for dementia, why not advocate for the drawing down of the American war machine?

There are *so many* opportunities to be organizationally bold and to act with courage. The last decade has shown that if you do this, it is not political suicide—people will follow those who stand on principle and respect them for acting in the direction of their values rather than just being shills who defend the status quo that is quite literally killing us. Right now, advocacy groups are so cagey and calculating. On one hand, I understand that they have a difficult line to walk in shaky financial times, but I also think they will win the PR battle by actually having a moral bearing and advocating for healthier societies and brains. There are good people in those organizations, and I hope they can start to break through and make a material difference.

What comes after neoliberalism, and how can it help our society and our brains?

PETER: Pay attention to the Great Derangement (our failure to think and act on climate change) and the Great Degeneration (the slow failure of our most important institutions, like health and education), which illustrate the American (and proliferated global) dementia. I also think that much of the current malaise is spiritual and ethical; hence, we are facing a Great Demoralization as well. The best answer is to educate, educate, and educate some more; in fact, we all need to wise up to design a course for the future (the title of my current intergenerational and transdisciplinary academic and community offering in Cleveland at Case Western Reserve University and in the community). Innovation in education is critical and needs to be infused with purpose, passion, and playfulness. Ultimately, we need to give everyone an opportunity for a decent life (meaningful employment, community belonging, healthy environment).

DANNY: I think some iteration of socialism (whatever we may call a more fair, humane, and egalitarian organization of our societies in the future) will be necessary to ensure the survival of civil society as we know it. We have to reorganize society—domestically and globally—in a way that prevents wealth from continuing to accrue to the wealthiest among us and pursue a healthier political formation that truly gives people the economic freedom and material resources they need to flourish. Our society is in disorder right now, with unfettered capitalism representing a system that seems predisposed to spasms of chaos and self-destruction. Democratic socialism is a necessary stabilizing force—a way of balancing chaos and order in our civilization—especially given our serious climatic and public health challenges. Can we get back to a similar type of egalitarian political order as we had after World War II but calibrate it to a world that is warming at dangerous levels? Can we do it quickly enough to mobilize our collective efforts and resources to avoid environmental cataclysm and mass suffering? These are the fundamental questions and existential crisis points of our era.

I honestly don't see how we make necessary progress without purging the mind worm of neoliberalism, which has put us on this runaway path to societal despair and species destruction. But I'm also not fatalistic about our situation. Humans are at their core nature an ever-adaptable animal, and we've faced more formidable existential crises in our time on this earth. But in order to manifest change and survive and thrive into the future, we need new (old) values and a spirit of enlightened collectivism that positions everyone to do well. We need to move beyond this despairing cultural moment by organizing our actions around better and more egalitarian ideas that reinforce our connection and commitment to one another (and to the natural world) and reduce unnecessary suffering. As we've argued in this book—hopefully convincingly—a healthier society will invariably result in healthier brains.

Given the current cultural discourse, I can anticipate some people arguing that our message of enlightened collectivism is dangerously subsuming the individual to group identity. But what we are really talking about is creating a political order that guarantees secure material conditions that allow individuals to actually be free, to realize their full human potential, and to find meaning in the collective striving to better the human condition.

In ten years from now, how might a new book look at things differently?

PETER: Thinking optimistically, we will be paying more attention to climate change and the quality of our environments. We will have more symbiotic intelligence with digital devices and networks that help us think about complex problems. We will be discussing more deeply ethical issues about our individual and collective legacies. We will reverse the imperial colonization of indigenous and other minority populations and relearn a more humble and balanced way of being in the world. But honestly, we may be beyond the point of fully reversing neoliberalism's damage to our souls and our planet. Mother Nature has an answer: fewer humans on the planet (and not by sending them to other planets as some superrich billionaires imagine). The deadly devastations of storms, droughts, floods, epidemics, heat waves, and perhaps wars will accelerate. Our best human capabilities, flexibility, and resilience will be challenged. And we will have to discover whether we can find the balance between cooperation and completion that led to our initial evolutionary success.

DANNY: The 2010s were disproportionately shaped by societal traumas, and this book was forged in the fires of what I believe will come to be viewed in retrospect as a lost decade. Can the 2020s be the decade where we start righting the ship and effectively turning from our current wealth/income inequality, austerity, precarity, despair, and climate crisis—the defining characteristics of our cultural moment—and toward a future that looks decidedly more hopeful?

If not, we may need to write a new book that also serves as a floatation device to navigate the rising oceans!

On a serious note, hopefully, a book written in 2030 will be come to be in a more positive juncture, when humanity, freshly having collectively reoriented itself and forged domestic and international values and practices that move us past the death drive of hyper-capitalism and give us a better chance at surviving into the future, asks, "If we can act together on something as major an existential threat as climate change, what else might we be able to do together to make life better on earth for everyone?"

What would a single sentence statement of your legacy be?

PETER: He loved learning and was always learning to love.

DANNY: Admittedly a tough question to answer in my mid-thirties. But, if I must offer something, I guess it'd be, "Though flawed, he was a fully feeling, thinking, loving human being who tried to act in the direction of helping others."

What have you learned about intergenerational collaboration from writing these two books and many other articles together?

PETER: Danny and I have different talents, so our work is not merely intergenerational but *intergenerative*. We are both disciplinarily broad but in different arenas that overlap in social sciences, humanities, and ethics. I am more experienced in the Alzheimer's field and an extroverted political actor. Danny is a better writer. I harbor more guilt for the state of the world as a baby boomer born at the beginning of the great acceleration and what will probably be the start of a new geological epoch, the so-called Anthropocene. Danny will very likely be around longer than I will to have an impact—he helps me align with a "younger" vision of the future and be a part of my legacy.

Priority setting and time management change with age. Danny was way ahead of me in thinking about neoliberalism and in pushing the book forward. I am still not caught up. He is the leader of this effort, as I was more of on our first book together. In some sense I am already "beyond" the book project—I just want to take action while I have energy. At 70 (rather than, say, closer to 50 when Danny and I first met) my life priorities are different. I have grown children Danny's age and four grandchildren. Yet I am also still expanding my academic profile by working at the University of Toronto and University of Oxford. I still have a form of attention deficit and hyperactivity disorder, which means I dance readily from one point to another trying to connect the dots but always running the risk of superficiality. Yet I seek the depth in breadth.

When I enter a room full of new people to meet, I used to seek out the elders (and still do), but now increasingly I look to talk with the younger people present—forget the adults. The bidirectional mentorship we see in our intergenerational schools has become more important. Danny and I take what we learned from each other into other relationships, intergenerational or not.

DANNY: I alluded to it earlier, but in writing this book, I've powerfully felt the way in which our worldviews have been shaped by our generational circumstance. I'm certainly guilty of being the one pushing the political message in this book, and with a fervor shared by many millennials. Over the last 15 years, I've learned an enormous amount from Peter as a mentee, but in undertaking this book, I do feel like I've been able to teach him, or at least guide him toward a different way of seeing the world and our field, which is kind of gratifying. Now, I don't know that I've won him to the side of democratic socialism, but I at least think he has embraced a critique of neoliberalism and that it's given him a vocabulary to clarify his thinking about the field and its ills.

It's also the case that his generational perspective, even when challenging to mine, is invaluable. Conversations with him (and with my parents) have helped me see the limitations in the substantive and tonal ways millennials tend to frame our political challenges and think of strategies to make democratic socialism (or whatever we ultimately call political manifestations of a more enlightened collectivism) more palatable to those who came of age in the Cold War, with a different and more "red scare"-inflected understanding of socialism. Specifically, linking the Bernie Sanders–era push for democratic socialism to FDR and the New Deal (rather than presenting it as a sui generis revolution) seems to be rhetorically useful, especially since working-class boomers largely enjoyed the fruits of post–World War II egalitarian policies. Also invoking the social democracies of modern thriving Scandinavian countries helps reframe the way people interpret the word *socialism* away from autocratic 20th-century totalitarianism, which abandoned the democratic aspects we know to be so critical to keeping a check on power.

PETER'S REPLY: I am being less concrete in my replies about which bills and which candidates for office to support. I thought I needed to understand the cultural currents underlying the 2020 elections and legislative process around Medicare for All and the Green New Deal a bit longer before choosing specific courses of action. Yet even as we have written this intergenerational dialogue for the conclusion of the book, my ideas have been influenced by Danny and the world at large. Reading Naomi Klein's 2019 book *On Fire: The (Burning) Case* *for a Green New Deal* has made me a more full-throated advocate for the GND, but attending the Extinction Rebellion occupation of the Westminster Bridge in London in October 2019 made me start using the *climate emergency* language and makes me think that more of a revolution than the GND represents may be coming.

Thinking back, I started the process believing that we needed to redress the imbalance in political life between Left and Right by learning to compromise again. I see Republicans as increasingly aligned with bad ideas and practices, like favoring the rich; being socially conservative, as in opposing abortion; encouraging white male supremacy and racism; denying climate heating; and fundamentally undermining democracy; as in voter suppression. I saw them more neoliberal than Democrats. But Danny was and is right, and I had the same intuition, that there is a larger force at work in both parties—market fundamentalism and excessive focus on individual rather than collective responsibility. Economics is dominating politics. I actually have strengthened my belief in social democracy through discussion with Danny because of its success in Scandinavian countries. I do think we are headed towards some form of more dramatic revolution because I don't believe our political system can respond quickly enough to the accelerating pace of climate heating. More actions to support resilience must occur in local communities.

I also have come to see the issue of time as a more critical aspect of intergenerational relationships. I work with Danny and lots of other young adults who will live longer than I will. In our intergenerational schools, I say all the time that the youth see the past through the eyes (lived experience) of the older people, and the elders can see the future (they will not see) through the imaginations of the children. I occasionally refer to myself as a baby boomer but most often in the context of saying that they are the group responsible for the great acceleration in impact on climate. I was born in 1949, about when we expect the Anthropocene, perhaps to be formally announced as an official geologic period soon, to have started. That said, I think it is a flawed term, as if all humans were equally responsible for the devastation we have wrought on the planet's geology, ecosystems, and ourselves.

DANNY'S REPLY: Peter and I agree that we are approaching crisis. To paraphrase W. B. Yeats's famous line in his portentous poem "The Second Coming," the neoliberal center cannot hold, and another reordering of our political economy feels inevitable. We also agree that neither political party, including the corporate Democrats, appears to have the capacity to initiate changes that will be necessary for our continued survival. With Bernie Sanders' moment now lost to history, I find myself a bit despairing about where meaningful change will come from, if it is possible at all. That said, I feel hopeful that the intergenerative convergence Peter and I have had in writing this book could model ways in which older and younger generations can find some common ground around visions for a healthier society. I hope it can happen fast enough.

PETER'S REPLY: So Danny is back to his (and our main) message—the needed revolution in our political and economic systems. I learned this from him: the power of a consistent powerful well-written message. But I think this is going to be a catastrophic revolution, where human civilization and populations will likely be decimated. Perhaps we can reborn as more genuinely progressive humans and societies than we are today. All I can do is take faith in the young people like Danny, who I try in some small way to guide while at the same time feeling regretful for the paths current generations have taken so far.

DANNY'S REPLY: I appreciate Peter's faith in younger generations. But I want to emphasize that boomers can and must be a part of the solution. It is true that their generation came of age during the so-called end of history, when global capitalism defeated communism. With the fall of the Berlin Wall, there seemed to be, as Margaret Thatcher famously proclaimed, "no alternative" to free markets, free trade, and globalization. While the dominance and internalization of this hyper-capitalist logic has gradually limited their generational political horizons across the American dementia era, it's also true that boomers have witnessed, participated in, and benefited from profound societal change. Just to name a few accomplishments, in less than 100 years, we have

- regulated lead;
- busted trusts and monopolies;
- sent men to moon;
- ended segregation and won sweeping civil rights victories;
- vaccinated whole populations and virtually eliminated polio and smallpox in the US;
- innovated crop yields to save millions of lives from widespread mass famine;
- reduced damage from HIV/AIDS;
- significantly lowered smoking rates;
- made major advances in motor vehicle and workplace safety;
- closed the hole in the ozone through an international ban on chlorofluorocarbons; and
- extended lifespan from 47 to 77 years between 1900 and 1999.

Now, we have reached a cultural watershed when, out of the wreckage of unfettered global capitalism, we need to build inclusive cross-generational movements toward a healthier society that unify people across race, gender, age, and class. Issues we've dealt with in this book—climate change, worker empowerment, living wage, demilitarization—can be rallying points for intergenerational solidarity, which is ultimately much more of a force than corporate power consolidated in our government, defending a failed and self-serving system. Put simply, there are more of us than there are of the elites, and we need for people across the generations to get involved in growing working-class movements (for instance, the Fight for $15 and Medicare for All), pool their collective talents, pressure structures of societal power, and help put humankind on a better course. That 2018 saw the biggest strike wave since 1987 is grounds for some encouragement.

Intergenerational tensions are growing, and the hugely popular generation Z meme we mentioned of "OK boomer"—which functions as a sort of collective eye roll at older generations and the broader decisions they've made as a voting bloc over the last several decades—is a warning signal of how things could go if we don't get boomer buy-in on things like creating a fairer political-economic order or acting decisively on climate change. We are going to have to rely on people power and the "wising up" of Boomers in a very small window of time.

In his *Peoples History of the United States,* Howard Zinn reminded us:

> The Constitution gave no rights to working people: no right to work less than twelve hours a day, no right to a living wage, no right to safe working conditions. Workers had to organize, go on strike, defy the law, the courts, the police, create a great movement which won the eight-hour day, and caused such commotion that Congress was forced to pass a minimum wage law, and Social Security, and unemployment insurance . . . [F]undamental change will depend, the experience of the past suggests, on the actions of an aroused citizenry, demanding that the promise of the Declaration of Independence—an equal right to life, liberty, and the pursuit of happiness—be fulfilled.

In other words, at this time of crisis, we have to band together, demanding and fighting for a future informed by new values that push humanity forward from this stagnant, precarious, and decidedly dangerous predicament we find ourselves in. A healthier society is there for us, if we want it and can find the fortitude to win it.

Finally, as we conclude this interview in May 2020, we find ourselves facing an uncertain future due to the COVID-19 pandemic. How has the reality of this deadly virus affected your thinking about a healthier society? And specifically, what does it mean for how we collectively approach brain health and care for our most vulnerable, including the elderly and those living with dementia?

PETER: COVID-19 is revealing how much a monster neoliberalism and its modes of thought have become by magnifying the same tears in our social fabric that dementia was more slowly unraveling. Ironically, the virus itself also causes cognitive impairment and is emerging as much more than a respiratory disease primarily of elders. Children are being affected by multisystem failure, and the virus is causing dementia in people of all ages through a variety of different mechanisms, including vascular damage (stroke) and inflammation (encephalitis). It also causes temporary states of confusion (delirium) and can precipitate psychiatric symptoms like depression and psychosis. So COVID-19 is, in many ways, impairing our ability to see individually and collectively the root causes and ways forward.

And with respect to neoliberalism, income inequity, environmental deterioration, market fundamentalism, public health disinvestment, and power in the hands of a few are all making the virus much worse than it might have been in the US. This also appears to be the case in countries like the UK that have similarly committed to the neoliberal project over the last 40 years. Physical distancing is challenging our ability to maintain social solidarity, which was already at a low ebb because of destructive polarities in our politics. Former President Trump was perhaps the caricature, but not the cause, of "American dementia"—a malignant narcissist, pathological liar, and business failure with poor executive functions and verbal communication skills. But the wealthy dominant white patriarchy (oligarchy) at the heart of neoliberalism is supporting his efforts to consolidate power among the few. Trump represented what you get when neoliberalism is taken to its extreme. Low-income elders who need care in nursing homes and in community, and children, who deserve quality education, are the most vulnerable.

Even before COVID-19 we needed a Green New Deal, or perhaps even more radical action in order to transform our communities and society. Now the choices are even clearer. We either band together during this pandemic to create a society more responsive and resilient to the intensifying climate change ahead or we make things worse. The virus is not only a magnifier of our troubles but a metaphor for them. SARS-CoV-2 is an individual player that only wants to grow its numbers. As a virus, it is barely defined as "alive" as it sucks life from others. It thrives on weakened hosts. It in many ways resembles zombie neoliberalism: a cultural virus even more destructive than a biological one. Our economic and political focus on the individual and economic growth, even on numbers, seems mirrored in the virus and our response to it.

We humans get to tell the story of the legacy of SARS-CoV-2. Years from now, will we be able to say we learned the lesson that our wealth should be measured by distributed happiness, not by out-of-balance individual economic gain? Whether we waste money on expensive ineffective biologics and drugs or reinvest in communities will determine how we respond to the problem of clinical dementia. We will require healthy brains and collective wisdom, including a large measure of humility, to make those decisions and to reimagine and reenchant our lives. The monstrous distortions in our thinking that have led to uncivil modern civilization must be challenged. We need to develop new ecologically based social contracts to ungird our societies. COVID-19 and dementia can help us rethink our lives together embedded within nature and with the huge but exciting job of creating new civilizations.

As we see our place in the inspiring story of life in the cosmos and act with sufficient courage, we can look forward to the new age of *cosmodernity*. That is the term that I have adopted to try to capture the depths of the necessary transitions in civilization we need to make. This is a time for renaissance and reformation, as other ages have been labeled. Cosmodernity is a label that invites the perspective of big history and deep time, extending back 13.8 billion years to the birth of the universe. It motivates humility about our role and responsibilities in relationship to life. It signals reenhancement with wonder, awe, and mystery and implies both the importance of science but also other forms of knowledge and sources of beauty and meaning. In the context of cosmodernity, we are all out of our purely intellectual depth and need to depend on values and intuitions to guide us. The rethinking and valuing of dementia can contribute to this growth of the wisdom needed to create new communities, societies, and even global human civilization.

DANNY: Shakespeare famously wrote in *Hamlet* that "Something is rotten in the state of Denmark." While I take pride in being a US citizen, in an age of COVID-19, it is impossible not to feel some resonance with this sentiment as an American.

I hope we have shown in this book how, over the last four decades, our political-economic system has become unbalanced, allowing greed, political corruption, corporatism, free-market dominance, excess individualism, austerity, and the gradual oligarchic rot of hyper-capitalism to weaken our shared commitment to one another, and thus leaving the country vulnerable to all manner of crises, including an opportunistic virus. Perhaps ironically, while the modern-day "state of Denmark" has preserved a social democratic system that has, as of May 2020, allowed the country to flatten the initial wave of the virus and lift its lockdown, the US remains mired in crisis. Neoliberalism may not be torn asunder by COVID-19, but the lethal consequences of the unhealthy society it has wrought have been laid bare for the world to see—from the bodies piling up in our overwhelmed hospitals, to the tens of millions unemployed, to the mile-long crush of cars lining up for food bank distribution.

That said, as Peter expressed, while things are murky in spring 2020, the story of the future is ours to tell. A healthier society will provide health care for all as a human right. It will bolster and fund public health programs and social safety nets that protect everyone, especially the neediest among us. People will be shielded in crisis by safeguards like job guarantees, universal basic incomes, rent controls, guaranteed access to food and water, and other measures that limit unnecessary suffering and loss of life. We will develop ways to automate some dangerous "essential" jobs and ensure the protection, proper remuneration, and labor power of those who assume greater risk. Such social organization will protect us against the worst ravages of viruses; however, as I hope we've shown in this book, so too will it support healthier brains, healthier minds, and place our society on a more life-affirming trajectory.

With respect to caring for our elders, the pandemic and its major death toll for those living and working in institutional care has deepened moral urgency to move toward more humane long-term care systems. For those who have survived the initial wave of the virus, the social costs have been severe: isolation from kids, grandkids, and other external visitors; reduced engagement with the arts and socialceuticals; daily care from depersonalized staff wearing clinical masks, face shields, and gloves; randomly losing friends and neighbors by the day. How do we prepare for the next crisis and ensure the dignity and quality of life of people living with dementia, and the safety, support, and proper remuneration of those who care for them? Can we use this tragedy to expedite progress toward truly age- and dementia-friendly communities and a universal long-term care insurance system to care for elders living in institutions and being cared for at home?

Right now, the precariousness and depth of suffering we face are near overwhelming. But overcoming American dementia requires that we confront our problems squarely, remembering the vital lessons of the past and moving assertively toward the more dignified society of the future that this unavoidably Shakespearean moment demands.

Notes

PREFACE

1. Joseph Lucco, "The Eisenhower Principle Applied to Business Strategy Management," ClearPoint Strategy, November 4, 2014, https://www.clearpointstrategy.com/eisenhower-principle-and-business-strategy-management/.

CHAPTER 1. OCCUPY ALZHEIMER'S!

1. See the tactical briefing that sparked Occupy Wall Street: "8th Anniversary of #Occupy WallStreet," A Billion People, September 16, 2019, http://abillionpeople.org/8th-anniversary-of-occupywallstreet/.
2. Publisher's description of *Giants: The Global Power Elite* by Peter Phillips, Seven Stories Press, accessed February 26, 2020, https://sevenstories.com/books/4097-giants.
3. Naomi Wolf, "Revealed: How the FBI Coordinated the Crackdown on Occupy," *Guardian*, December 29, 2012, sec. Opinion, https://www.theguardian.com/commentisfree/2012/dec/29/fbi-coordinated-crackdown-occupy.
4. Sarah Jaffe, *Necessary Trouble: Americans in Revolt* (New York: Bold Type, 2017), 35.
5. Naomi Klein, *No Is Not Enough: Resisting Trump's Shock Politics and Winning the World We Need* (London: Penguin, 2017).
6. John Maynard Keynes, *The General Theory of Employment, Interest, and Money* (New York: Palgrave Macmillan, 1936).
7. Brandon Richard, "WTF Is Neoliberalism?" Democratic Socialists of America (DSA), April 20, 2017, https://www.dsausa.org/democratic-left/wtf_is_neoliberalism_dl/.
8. Judith Stein, *The Pivotal Decade: How the United States Traded Factories for Finance in the Seventies* (New Haven, CT: Yale University Press, 2010).
9. Thomas Frank, *Listen Liberal: What Ever Happened to the Party of the People?* (New York: Metropolitan Books, 2015).
10. Stein, *Pivotal Decade*, xii.
11. Tim Barker, "Other People's Blood," *n+1*, May 1, 2019, https://nplusonemag.com/issue-34/reviews/other-peoples-blood-2/.
12. As Volcker said in 1979 about his "Volcker shock," "the standard of living of the average American has to decline." See Steven Rattner, "Volcker Asserts U.S. Must Trim Living Standard," *New York Times*, October 18, 1979, sec. Archives, https://www.nytimes.com/1979/10/18/archives/volcker-asserts-us-must-trim-living-standard-warns-of-inflation.html.
13. "Thatcher's Legacy," *Guardian*, May 3, 1999, sec. Politics, https://www.theguardian.com/politics/1999/may/03/thatcher.uk.
14. " 'Turn the Bull Loose,' Reagan Says on Exchange Floor: President Gives Bullish Wall St. Pep Talk," *Los Angeles Times*, March 29, 1985, https://www.latimes.com/archives/la-xpm-1985-03-29-mn-20409-story.html.
15. Milton Friedman, "The Social Responsibility of a Business Is to Increase Its Profits," *New York Times Magazine*, May 13, 1970.

16. William C. Berman, *From the Center to the Edge: The Politics and Policies of the Clinton Presidency* (Lanham, MD: Rowman and Littlefield, 2001), i.
17. "Personal Responsibility and Work Opportunity Act," *Wikipedia*, last updated February 14, 2020, https://en.wikipedia.org/w/index.php?title=Personal_Responsibility_and_Work_Opportunity_Act&oldid=940832741.
18. "Gramm–Leach–Bliley Act," *Wikipedia*, last updated February 20, 2020, https://en.wikipedia.org/w/index.php?title=Gramm%E2%80%93Leach%E2%80%93Bliley_Act&oldid=941666735.
19. Barker, "Other People's Blood."
20. Lawrence H. Summers, "Opinion: The Great Liberator," *New York Times*, November 19, 2006, sec. Opinion, https://www.nytimes.com/2006/11/19/opinion/19summers.html.
21. Ted Schrecker and Clare Bambra, *How Politics Makes Us Sick: Neoliberal Epidemics* (New York: Palgrave Macmillan, 2015), 12.
22. Paul S. Teller, "Pro-Free-Market Ideas for Responding to Hurricane Katrina and High Gas," *Shock Doctrine*, September 13, 2005, http://www.naomiklein.org/shock-doctrine/resources/part7/chapter20/pro-market-ideas-katrina.
23. Naomi Klein, *The Shock Doctrine: The Rise of Disaster Capitalism* (New York: Metropolitan Books / Henry Holt, 2007).
24. Noam Chomsky, "Neoliberalism: An Accounting," streamed live as "Noam Chomsky Speaks at Crotty Hall," by UMassEconomics, video, 1:17:49, April 13, 2017, https://www.youtube.com/watch?v=PbjtRgYhLzU&feature=youtu.be.
25. John Quiggan, *Zombie Economics: How Dead Ideas Still Walk among Us* (Princeton, NJ: Princeton University Press, 2010).
26. Stein, *Pivotal Decade*, xii.
27. "Margaret Thatcher: A Life in Quotes," *Guardian*, April 8, 2013, sec. Politics, https://www.theguardian.com/politics/2013/apr/08/margaret-thatcher-quotes.
28. David Harvey, *A Brief History of Neoliberalism* (Oxford: Oxford University Press, 2005).
29. "George Carlin—The Big Club," uploaded by Gábor Hényel, video, 3:14, May 4, 2014, https://www.youtube.com/watch?v=cKUaqFzZLxU.
30. Globally, the 1% are on track to own two-thirds of all wealth by 2030.
31. "Distributional Financial Accounts Overview," Board of Governors of the Federal Reserve System, last updated March 20, 2020, https://www.federalreserve.gov/releases/z1/dataviz/dfa/.
32. Richard Blundell, Robert Joyce, Agnes Norris Keiller, and James P. Ziliak, "Income Inequality and the Labour Market in Britain and the US," *Journal of Public Economics* 162 (June 2018): 48–62, https://doi.org/10.1016/j.jpubeco.2018.04.001.
33. Martha Ross and Nicole Bateman, "Low-Wage Work Is More Pervasive than You Think, and There Aren't Enough 'Good Jobs' to Go Around," *Brookings* (blog), November 21, 2019, https://www.brookings.edu/blog/the-avenue/2019/11/21/low-wage-work-is-more-pervasive-than-you-think-and-there-arent-enough-good-jobs-to-go-around/.
34. Taylor Telford, "Income Inequality in America Is the Highest It's Been since Census Bureau Started Tracking It, Data Shows," *Washington Post*, September 26, 2019, https://www.washingtonpost.com/business/2019/09/26/income-inequality-america-highest-its-been-since-census-started-tracking-it-data-show/.
35. Joseph E. Stiglitz, "Opinion: Progressive Capitalism Is Not an Oxymoron," *New York Times*, April 19, 2019, sec. Opinion, https://www.nytimes.com/2019/04/19/opinion/sunday/progressive-capitalism.html.
36. Paul Buchheit, "The Evidence Pours In: Poverty Getting Much Worse in America," Common Dreams, November 5, 2018, https://www.commondreams.org/views/2018/11/05/evidence-pours-poverty-getting-much-worse-america.
37. R. Chetty, M. Stepner, and S. Abraham, "The Association between Income and Life Expectancy in the United States, 2001–2014," *JAMA* 315 (2016): 1750–66.

38. National Center for Health Statistics, ed., *National Center for Health Statistics Data Presentation Standards for Proportions*. Vital and Health Statistics, series 2, Data Evaluation and Methods Research, no. 175. Hyattsville, Maryland: U.S. Department of Health and Human Services, Centers for Disease Control and Prevention, National Center for Health Statistics, 2017.
39. "Socialism for the Rich and Capitalism for the Poor," *Wikipedia*, last updated February 24, 2020, https://en.wikipedia.org/w/index.php?title=Socialism_for_the_rich_and_capitalism_for_the_poor&oldid=942470230.
40. "Social Spending," OECD Data, accessed February 26, 2020, http://data.oecd.org/socialexp/social-spending.htm.
41. Career Builder, "Living Paycheck to Paycheck Is a Way of Life for Majority of U.S. Workers, According to New CareerBuilder Survey," press release, August 24, 2017, http://press.careerbuilder.com/2017-08-24-Living-Paycheck-to-Paycheck-is-a-Way-of-Life-for-Majority-of-U-S-Workers-According-to-New-CareerBuilder-Survey.
42. Howard Schneider, "Fed's Brainard: Middle-Class Wealth Still Less than before Great Recession," *Reuters*, May 10, 2019, https://www.reuters.com/article/us-usa-fed-brainard-idUSKCN1SG1BR.
43. J. Larrimore, A. Durante, C. Park, and A. Tranfaglia. *Report on the Economic Well-Being of US Households in 2016* (Washington, DC: Board of Governors of the Federal Reserve System, 2017).
44. The crowd-funding site GoFundMe has reported that one-third of its campaigns are aimed at paying medical bills. Over $650 million was raised in 2018 alone. Overall, Americans own more than $1 trillion in unpaid medical debt (Morgan Haefner, "Medical Bills Account for 1 in 3 GoFundMe Campaigns," Becker's Hospital CFO Report, July 3, 2018, https://www.beckershospitalreview.com/finance/medical-bills-account-for-1-in-3-gofundme-campaigns.html). Americans have died from lack of or inadequate fundraising; see Dan Evon, "Fact Check: Did Shane Patrick Boyle Die After Starting a GoFundMe Campaign for Insulin?" Snopes, November 27, 2017, https://www.snopes.com/fact-check/shane-patrick-boyle-died-after-starting-a-gofundme-campaign-for-insulin/.
45. "Nearly 44 Million in United States without Health Insurance in 2008," CDC, press release, July 1, 2009, https://www.cdc.gov/media/pressrel/2009/r090701.htm.
46. David Cecere, "New Study Finds 45,000 Deaths Annually Linked to Lack of Health Coverage," *Harvard Gazette*, September 17, 2009, https://news.harvard.edu/gazette/story/2009/09/new-study-finds-45000-deaths-annually-linked-to-lack-of-health-coverage/.
47. K. Robin Yabroff, Jingxuan Zhao, Xuesong Han, and Zhiyuan Zheng, "Prevalence and Correlates of Medical Financial Hardship in the USA," *Journal of General Internal Medicine* 34, no. 8 (2019): 1494-1502, https://doi.org/10.1007/s11606-019-05002-w.
48. Michael Marmot, "Health Equity in England: The Marmot Review 10 Years On," *BMJ* 368 (2020): m693, https://doi.org/10.1136/bmj.m693.
49. Michael Chui, James Manyika, and Mehdi Miremadi, "Where Machines Could Replace Humans—and Where They Can't (Yet)," McKinsey Digital, July 8, 2016, https://www.mckinsey.com/business-functions/mckinsey-digital/our-insights/where-machines-could-replace-humans-and-where-they-cant-yet.
50. Julie Ray, "Americans' Stress, Worry and Anger Intensified in 2018," Gallup, April 25, 2019, https://news.gallup.com/poll/249098/americans-stress-worry-anger-intensified-2018.aspx.
51. CDC/NCHS, National Vital Statistics System, Mortality, 2018, CDC WONDER, U.S. Department of Health and Human Services, CDC, Atlanta, Georgia, https://wonder.cdc.gov.
52. Sherry L. Murphy, Jiaquan Xu, Kenneth D. Kochanek, and Elizabeth Arias, *Mortality in the United States, 2017* (Hyattsville, MD: U.S. Department of Health and Human Services, Centers for Disease Control and Prevention, National Center for Health Statistics, 2018).

Kamran Abassi, Steven H. Woolf, Derek A. Chapman, Jeanine M. Buchanich, Kendra J. Bobby, Emily B. Zimmerman, and Sarah M. Blackburn, "Changes in Midlife Death Rates across Racial and Ethnic Groups in the United States: Systematic Analysis of Vital Statistics," *BMJ* 362 (2018): k3096.

53. "Life Expectancy at Birth—Country Comparison, TOP 100," *CIA World Factbook*, accessed June 20, 2020, https://www.indexmundi.com/g/r.aspx?t=100&v=30.
54. Reid Davenport, "Wall Street Funds Down from Obama's Inaugural Run," *Open Secrets News*, October 25, 2012, https://www.opensecrets.org/news/2012/10/wall-street-funds-down-from-obamas/.
55. Martin Gilens and Benjamin I. Page, "Testing Theories of American Politics: Elites, Interest Groups, and Average Citizens," *Perspectives on Politics* 12, no. 3 (2014): 564–81.
56. "Five Lobbyists for Each Member of Congress on Financial Reforms," Center for Public Integrity, May 21, 2010, https://publicintegrity.org/politics/five-lobbyists-for-each-member-of-congress-on-financial-reforms/.
57. Noah Barkin, "Trust in US Institutions Plunges in Trump's First Year," *Reuters* January 21, 2018, https://www.reuters.com/article/us-davos-meeting-trust/trust-in-u-s-institutions-plunges-in-trumps-first-year-idUSKBN1FB08T.
58. Betsy Cooper, Daniel Cox, Rachel Lienesch, and Robert P. Jones, "The Divide over America's Future: 1950 or 2050?" PRRI, October 25, 2016, https://www.prri.org/research/poll-1950s-2050-divided-nations-direction-post-election/.
59. Terry Lynn Karl, "Extreme Inequality and State Capture: The Crisis of Liberal Democracy in the United States," *Chinese Political Science Review* 4, no. 2 (2019): 164–87.
60. Thirty-six of the world's 100 wealthiest billionaires are US citizens and—thanks to Citizens United—eligible to contribute politically at a large scale. A 2017 investigation by Open Secrets found that 30 of these billionaires contributed $184.4 million to candidates and political action committees. See Ashley Balcerzak, "Richest Billionaires Are also Top Political Spenders," *Open Secrets News*, March 31, 2017, https://www.opensecrets.org/news/2017/03/richest-billionaires-are-top-political-spenders.
61. Of course, voter suppression and redistricting efforts led by Republicans denied hundreds of thousands of people a right to vote in the 2016 election.
62. Noam Chomsky has summed up our current predicament quite forthrightly: "The two parties are two factions of the business party. Most of the population doesn't even bother voting because it looks meaningless. They're marginalized and properly distracted. At least that's the goal." See Noam Chomsky, *Media Control: The Spectacular Achievements of Propaganda*, 2nd ed. (New York: Seven Stories Press, 2002), 29.
63. Tara Golshan, "Read: Bernie Sanders Defines His Vision for Democratic Socialism in the United States," *Vox*, June 12, 2019, https://www.vox.com/2019/6/12/18663217/bernie-sanders-democratic-socialism-speech-transcript.
64. Albert Einstein, "Why Socialism?" *Monthly Review* (blog), [May 1949] May 1, 2009, https://monthlyreview.org/2009/05/01/why-socialism/.
65. Lucy Diavolo, "Bernie Sanders Explained What Democratic Socialism Means to Him," *Teen Vogue*, February 26, 2019, https://www.teenvogue.com/story/bernie-sanders-explained-democratic-socialism-cnn-town-hall.
66. "Ocasio-Cortez Impresses 'The View' with Democratic Socialism,"video, 12:00, the Rational National, June 29, 2018, https://www.youtube.com/watch?v=L8zd4L57esY.
67. Thomas Piketty, *Capital in the Twenty-First Century* (Cambridge, MA: Belknap Press of Harvard University, 2014).
68. Seymour Martin Lipset and Gary Marks, "How FDR Saved Capitalism," *Hoover Digest*, January 30, 2001, https://www.hoover.org/research/how-fdr-saved-capitalism.
69. Such a system is, ironically, much closer to what Adam Smith articulated in his famous treatise *The Wealth of Nations*. See Paul Sagar, "The Real Adam Smith," *Aeon*, January 16, 2018, https://aeon.co/essays/we-should-look-closely-at-what-adam-smith-actually-believed.
70. Stein, *Pivotal Decade*, 1–2.

71. "Historical Highest Marginal Income Tax Rates," Tax Policy Center, February 4, 2020, https://www.taxpolicycenter.org/statistics/historical-highest-marginal-income-tax-rates.
72. "Nixon Reportedly Says He Is Now a Keynesian," *New York Times*, January 7, 1971, sec. Archives, https://www.nytimes.com/1971/01/07/archives/nixon-reportedly-says-he-is-now-a-keynesian.html.
73. Schrecker and Bambra, *How Politics Makes Us Sick*, 5.
74. Claudia Goldin and Robert A. Margo, "The Great Compression: The Wage Structure in the United States at Mid-Century," *Quarterly Journal of Economics* 107, no. 1 (1992): 1–34.
75. In 2019, the top 10 included all Scandinavian countries, including 4 of the top 5: (1) Finland, (2) Denmark, (3) Norway, (4) Iceland, (5) Netherlands, (6) Switzerland, (7) Sweden, (8) New Zealand, (9) Canada, (10) Austria (United States is 19th). See "Changing World Happiness," *World Happiness Report 2019*, accessed February 26, 2020, http://worldhappiness.report/.
76. George Lakey, "Why Are the Danes so Happy? Because Their Economy Makes Sense," openDemocracy, August 31, 2017, https://www.opendemocracy.net/en/transformation/why-are-danes-so-happy-because-their-economy-makes-sense/.
77. "Best Countries for Business," *Forbes*, 2018 Ranking, accessed February 26, 2020, https://www.forbes.com/best-countries-for-business/list/.
78. Peter Dreier, "Martin Luther King Was a Democratic Socialist," *HuffPost*, January 18, 2016, https://www.huffpost.com/entry/martin-luther-king-was-a-democratic-socialist_b_9008990.
79. Andreas Møller Mulvad and Rune Møller Stahl, "The Real Denmark," *Jacobin*, October 14, 2018, https://jacobinmag.com/2018/10/denmark-welfare-state-socialism-nordic-model-regan.
80. "Harry S. Truman Quotes," *Notable Quotes*, accessed February 26, 2020, http://www.notable-quotes.com/t/truman_harry_s.html.
81. Schrecker and Bambra, *How Politics Makes Us Sick*, 120.
82. Stiglitz, "Progressive Capitalism."
83. Bernie Sanders, "The Failed Prophet," *In These Times*, February 6, 2009, http://inthesetimes.com/article/4193/the_failed_prophet.
84. Mohamed Younis, "Four in 10 Americans Embrace Some Form of Socialism," Gallup, May 20, 2019, https://news.gallup.com/poll/257639/four-americans-embrace-form-socialism.aspx.
85. Max Ehrenfreund, "A Majority of Millennials Now Reject Capitalism, Poll Shows," *Washington Post*, April 26, 2016, https://www.washingtonpost.com/news/wonk/wp/2016/04/26/a-majority-of-millennials-now-reject-capitalism-poll-shows/.
86. Lydia Saad, "Socialism as Popular as Capitalism among Young Adults in U.S.," Gallup, November 25, 2019, https://news.gallup.com/poll/268766/socialism-popular-capitalism-among-young-adults.aspx.
87. Martin Luther King Jr., "The Three Evils of Society," August 31, 1967, Scribd, https://www.scribd.com/doc/134362247/Martin-Luther-King-Jr-The-Three-Evils-of-Society-1967.
88. Schrecker and Bambra, *How Politics Makes Us Sick*, 5.
89. Clayton Dalton, "Lifestyle Changes, Not a Magic Pill, Can Reverse Alzheimer's," *Aeon*, May 3, 2017, https://aeon.co/ideas/lifestyle-changes-not-a-magic-pill-can-reverse-alzheimers.
90. Mark Moran, "Several Theories Try to Explain Rise in Bipolar Diagnoses," *Psychiatric News*, October 5, 2007, https://doi.org/10.1176/pn.42.19.0018.
91. "This Is Water," *Kenyon College Alumni Bulletin*, accessed February 26, 2020, http://bulletin-archive.kenyon.edu/x4280.html.
92. Schrecker and Bambra, *How Politics Makes Us Sick*.
93. Thomas S. Kuhn, *The Structure of Scientific Revolutions*, 2nd ed. (Chicago: University of Chicago Press, 1970).
94. Patricia L. Price, "Cultural geography and the stories we tell ourselves," *Cultural Geographies* 17, no. 2 (2010): 203–10.

95. Daniel Smith, Philip Schlaepfer, Katie Major, Mark Dyble, Abigail E. Page, James Thompson, Nikhil Chaudhary, Gul Deniz Salali, Ruth Mace, Leonora Astete, Marilyn Ngales, Lucio Vinicius, and Andrea Bamberg Migliano, “Cooperation and the Evolution of Hunter-Gatherer Storytelling,” *Nature Communications* 8, no. 1 (2017): 1–9, https://doi.org/10.1038/s41467-017-02036-8.
96. In Jonathan White, *Talking on the Water: Conversations about Nature and Creativity* (Dublin: Trinity University Press, 2016).
97. Margaret Lock, *The Alzheimer Conundrum: Entanglements of Dementia and Aging* (Princeton, NJ: Princeton University Press, 2013), 4.

CHAPTER 2. ALZHEIMER’S AND THE NEOLIBERAL TURN

1. Alois Alzheimer, “Über eigenartige Krankheitsfälle des späteren Alters,” *Zeitschrift für die gesamte Neurologie und Psychiatrie* 4, no. 1 (December 1911): 356–85, https://doi.org/10.1007/BF02866241.
2. Daniel R. George, Peter J. Whitehouse, Simon D’Alton, and Jesse Ballenger, “Through the Amyloid Gateway,” *Lancet* 380, no. 9858 (December 2012): 1986–87, https://doi.org/10.1016/S0140-6736(12)62145-X.
3. H-J. Möller and M. B. Graeber, “The Case Described by Alois Alzheimer in 1911,” *European Archives of Psychiatry and Clinical Neuroscience* 248, no. 3 (1998): 111–22.
4. Alzheimer, “Über eigenartige Krankheitsfälle.” See also Hans H. Klünemann, Wolfgang Fronhöfer, Herbert Wurster, Wolfgang Fischer, Bernd Ibach, and Helmfried E. Klein, “Alzheimer’s Second Patient: Johann F. and His Family,” *Annals of Neurology: Official Journal of the American Neurological Association and the Child Neurology Society* 52, no. 4 (2002): 520–23.
5. Alois Alzheimer, “Über eigenartige Krankheitsfälle des späteren Alters,” *Zeitschrift für die Gesamte Neurologie und Psychiatrie* 4 (1911): 356–85.
6. Emil Kraepelin, *Psychiatry: A Textbook for Students and Physicians* (Canton, MA: Science History Press, 1991).
7. Ulrich Müller, Pia Winter, and Manuel B. Graeber, “A Presenilin 1 Mutation in the First Case of Alzheimer’s Disease,” *Lancet Neurology* 12, no. 2 (2013): 129–30.
8. Kieran Keohane and Victoria Grace, “What Is ‘Alzheimer’s Disease’? The Auguste D’Case Re-opened,” *Culture, Medicine, and Psychiatry* 43, no. 2 (2019): 336–59. Note: In this article, the authors argue that Auguste D. may not have carried a genetic mutation but rather may have been suffering the effects of tertiary syphilis given to her by a husband who could have been unfaithful and contracted the STI from a prostitute. They reason that Auguste D’s husband was a rail clerk working next to a red light district, and, at that time, there was an epidemic of “demise maladies,” a euphemism whereby doctors colluded with husbands to protect men’s and family’s reputations.
9. Margaret Lock, *The Alzheimer Conundrum: Entanglements of Dementia and Aging* (Princeton, NJ: Princeton University Press, 2013).
10. G. E. Berrios, “Alzheimer’s Disease: A Conceptual History,” *International Journal of Geriatric Psychiatry* 5, no. 6 (November 1990): 355–65, https://doi.org/10.1002/gps.930050603.
11. Douglas C. Ewbank and Samuel H. Preston, “Personal Health Behaviour and the Decline in Infant and Child Mortality: The United States, 1900-1930,” in *What We Know about Health Transition: The Culture, Social and Behavioural Determinants of Health*, ed. John C. Caldwell (Canberra: Health Transition Centre, 1990), 116–50.
12. Tommy Bengtsson, Cameron Campbell, and James Z. Lee, *Life under Pressure: Mortality and Living Standards in Europe and Asia, 1700-1900* (Cambridge, MA: MIT Press, 2004).
13. Frans Van Poppel and Cor Van der Heijden, “The Effects of Water Supply on Infant and Childhood Mortality: A Review of Historical Evidence,” *Health Transition Review* (1997): 113–48.

14. Thomas McKeown, *The Modern Rise of Populations* (New York: Academic Press, 1976).
15. John E. Murray, "Standards of the Present for People of the Past: Height, Weight, and Mortality among Men of Amherst College, 1834-1949," *Journal of Economic History* 57, no. 3 (1997): 585–606.
16. Richard H. Steckel, "Stature and the Standard of Living," *Journal of Economic Literature* 33, no. 4 (1995): 1903–40.
17. McKeown, *Modern Rise of Populations.*
18. Esme Fuller-Thomson and Sydney A. Jopling, "Could the Adoption of Unleaded Gasoline in the 1970s Play a Role in the Precipitous Decline in Dementia Prevalence?" *JAMA Internal Medicine* 177, no. 6 (June 1, 2017): 892–93, https://doi.org/10.1001/jama internmed.2017.1074.
19. Werner Troesken, *The Great Lead Water Pipe Disaster* (Cambridge, MA: MIT Press, 2008), 22.
20. Mark A. S. Laidlaw, Arthur E. Poropat, Andy Ball, and Howard W. Mielke, "Exposure to Lead in Petrol and Increased Incidence of Dementia," *Lancet* 389, no. 10087 (2017): 2371–72.
21. Joshua T. Cohen and Peter J. Neumann, "The Cost Savings and Cost-Effectiveness of Clinical Preventive Care," *POLICY* 1 (2009): 6.
22. Robert Butler, *The Longevity Revolution* (New York: Public Affairs, 2008).
23. US Bureau of the Census, *Statistical Abstract of the United States: 1970*, 91st ed. (Washington, DC: US GPO, 1970).
24. Marja Ylönen and Luigi Pellizzoni, *Neoliberalism and Technoscience: Critical Assessments* (London: Taylor and Francis, 2016).
25. Patrick Fox, "From Senility to Alzheimer's Disease: The Rise of the Alzheimer's Disease Movement," *Milbank Quarterly* 67, no. 1 (1989): 82.
26. Robert Katzman, "The Prevalence and Malignancy of Alzheimer Disease: A Major Killer," *Archives of Neurology* 33, no. 4 (1976): 217–18.
27. US Senate, *Endless Night, Endless Mourning: Living with Alzheimer's—Hearing before the Special Committee on Aging*, 97th Cong., 1st sess. (Washington, DC: US GPO, 1983), 48.
28. Jesse F. Ballenger, *Self, Senility, and Alzheimer's Disease in Modern America: A History* (Baltimore, MD: Johns Hopkins University Press, 2006), 183.
29. Fox, "From Senility to Alzheimer's Disease."
30. U.S. Congress, *Congressional Record* (Washington D.C.: GPO, 1983), 24327–29.
31. James D. Watson, *Avoid Boring People: Lessons from a Life in Science* (New York: Vintage, 2009).
32. Eilon Caspi, "Trust at Stake: Is the 'Dual Mission' of the US Alzheimer's Association out of Balance?" *Dementia* 18, no. 5 (2019): 1629–50.
33. Robert Pear, "New Reagan Policy to Cut Benefits for the Aged, Blind and Disabled," *New York Times*, October 16, 1987, sec. U.S., https://www.nytimes.com/1987/10/16 /us/new-reagan-policy-to-cut-benefits-for-the-aged-blind-and-disabled.html.
34. Internal Revenue Service, U.S. Dept. of the Treasury, Tax Rate Schedules, Instructions for 1988 Form 1040, p. 51.
35. Ballenger, *Self, Senility, and Alzheimer's Disease*, 122.
36. Walter D. Valdivia, "The Stakes in Bayh-Dole: Public Values beyond the Pace of Innovation," *Minerva* 49, no. 1 (March 2011): 25–46, https://doi.org/10.1007/s11024-011-9162-6.
37. This reflected a long tradition in academic science. It is often pointed out that Jonas Salk famously turned down a patent for his polio vaccine so that it could be made available around the world.
38. "Aricept," video, 1:01, Andy, June 27, 2009, https://www.youtube.com/watch?v=6LeD E9Zpbnc.
39. "H. G. Wells Quotes," BrainyQuote, accessed February 26, 2020, https://www.brainy quote.com/quotes/h_g_wells_102994.

40. C. Lee Ventola, "Direct-to-Consumer Pharmaceutical Advertising," *Pharmacy and Therapeutics* 36, no. 10 (October 2011): 669–84.
41. See George G. Glenner and Caine W. Wong, "Alzheimer's Disease and Down's Syndrome: Sharing of a Unique Cerebrovascular Amyloid Fibril Protein," *Biochemical and Biophysical Research Communications* 122, no. 3 (1984): 1131–35; John Hardy and Dennis J. Selkoe, "The Amyloid Hypothesis of Alzheimer's Disease: Progress and Problems on the Road to Therapeutics," *Science* 297, no. 5580 (2002): 353–56.
42. Alzheimer's Impact Movement, Alzheimer's Association, "Fiscal Year 2021 Alzheimer's Research Funding," March 2020, https://act.alz.org/site/DocServer/2015_Appropriations_Fact_Sheet__FY16_.pdf?docID=3641.
43. Sharon Begley, "The Maddening Saga of How an Alzheimer's 'Cabal' Thwarted Progress toward a Cure for Decades," *STAT*, June 25, 2019, https://www.statnews.com/2019/06/25/alzheimers-cabal-thwarted-progress-toward-cure/.
44. Ibid.
45. Jeffrey L. Cummings, Travis Morstorf, and Kate Zhong, "Alzheimer's Disease Drug-Development Pipeline: Few Candidates, Frequent Failures," *Alzheimer's Research and Therapy* 6, no. 4 (2014): 37.
46. James E. Galvin, "Prevention of Alzheimer's Disease: Lessons Learned and Applied," *Journal of the American Geriatrics Society* 65, no. 10 (2017): 2128–33.
47. Suzanne Hendrix and Noel Ellison, "Are Alzheimer's Drug Failures Due to Inactive Compounds or Are We Doing Something Wrong?" *Alzheimer's and Dementia: The Journal of the Alzheimer's Association* 13, no. 7 (2017): P617.
48. Tim Erickson, "Biogen's Statistical Gymnastics and PR Maneuvering Will Likely Turn Aducanumab Straw into Mega Blockbuster Gold (NASDAQ:BIIB)," *Seeking Alpha*, June 24, 2020, https://seekingalpha.com/article/4355504-biogens-statistical-gymnastics-and-pr-maneuvering-will-likely-turn-aducanumab-straw-mega.
49. J. Karlawish, "Aducanumab Isn't the Simple Solution to the Alzheimer's Crisis," *STAT*, December 20, 2019, https://www.statnews.com/2019/12/20/aducanumab-isnt-simple-solution-complicated-alzheimers-crisis/.
50. Alex Keown, "Approximately 100 COVID-19 Cases Stem from Biogen Meeting," BioSpace, March 17, 2020, https://www.biospace.com/article/approximately-100-covid-19-cases-stem-from-biogen-meeting/.
51. Peter J. Whitehouse and Daniel R. George, "A Tale of Two Reports: What Recent Publications from the Alzheimer's Association and Institute of Medicine Say about the State of the Field," *Journal of Alzheimer's Disease* 49, no. 1 (2016): 21–25.
52. "Amyloid PET," CMS, last updated January 30, 2020, https://www.cms.gov/Medicare/Coverage/Coverage-with-Evidence-Development/Amyloid-PET.
53. Imaging Dementia—Evidence for Amyloid Scanning (IDEAS) home page, accessed February 26, 2020, https://www.ideas-study.org/.

CHAPTER 3. ALZHEIMER'S TODAY

1. Daniel R. George and Peter J. Whitehouse, "Marketplace of Memory: What the Brain Fitness Technology Industry Says about Us and How We Can Do Better," *Gerontologist* 51, no. 5 (2011): 590–96.
2. Our colleague George Perry is a leading proponent of the oxidative stress hypothesis of Alzheimer's, which holds that amyloid is a protective response to age-related metabolic pressures in the cell, specifically dysfunction of the mitochondria, the cell's energy-producing organelles. Energy shortages have been shown to alter the processing of amyloid. There is also evidence that amyloid-beta can reduce oxidative stress in brains. Indeed, amyloid binds tightly to copper and blocks the production of free radicals that can cause oxidative damage.

3. Our colleague Rudy Tanzi has been a leading proponent of this theory. He has published evidence that beta-amyloid can protect human cells, worms, and mice from bacterial infections. Tanzi believes amyloid has antimicrobial properties, and that the clumping of beta-amyloid into oligomers and fibrils are a means of trapping infectious agents such as the herpes virus (HSV, HHV).
4. Deepak Kumar Vijaya Kumar, Se Hoon Choi, Kevin J. Washicosky, William A. Eimer, Stephanie Tucker, Jessica Ghofrani, Aaron Lefkowitz, et al., "Amyloid-β Peptide Protects against Microbial Infection in Mouse and Worm Models of Alzheimer's Disease," *Science Translational Medicine* 8, no. 340 (May 25, 2016): 340ra72-340ra72, https://doi.org/10.1126/scitranslmed.aaf1059.
5. George M. Savva, Stephen B. Wharton, Paul G. Ince, Gillian Forster, Fiona E. Matthews, and Carol Brayne, "Age, Neuropathology, and Dementia," *New England Journal of Medicine* 360, no. 22 (2009): 2302–9.
6. David A. Snowdon, "Healthy Aging and Dementia: Findings from the Nun Study," *Annals of Internal Medicine* 139, no. 5, part 2 (2003): 450–54.
7. See Willemijn J. Jansen, Rik Ossenkoppele, Dirk L. Knol, Betty M. Tijms, Philip Scheltens, Frans R. J. Verhey, Pieter Jelle Visser, et al., "Prevalence of Cerebral Amyloid Pathology in Persons without Dementia: A Meta-analysis," *Journal of the American Medical Association* 313, no. 19 (2015): 1924–38; Thomas G. Beach, Sarah E. Monsell, Leslie E. Phillips, and Walter Kukull, "Accuracy of the Clinical Diagnosis of Alzheimer Disease at National Institute on Aging Alzheimer Disease Centers, 2005-2010," *Journal of Neuropathology and Experimental Neurology* 71, no. 4 (2012): 266-73; Alberto Serrano-Pozo, Jing Qian, Sarah E. Monsell, Deborah Blacker, Teresa Gómez-Isla, Rebecca A. Betensky, John H. Growdon, et al., "Mild to Moderate Alzheimer Dementia with Insufficient Neuropathological Changes," *Annals of Neurology* 75, no. 4 (2014): 597–601.
8. Sarah E. Monsell, Walter A. Kukull, Alex E. Roher, Chera L. Maarouf, Geidy Serrano, Thomas G. Beach, Richard J. Caselli, Thomas J. Montine, and Eric M. Reiman, "Characterizing Apolipoprotein E ε4 Carriers and Noncarriers with the Clinical Diagnosis of Mild to Moderate Alzheimer Dementia and Minimal β-Amyloid Peptide Plaques," *JAMA Neurology* 72, no. 10 (2015): 1124–31.
9. Stephen Salloway, Reisa Sperling, Keith Gregg, Peng Yu, Abhinay Joshi, Ming Lu, Mark Mintun, et al., "P4-417: Incidence and Clinical Progression of Placebo-Treated Amyloid-Negative Subjects with Mild-to-Moderate Alzheimer's Disease (AD): Results from the Phase III PET Substudies of Bapineuzumab and Solanezumab," *Alzheimer's and Dementia* 9 (2013): P888–P889.
10. Vincent van Gogh, *Prisoners Exercising (after Dore)*, Van Gogh Paintings, accessed February 27, 2020, http://www.vggallery.com/painting/p_0669.htm.
11. Ironically, as Bob Butler himself aged, one of us (Peter) who knew him well saw changes in his attitudes about Alzheimer's as a heterogeneous entity. In one of his last books, *The Longevity Revolution*, he says twice that he no longer believed that Alzheimer's disease was a single disorder. This change of position, however, is hidden in footnotes in the back of the book, and he never lost his enthusiasm for medical approaches to addressing the challenges.
12. Julie A. Schneider, Zoe Arvanitakis, Woojeong Bang, and David A. Bennett, "Mixed Brain Pathologies Account for Most Dementia Cases in Community-Dwelling Older Persons," *Neurology* 69, no. 24 (2007): 2197–2204.
13. Fiona E. Matthews, Carol Brayne, James Lowe, Ian McKeith, Stephen B. Wharton, and Paul Ince, "Epidemiological Pathology of Dementia: Attributable-Risks at Death in the Medical Research Council Cognitive Function and Ageing Study," *PLoS Medicine* 6, no. 11 (2009), https://doi.org/10.1371/journal.pmed.1000180.
14. Jon B. Toledo, Steven E. Arnold, Kevin Raible, Johannes Brettschneider, Sharon X. Xie, Murray Grossman, Sarah E. Monsell, Walter A. Kukull, and John Q. Trojanowski,

"Contribution of Cerebrovascular Disease in Autopsy Confirmed Neurodegenerative Disease Cases in the National Alzheimer's Coordinating Centre," *Brain* 136, no. 9 (2013): 2697–2706.

15. Matthews et al., "Epidemiological Pathology of Dementia."
16. Robert E. Mrak and W. Sue T. Griffin, "Dementia with Lewy Bodies: Definition, Diagnosis, and Pathogenic Relationship to Alzheimer's Disease," *Neuropsychiatric Disease and Treatment* 3, no. 5 (2007): 619.
17. Julie A. Schneider, Zoe Arvanitakis, Sue E. Leurgans, and David A. Bennett, "The Neuropathology of Probable Alzheimer Disease and Mild Cognitive Impairment," *Annals of Neurology: Official Journal of the American Neurological Association and the Child Neurology Society* 66, no. 2 (2009): 200–208.
18. Catalina Amador-Ortiz, Wen-Lang Lin, Zeshan Ahmed, David Personett, Peter Davies, Ranjan Duara, Neill R. Graff-Radford, Michael L. Hutton, and Dennis W. Dickson, "TDP-43 Immunoreactivity in Hippocampal Sclerosis and Alzheimer's Disease," *Annals of Neurology: Official Journal of the American Neurological Association and the Child Neurology Society* 61, no. 5 (2007): 435–45.
19. Shinji Higashi, Eizo Iseki, Ryoko Yamamoto, Michiko Minegishi, Hiroaki Hino, Koshiro Fujisawa, Takashi Togo, et al., "Concurrence of TDP-43, Tau and α-Synuclein Pathology in Brains of Alzheimer's Disease and Dementia with Lewy Bodies," *Brain Research* 1184 (2007): 284–94.
20. Patricia A. Boyle, Lei Yu, Robert S. Wilson, Sue E. Leurgans, Julie A. Schneider, and David A. Bennett, "Person-Specific Contribution of Neuropathologies to Cognitive Loss in Old Age," *Annals of Neurology* 83, no. 1 (2018): 74–83.
21. John L. Robinson, Edward B. Lee, Sharon X. Xie, Lior Rennert, EunRan Suh, Colin Bredenberg, Carrie Caswell, et al., "Neurodegenerative Disease Concomitant Proteinopathies Are prevalent, Age-Related and APOE4-Associated," *Brain* 141, no. 7 (2018): 2181–93.
22. Lidia Sarro, Nirubol Tosakulwong, Christopher G. Schwarz, Jonathan Graff-Radford, Scott A. Przybelski, Timothy G. Lesnick, Samantha M. Zuk, et al., "An Investigation of Cerebrovascular Lesions in Dementia with Lewy Bodies Compared to Alzheimer's Disease," *Alzheimer's and Dementia* 13, no. 3 (2017): 257–66.
23. Elizabeth J. Coulthard and Seth Love, "A Broader View of Dementia: Multiple Copathologies Are the Norm," *Brain* 141, no. 7 (2018): 1894–97.
24. Simon D'Alton, Sally Hunter, Peter Whitehouse, Carol Brayne, and Daniel George, "Adapting to Dementia in Society: A Challenge for Our Lifetimes and a Charge for Public Health," *Journal of Alzheimer's Disease* 42, no. 4 (2014): 1151–63.
25. Dale Bredesen, *The End of Alzheimer's: The First Program to Prevent and Reverse Cognitive Decline* (New York: Penguin, 2017).
26. Gina Kolata, "The Diagnosis Is Alzheimer's: But That's Probably Not the Only Problem," *New York Times*, April 8, 2019, sec. Health, https://www.nytimes.com/2019/04/08/health/alzheimers-dementia-stroke.html.
27. Margaret Lock, *The Alzheimer Conundrum: Entanglements of Dementia and Aging* (Princeton, NJ: Princeton University Press, 2017).
28. Carol Brayne and Daniel Davis, "Making Alzheimer's and Dementia Research Fit for Populations," *Lancet* 380, no. 9851 (2012): 1441–43.
29. George M. Savva, Stephen B. Wharton, Paul G. Ince, Gillian Forster, Fiona E. Matthews, and Carol Brayne, "Age, Neuropathology, and Dementia," *New England Journal of Medicine* 360, no. 22 (2009): 2302–9.
30. Margaret Lock, *The Alzheimer Conundrum: Entanglements of Dementia and Aging* (Princeton, NJ: Princeton University Press, 2017), 41.
31. Newt Gingrich and Michelle Stein, "Alzheimer's: The Fight that Matters," *Minneapolis Star Tribune*, September 21, 2009.

32. Sandra Day O'Connor, Stanley Prusiner, and Ken Dychtwald, "Opinion: The Age of Alzheimer's," *New York Times*, October 27, 2010, sec. Opinion, https://www.nytimes.com/2010/10/28/opinion/28oconnor.html.
33. "Team Develops Plan to Globally Crowdsource Breakthrough Innovations to End Alzheimer's," Business Wire, press release, September 7, 2017, https://www.businesswire.com/news/home/20170907005232/en/Team-Develops-Plan-Globally-Crowdsource-Breakthrough-Innovations.
34. Kolata, "Diagnosis Is Alzheimer's."
35. Francesca Mangialasche, Alina Solomon, Bengt Winblad, Patrizia Mecocci, and Miia Kivipelto, "Alzheimer's Disease: Clinical Trials and Drug Development," *Lancet Neurology* 9, no. 7 (2010): 702–16.
36. Some now worry that the Alzheimer's field is thus beginning to resemble the antiaging medicine quacks who promise the public that we will soon cure aging itself.
37. Bill Gates, "Why I'm Digging Deep into Alzheimer's," *Gates Notes* (blog), November 13, 2017, https://www.gatesnotes.com/Health/Digging-Deep-Into-Alzheimers.
38. Sanjay Gupta, "Bill Gates' Newest Mission: Curing Alzheimer's," CNN, November 14, 2017, https://www.cnn.com/2017/11/13/health/bill-gates-announcement-alzheimers/index.html.
39. Howard Fillit, "Pfizer Ends Its Neuroscience Program—What Does It Mean for Alzheimer's?" *HuffPost*, January 10, 2018, https://www.huffpost.com/entry/pfizer-ends-its-neuroscience-programwhat-does-it-mean_b_5a5521a1e4b0f9b24bf31b53.
40. Atul Gawande, "Testing, Testing: The Healthcare Bill Has No Master Plan for Curbing Costs. Is That a Bad Thing?" *New Yorker*, December 7, 2009.
41. Nathaniel Popper and Bill Vlasic, "Quiet Doctor, Lavish Insider: A Parallel Life," *New York Times*, December 15, 2012, sec. Business, https://www.nytimes.com/2012/12/16/business/sidney-gilmans-shift-led-to-insider-trading-case.html.
42. See excellent reporting in the *Ann Arbor Observer*: Michael Betzold, "The Corruption of Sid Gilman: How a Top U-M Doctor Lost His Way," *Ann Arbor Observer*, January 2013, https://annarborobserver.com/articles/the_corruption_of_sid_gilman.html#.Xlfd4hNKiL5.
43. R. A. Sperling, P. S. Aisen, L. A. Beckett, D. A. Bennett, S. Craft, A. M. Fagan, T. Iwatsubo, et al., "Toward Defining the Preclinical Stages of Alzheimer's Disease: Recommendations from the National Institute on Aging—Alzheimer's Association Workgroups on Diagnostic Guidelines for Alzheimer's Disease," *Alzheimer's and Dementia* 7(2011): 280–92, doi:10.1016/j.jalz.2011.03.003.
44. Search results for "mild cognitive impairment," ClinicalTrials.gov, accessed February 27, 2020, https://clinicaltrials.gov/ct2/results?cond=Mild+Cognitive+Impairment&term=&cntry=&state=&city=&dist=.
45. Seema Y. Pandya, Laura H. Lacritz, Myron F. Weiner, Martin Deschner, and Fu L. Woon, "Predictors of Reversion from Mild Cognitive Impairment to Normal Cognition," *Dementia and Geriatric Cognitive Disorders* 43, nos. 3-4 (2017): 204–14.
46. See Mary Ganguli, Hiroko H. Dodge, Changyu Shen, and Steven T. DeKosky, "Mild Cognitive Impairment, Amnestic Type: An Epidemiologic Study," *Neurology* 63, no. 1 (2004): 115–21; Sujuan Gao, Frederick W. Unverzagt, Kathleen S. Hall, Kathleen A. Lane, Jill R. Murrell, Ann M. Hake, Valerie Smith-Gamble, and Hugh C. Hendrie, "Mild Cognitive Impairment, Incidence, Progression, and Reversion: Findings from a Community-Based Cohort of Elderly African Americans," *American Journal of Geriatric Psychiatry* 22, no. 7 (2014): 670–81; Hanna Kaduszkiewicz, Marion Eisele, Birgitt Wiese, Jana Prokein, Melanie Luppa, Tobias Luck, Frank Jessen, et al., "Prognosis of Mild Cognitive Impairment in General Practice: Results of the German AgeCoDe Study," *Annals of Family Medicine* 12, no. 2 (2014): 158–65; Jennifer J. Manly, Ming-X. Tang, Nicole Schupf, Yaakov Stern, Jean-Paul G.

Vonsattel, and Richard Mayeux, "Frequency and Course of Mild Cognitive Impairment in a Multiethnic Community," *Annals of Neurology: Official Journal of the American Neurological Association and the Child Neurology Society* 63, no. 4 (2008): 494–506.

47. Paula Span, "A Brain Scan May Predict Alzheimer's: Should You Get One?" *New York Times*, August 2, 2019, sec. Health, https://www.nytimes.com/2019/08/02/health/alzheimers-brain-scan.html.
48. Stephen Katz, Kevin Peters, and Peri Ballantyne, "Narrative Practices and Ethical Fallout: The Case of Mild Cognitive Impairment (MCI) Diagnosis." Presented at "Mapping a Critical Ethical Landscape for Dementia Research, Policy and Practice," Joint Conference of the International Association of Gerontology and Geriatrics World Congress and The Gerontology Society of America, July 23-27, 2017, San Francisco, California.
49. Lock, *Alzheimer Conundrum*, 91.
50. Renee Beard, *Living with Alzheimer's: Managing Memory Loss, Identity, and Illness* (New York: New York University Press, 2016).
51. Stina Saunders, Karen Ritchie, Tom C. Russ, Graciela Muniz-Terrera, and Craig W. Ritchie, "Evolution and Future Directions for the Concept of Mild Cognitive Impairment," *International Psychogeriatrics* 30, no. 10 (2018): 1431–34.
52. "Aging Mother Knows Any Wrong Move Could Be Taken for Telltale Sign of Dementia," *Onion*, October 13, 2015, https://www.theonion.com/aging-mother-knows-any-wrong-move-could-be-taken-for-te-1819578320.
53. George and Whitehouse, "Marketplace of Memory."
54. Global Council on Brain Health, "The Real Deal on Brain Health Supplements: GCBH Recommendations on Vitamins, Minerals, and Other Dietary Supplements," Global Council on Brain Health, June 11, 2019, https://www.aarp.org/content/dam/aarp/health/brain_health/2019/06/gcbh-supplements-report-english.doi.10.26419-2Fpia.00094.001.pdf.
55. For a great read on the nootropic marketplace, see Kaitlyn Tiffany, "The All-Too-Understandable Urge to Buy a Better Brain," *Vox*, July 8, 2019, https://www.vox.com/the-goods/2019/7/8/18772467/nootropics-silicon-valley-brain-fitness-goop-smart-drugs.
56. "BrainGear Brain Booster Natural Nootropic Supplement," Amazon, accessed February 27, 2020, https://www.amazon.com/BrainGear-Brain-Nutrition-Drink-BlackBerry/dp/B07JJMGG4B?th=1.
57. Ibid.
58. Drew DeMartinis, "Nerd Alert: A Chew that Gives You a Mental Boost," Goop, February 24, 2019, https://goop.com/wellness/health/nerd-alert-mental-boost-chew-review/.
59. "Genius Consciousness," the Genius Brand, accessed February 27, 2020, https://thegeniusbrand.com/products/genius-consciousness.
60. "Alpha Brain," Onnit, accessed February 27, 2020, https://www.onnit.com/alphabrain/.
61. Global Council on Brain Health, "Real Deal on Brain Health Supplements."
62. Christina Farr, "This Start-up Raised Millions to Sell 'Brain Hacking' Pills, but Its Own Study Found Coffee Works Better," CNBC, November 30, 2017, https://www.cnbc.com/2017/11/30/hvmn-nootrobox-study-smart-pill-less-effective-than-caffeine.html.
63. "FDA Takes Action against 17 Companies for Illegally Selling Products Claiming to Treat Alzheimer's Disease," FDA, press release, February 11, 2019, http://www.fda.gov/news-events/press-announcements/fda-takes-action-against-17-companies-illegally-selling-products-claiming-treat-alzheimers-disease.
64. Paula Span, "Supplements Won't Prevent Dementia, But These Steps Might," *New York Times*, March 1, 2019, sec. Health, https://www.nytimes.com/2019/03/01/health/dementia-prevention-supplements.html.
65. Pieter A. Cohen, Igor Zakharevich, and Roy Gerona, "Presence of Piracetam in Cognitive Enhancement Dietary Supplements," *JAMA Internal Medicine* 180, no. 3 (2020): 458–59.
66. Research and Markets, "Global Cognitive Assessment and Training Market 2017-2021: Aging Population, Increasing Awareness for Brain Fitness and Advancement in

Technology Drive the $8.06 Billion Market—Research and Markets," CISION PR Newswire, press release, April 21, 2017, https://www.prnewswire.com/news-releases/global-cognitive-assessment-and-training-market-2017-2021-aging-population-increasing-awareness-for-brain-fitness—advancement-in-technology-drive-the-806-billion-market-research-and-markets-300443424.html.

67. George and Whitehouse, "Marketplace of Memory."
68. "Nintendo Brain Age 2: More Training in Minutes a Day," Amazon, accessed June 4, 2020, https://www.amazon.it/Nintendo-Brain-Age-Training-Educational/dp/B06Y2C4BRP.
69. Big Brain Academy: Wii Degree, "Flex Your Brain the Fun Way with Family and Friends, GameSpot, June 7, 2008, https://www.gamespot.com/big-brain-academy-wii-degree/user-reviews/2200-102918/.
70. Brain HQ, "Social Life and Brain Fitness," https://www.brainhq.com/brain-resources/everyday-brain-fitness/social-life-brain-fitness. Elevate—Your Personal Brain Trainer, accessed June 4, 2020, https://www.elevateapp.com.
71. *Brain Age: Train Your Brain in Minutes a Day!* instruction booklet, accessed June 4, 2020, https://www.nintendo.com/consumer/gameslist/manuals/DS_Brain_Age.pdf.
72. Robert L. Kane, Mary Butler, Howard A. Fink, Michelle Brasure, Heather Davila, Priyanka Desai, Eric Jutkowitz, et al., *Interventions to Prevent Age-Related Cognitive Decline, Mild Cognitive Impairment, and Clinical Alzheimer's-Type Dementia* (Rockville, MD: Agency for Healthcare Research and Quality, 2017).
73. Adrian M. Owen, Adam Hampshire, Jessica A. Grahn, Robert Stenton, Said Dajani, Alistair S. Burns, Robert J. Howard, and Clive G. Ballard, "Putting Brain Training to the Test," *Nature* 465, no. 7299 (2010): 775–78.
74. Kathryn V. Papp, Stephen J. Walsh, and Peter J. Snyder, "Immediate and Delayed Effects of Cognitive Interventions in Healthy Elderly: A Review of Current Literature and Future Directions," *Alzheimer's and Dementia* 5, no. 1 (2009): 50–60.
75. "The ACTIVE Study," BrainHQ, Posit Science, accessed February 27, 2020, https://www.brainhq.com/world-class-science/published-research/active-study.
76. "A Consensus on the Brain Training Industry from the Scientific Community," Stanford Center on Longevity, October 20, 2014, http://longevity.stanford.edu/a-consensus-on-the-brain-training-industry-from-the-scientific-community-2/.
77. Ibid.
78. "Lumosity to Pay $2 Million to Settle FTC Deceptive Advertising Charges for Its 'Brain Training' Program," Federal Trade Commission, press release, January 5, 2016, https://www.ftc.gov/news-events/press-releases/2016/01/lumosity-pay-2-million-settle-ftc-deceptive-advertising-charges.
79. Edward Ratner and David Atkinson, "Why Cognitive Training and Brain Games Will Not Prevent or Forestall Dementia," *Journal of the American Geriatrics Society* 3, no. 12 (2015): 2612–14.
80. Sabrina Weiss, "Brain Training Apps Don't Really Work: So Why Do We Love Them?" *Wired UK*, October 6, 2019, https://www.wired.co.uk/article/nintendo-brain-training-switch.
81. See Sharp Brains website, accessed June 4, 2020, http://www.SharpBrains.com. Note: Peter has worked with Sharp Brains (unpaid).
82. Apollo Health, "ReCODE Report Delivers Personalized Information that Helps Prevent and Reverse Cognitive Decline," accessed May 27, 2020, https://www.apollohealthco.com/solution/recode/.
83. Bredesen, *End of Alzheimer's*.
84. "Blair Calls for Lifestyle Change," BBC News, July 26, 2006, http://news.bbc.co.uk/2/hi/uk_news/politics/5215548.stm.
85. Charlie Boothe, "Potential Teacher Strike Looms over West Virginia," *Bluefield (WV) Daily Telegraph*, January 29, 2018, https://www.bdtonline.com/news/potential-teacher-strike-looms-over-west-virginia/article_32f4a9f4-04a1-11e8-99f2-7f31dc816267.html.

86. Lock, *Alzheimer Conundrum.*
87. WHO and Alzheimer's Disease International, *Dementia: A Public Health Priority* (Geneva: WHO, 2012), http://www.who.int/mental_health/publications/dementia_report_2012/en/.
88. Alzheimer's Association and CDC, "Making Alzheimer's Our Next Public Health Success Story," Healthy Brain Initiative, 2018, https://www.cdc.gov/aging/pdf/executive-brief-HBI-2018-road-map-final-508.pdf.
89. "Why People in Finland Are so Much Happier than Americans," Davidson Home Group, March 20, 2019, https://www.davidsonhomegroup.com/2019/03/20/why-people-in-finland-are-so-much-happier-than-americans/.
90. Peter Reed, Jennifer Carson, and Zebbedia Gibb, "Transcending the Tragedy Discourse of Dementia: An Ethical Imperative for Promoting Selfhood, Meaningful Relationships, and Well-Being," *AMA Journal of Ethics* 19, no. 7 (2017): 693–703.
91. "NIH State-of-the-Science Conference: Preventing Alzheimer's Disease and Cognitive Decline, Day 3," video, 2:01:20, Bill Thies at 93:40, http://videocast.nih.gov/summary.asp?Live=8412.
92. Susan M. Behuniak, "The Living Dead? The Construction of People with Alzheimer's Disease as Zombies," *Ageing and Society* 31, no. 1 (2011): 70–92.
93. Nacho Gayan, dir., "Alzheimer 'Heureusement,'" video, 0:46, flouze1, May 6, 2009, https://www.youtube.com/watch?v=C8EWWCNhFao.
94. Carol Bryden, *Nothing about Us without Us: 20 Years of Dementia Advocacy* (London: Jessica Kingsley, 2016), 138.
95. Alzheimer Autrement petition, August 2009, http://www.alzheimer-autrement.org/petition.php3.
96. Newt Gingrich, *Winning the Future: A 21st Century Contract with America*, rev. ed. (Lanham, MD: Regnery, 2006), 132.
97. Robin Marantz Henig, "The Last Day of Her Life," *New York Times*, May 14, 2015, sec. Magazine, https://www.nytimes.com/2015/05/17/magazine/the-last-day-of-her-life.html.
98. Comedian Norm MacDonald provides an utterly brilliant critique of our tendency to use war metaphors in understanding chronic disease: "Norm Macdonald—Battling Cancer," season 1, ep. 1, *Norm Macdonald: Me Doing Stand-Up*, Comedy Central, March 25, 2011, video clip, 2:34, http://www.cc.com/video-clips/8kgu68/battling-cancer.
99. James Geary, *I Is an Other: The Secret Life of Metaphor and How It Shapes the Way We See the World* (New York: Harper Collins, 2011).

CHAPTER 4. TREATING POPULATIONS

1. Ken M. Langa, Eric B. Larson, and E. Crimmins, "A Comparison of the Prevalence of Dementia in the United States in 2000 and 2012," *JAMA Internal Medicine* 177 (2017): 51–58.
2. K. G. Manton, X. L. Gu, and S. V. Ukraintseva, "Declining Prevalence of Dementia in the US Elderly Population," *Advanced Gerontology* 16 (2005): 30–37.
3. Claudia L. Satizabal, Alexa S. Beiser, Vincent Chouraki, Geneviève Chêne, Carole Dufouil, and Sudha Seshadri, "Incidence of Dementia over Three Decades in the Framingham Heart Study," *New England Journal of Medicine* 374, no. 6 (2016): 523–32.
4. Kenneth M. Langa, Eric B. Larson, Jason H. Karlawish, David M. Cutler, Mohammed U. Kabeto, Scott Y. Kim, and Allison B. Rosen, "Trends in the Prevalence and Mortality of Cognitive Impairment in the United States: Is There Evidence of a Compression of Cognitive Morbidity?" *Alzheimer's and Dementia* 4, no. 2 (2008): 134–44.
5. Chengxuan Qiu, Eva von Strauss, Lars Bäckman, Bengt Winblad, and Laura Fratiglioni, "Twenty-Year Changes in Dementia Occurrence Suggest Decreasing Incidence in Central Stockholm, Sweden," *Neurology* 80, no. 20 (2013): 1888–94.
6. Elisabeth M. C. Schrijvers, Benjamin F. J. Verhaaren, Peter J. Koudstaal, Albert Hofman, M.Arfan Ikram, and Monique M. B. Breteler, "Is Dementia Incidence Declining?: Trends

in Dementia Incidence since 1990 in the Rotterdam Study," *Neurology* 78, no. 19 (2012): 1456–63.

7. See Fiona E. Matthews, Antony Arthur, Linda E. Barnes, John Bond, Carol Jagger, Louise Robinson, Carol Brayne, and Medical Research Council Cognitive Function and Ageing Collaboration, "A Two-Decade Comparison of Prevalence of Dementia in Individuals Aged 65 Years and Older from Three Geographical Areas of England: Results of the Cognitive Function and Ageing Study I and II," *Lancet* 382, no. 9902 (2013): 1405–12; Fiona E. Matthews, Blossom C. M. Stephan, Louise Robinson, Carol Jagger, Linda E. Barnes, Antony Arthur, and Carol Brayne, "A Two Decade Dementia Incidence Comparison from the Cognitive Function and Ageing Studies I and II," *Nature Communications* 7, no. 1 (2016): 1–8.
8. Gill Livingston, Andrew Sommerlad, Vasiliki Orgeta, Sergi G. Costafreda, Jonathan Huntley, David Ames, Clive Ballard, et al., "Dementia Prevention, Intervention, and Care," *Lancet* 390, no. 10113 (2017): 2673–2734.
9. Leslie Grasset, Carol Brayne, Pierre Joly, Hélène Jacqmin-Gadda, Karine Peres, Alexandra Foubert-Samier, Jean-François Dartigues, and Catherine Helmer, "Trends in Dementia Incidence: Evolution over a 10-Year Period in France," *Alzheimer's and Dementia* 12, no. 3 (2016): 272–80.
10. Sujuan Gao, Heather N. Burney, Chris M. Callahan, Christianna E. Purnell, and Hugh C. Hendrie, "Incidence of Dementia and Alzheimer Disease over Time: A Meta-analysis," *Journal of the American Geriatrics Society* 67, no. 7 (2019): 1361–69.
11. Yu-Tzu Wu, Alexa S. Beiser, Monique M. B. Breteler, Laura Fratiglioni, Catherine Helmer, Hugh C. Hendrie, Hiroyuki Honda, et al., "The Changing Prevalence and Incidence of Dementia over Time—Current Evidence," *Nature Reviews Neurology* 13, no. 6 (2017): 327.
12. Frank J. Wolters, Lori B. Chibnik, Reem Waziry, Roy Anderson, Claudine Berr, Alexa Beiser, Joshua C. Bis et al. "Twenty-seven-year time trends in dementia incidence in Europe and the United States: The Alzheimer Cohorts Consortium." Neurology 95, no. 5 (2020): e519–e531.
13. Even the most conservative estimates suggest such societies have, at worst, tended to possess a "moderate" level of inequality comparable to that of the modern-day social democracy of Denmark. See Eric Alden Smith, Kim Hill, Frank W. Marlowe, David Nolin, Polly Wiessner, Michael Gurven, Samuel Bowles, Monique Borgerhoff Mulder, Tom Hertz, and Adrian Bell, "Wealth Transmission and Inequality among Hunter-Gatherers," *Current Anthropology* 51, no. 1 (2010): 19–34.
14. Christopher Boehm, *Hierarchy in the Forest: The Evolution of Egalitarian Behavior* (Cambridge, MA: Harvard University Press, 2001), 12.
15. Yuval Noah Harari, *Homo Deus: A Brief History of Tomorrow* (New York: Random House, 2016), 141.
16. Daniel Smith, Philip Schlaepfer, Katie Major, Mark Dyble, Abigail E. Page, James Thompson, Nikhil Chaudhary, et al., "Cooperation and the Evolution of Hunter-Gatherer Storytelling," *Nature Communications* 8, no. 1 (December 5, 2017): 1-9, https://doi.org/10.1038/s41467-017-02036-8.
17. Jordan B. Peterson, Norman Doidge, and Ethan Van Sciver, *12 Rules for Life: An Antidote to Chaos* (Toronto: Random House Canada, 2018).
18. Boehm, *Hierarchy in the Forest*, 231.
19. Ibid., 41.
20. There is some evidence of fishing villages in the Indonesian Islands around 45,000 years ago, which would predate agricultural settlements.
21. Yuval Noah Harari, *Sapiens: A Brief History of Humankind* (New York: Random House, 2014), 77.
22. Jared Diamond, "The Worst Mistake in the History of the Human Race," *Discover*, May 1, 1999, https://www.discovermagazine.com/planet-earth/the-worst-mistake-in-the-history-of-the-human-race.

23. Mark Nathan Cohen, "The Emergence of Health and Social Inequalities in the Archaeological Record," in *Human Biology and Social Inequality*, ed. S. S. Strickland and P. S. Shetty (Cambridge: Cambridge University Press, 1998), 249–71.
24. While the New Deal in the United States largely succeeded in extending benefits to the whole population based on an ethos of inclusivity and equality, its implementation was challenged by the discrimination, bigotry, and hierarchies rooted in American society during the early 20th century. As a result, marginalized and racialized Americans were less able to enjoy its benefits and protections. For more, see "New Deal Inclusion," the Living New Deal, accessed May 27, 2020, https://livingnewdeal.org/what-was-the-new-deal/new-deal-inclusion/.
25. Diane Coyle, *The Weightless World: Strategies for Managing the Digital Economy* (Cambridge, MA: MIT Press, 1998).
26. Boehm, *Hierarchy in the Forest.*
27. "Social Spending," OECD Data, accessed February 27, 2020, http://data.oecd.org/socialexp/social-spending.htm.
28. Facundo Alvaredo, Lucas Chancel, Thomas Piketty, Emmanuel Saez, and Gabriel Zucman, eds., *World Inequality Report 2018* (Cambridge, MA: Belknap Press, 2018), http://wir2018.wid.world/files/download/wir2018-full-report-english.pdf.
29. "At DNC, Bernie Sanders Repeats Claim that Top One-Tenth of 1% Owns as Much Wealth as Bottom 90%," *Politifact*, July 26, 2016, https://www.politifact.com/factchecks/2016/jul/26/bernie-sanders/dnc-bernie-sanders-repeats-claim-top-one-tenth-1-o/.
30. Katie Hope, "'World's Richest 1% Get 82% of the Wealth,' Says Oxfam," *BBC News*, January 22, 2018, sec. Business, https://www.bbc.com/news/business-42745853.
31. Catherine Clifford, "Bill Gates, Jeff Bezos and Warren Buffett Have More Wealth than Half the Population of the US Combined," *CNBC*, November 9, 2017, https://www.cnbc.com/2017/11/09/gates-bezos-buffett-have-more-wealth-than-half-the-us-combined.html.
32. "Making the Rich Pay Their Fair Share in Taxes," Bernie Sanders official campaign website, accessed May 27, 2020, https://berniesanders.com/en/issues/tax-increases-for-the-rich/.
33. Prachi Bhardwaj, "Jeff Bezos Got So Rich in 2018 that He Now Makes More per Minute than Most People Do in a Year," *Business Insider*, December 19, 2018, https://www.businessinsider.com/how-much-jeff-bezos-makes-per-minute-2018-12.
34. Emily Wells, "'Paradise Papers' Show How Wealthy Stash Riches, Dodge Taxes," *Truthdig*, November 6, 2017, https://www.truthdig.com/articles/paradise-papers-show-wealthy-stash-riches-dodge-taxes/.
35. Jose Pagliery, "You Can Now Search the Panama Papers Database Online," *CNNMoney*, May 6, 2016, https://money.cnn.com/2016/05/06/technology/panama-papers-search/index.html.
36. Anne Case and Angus Deaton, "Rising Morbidity and Mortality in Midlife among White Non-Hispanic Americans in the 21st Century," *Proceedings of the National Academy of Sciences* 112, no. 49 (2015): 15078–83.
37. Adeel Hassan, "Deaths from Drugs and Suicide Reach a Record in the U.S," *New York Times*, March 7, 2019, sec. U.S., https://www.nytimes.com/2019/03/07/us/deaths-drugs-suicide-record.html.
38. Steven H. Woolf and Heidi Schoomaker, "Life Expectancy and Mortality Rates in the United States, 1959-2017," *JAMA* 322, no. 20 (November 26, 2019): 1996-2016, https://doi.org/10.1001/jama.2019.16932.
39. Sherry L. Murphy, Jiaquan Xu, Kenneth D. Kochanek, and Elizabeth Arias, *Mortality in the United States, 2017* (Hyattsville, MD: U.S. Department of Health and Human Services, Centers for Disease Control and Prevention, National Center for Health Statistics, 2018).
40. Elizabeth M. Stein, Keith P. Gennuso, Donna C. Ugboaja, and Patrick L. Remington, "The Epidemic of Despair among White Americans: Trends in the Leading Causes of Premature Death, 1999–2015," *American Journal of Public Health* 107, no. 10 (2017): 1541–47.

41. Usama Bilal and Ana V. Diez-Roux, "Troubling Trends in Health Disparities," *New England Journal of Medicine* 378, no. 16 (2018): 1557–58.
42. Anne Case and Angus Deaton, "Mortality and Morbidity in the 21st Century," *Brookings Papers on Economic Activity* 1 (2017): 397–476, esp. 409.
43. Matthew Goodwin, "'Deaths of Despair' Aren't Just a U.S. Problem," *Yahoo Finance*, January 22, 2020, https://finance.yahoo.com/news/deaths-despair-aren-t-just-085546457.html.
44. "'Deaths of Despair' Could Cause Life Expectancy to Decline: Experts," *HuffPost Canada*, November 5, 2018, https://www.huffingtonpost.ca/2018/11/05/canadian-life-expectancy-declines_a_23580643/.
45. Kate Aubusson, "More Women Suffering 'Deaths of Despair' but Wealthiest Are Shielded, Study Shows," *Sydney Morning Herald*, July 19, 2019, https://www.smh.com.au/healthcare/more-women-suffering-deaths-of-despair-but-wealthiest-are-shielded-study-shows-20190718-p528dp.html.
46. Matthew J. Loe and William D. Edwards, "A Light-Hearted Look at a Lion-Hearted Organ (or, a Perspective from Three Standard Deviations beyond the Norm), Part 1 (of Two Parts)," *Cardiovascular Pathology* 13, no. 5 (September 1, 2004): 282–92, https://doi.org/10.1016/j.carpath.2004.05.001.
47. "Blood Vessels," the Franklin Institute, accessed June 2, 2015, https://www.fi.edu/heart/blood-vessels.
48. Rebecca F. Gottesman, Andrea L. C. Schneider, Yun Zhou, Josef Coresh, Edward Green, Naresh Gupta, David S. Knopman, et al., "Association between Midlife Vascular Risk Factors and Estimated Brain Amyloid Deposition," *Journal of the American Medical Association* 317, no. 14 (2017): 1443–50.
49. Bridget M. Kuehn, "In Alzheimer Research, Glucose Metabolism Moves to Center Stage," *Journal of the American Medical Association* 323, no. 4 (2020): 297.
50. Pauline Anderson, "Heart Function Tied to Brain Function," Medscape, November 8, 2017, http://www.medscape.com/viewarticle/888207.
51. Jennifer S. Rabin, Aaron P. Schultz, Trey Hedden, Anand Viswanathan, Gad A. Marshall, Emily Kilpatrick, Hannah Klein, et al., "Interactive Associations of Vascular Risk and β-Amyloid Burden with Cognitive Decline in Clinically Normal Elderly Individuals: Findings from the Harvard Aging Brain Study," *JAMA Neurology* 75, no. 9 (September 1, 2018): 1124–31, https://doi.org/10.1001/jamaneurol.2018.1123.
52. David A. Snowdon, Lydia H. Greiner, James A. Mortimer, Kathryn P. Riley, Philip A. Greiner, and William R. Markesbery, "Brain Infarction and the Clinical Expression of Alzheimer Disease: The Nun Study," *Journal of the American Medical Association* 277, no. 10 (1997): 813–17.
53. Margaret M. Esiri, Zsuzsanna Nagy, Maria Z. Smith, Lin Barnetson, and A. David Smith, "Cerebrovascular Disease and Threshold for Dementia in the Early Stages of Alzheimer's Disease," *Lancet* 354, no. 9182 (1999): 919–20.
54. Dina Zekry, Charles Duyckaerts, Robert Moulias, Joël Belmin, Caroline Geoffre, François Herrmann, and Jean-Jacques Hauw, "Degenerative and Vascular Lesions of the Brain Have Synergistic Effects in Dementia of the Elderly," *Acta Neuropathologica* 103, no. 5 (2002): 481–87.
55. J. A. Schneider, R. S. Wilson, J. L. Bienias, D. A. Evans, and D. A. Bennett, "Cerebral Infarctions and the Likelihood of Dementia from Alzheimer Disease Pathology," *Neurology* 62, no. 7 (2004): 1148–55.
56. Jens Sundbøll, Erzsébet Horváth-Puhó, Kasper Adelborg, Morten Schmidt, Lars Pedersen, Hans Erik Bøtker, Victor W. Henderson, and Henrik Toft Sørensen, "Higher Risk of Vascular Dementia in Myocardial Infarction Survivors," *Circulation* 137, no. 6 (February 6, 2018): 567–77.
57. M. F. Elias, P. K. Elias, L. M. Sullivan, P. A. Wolf, and R. B. D'Agostino, "Lower Cognitive Function in the Presence of Obesity and Hypertension: The Framingham Heart Study," *International Journal of Obesity* 27, no. 2 (2003): 260–68.

58. Sara Kaffashian, Aline Dugravot, Hermann Nabi, G. David Batty, Eric Brunner, Mika Kivimäki, and Archana Singh-Manoux, "Predictive Utility of the Framingham General Cardiovascular Disease Risk Profile for Cognitive Function: Evidence from the Whitehall II Study," *European Heart Journal* 32, no. 18 (2011): 2326–32.
59. Deborah E. Barnes and Kristine Yaffe, "The Projected Effect of Risk Factor Reduction on Alzheimer's Disease Prevalence," *Lancet Neurology* 10, no. 9 (2011): 819–28.
60. J. A. Luchsinger, Christiane Reitz, Larry S. Honig, Ming-Xin Tang, Steven Shea, and Richard Mayeux, "Aggregation of Vascular Risk Factors and Risk of Incident Alzheimer Disease," *Neurology* 65, no. 4 (2005): 545–51.
61. Rebecca F. Gottesman, Marilyn S. Albert, Alvaro Alonso, Laura H. Coker, Josef Coresh, Sonia M. Davis, Jennifer A. Deal, et al., "Associations between Midlife Vascular Risk Factors and 25-Year Incident Dementia in the Atherosclerosis Risk in Communities (ARIC) Cohort." *JAMA Neurology* 74, no. 10 (2017): 1246–54.
62. Kristine Yaffe, "Prevention of Cognitive Impairment with Intensive Systolic Blood Pressure Control," *JAMA* 321, no. 6 (2019): 548–49.
63. Jennifer S. Rabin, Hannah Klein, Dylan R. Kirn, Aaron P. Schultz, Hyun-Sik Yang, Olivia Hampton, Shu Jiang, et al., "Associations of Physical Activity and β-Amyloid with Longitudinal Cognition and Neurodegeneration in Clinically Normal Older Adults," *JAMA Neurology* 76, no. 10 (October 1, 2019): 1203–10.
64. Keenan A. Walker, A. Richey Sharrett, Aozhou Wu, Andrea L. C. Schneider, Marilyn Albert, Pamela L. Lutsey, Karen Bandeen-Roche, et al., "Association of Midlife to Late-Life Blood Pressure Patterns with Incident Dementia," *JAMA* 322, no. 6 (August 13, 2019): 535–45, https://doi.org/10.1001/jama.2019.10575.
65. "Hypertension and Dementia," JN Learning, JAMA Network, video, 7:36, August 13, 2019, https://edhub.ama-assn.org/jn-learning/video-player/17795085.
66. Emer R. McGrath, Alexa S. Beiser, Charles DeCarli, Kendra L. Plourde, Ramachandran S. Vasan, Steven M. Greenberg, and Sudha Seshadri, "Blood Pressure from Mid- to Late Life and Risk of Incident Dementia," *Neurology* 89, no. 24 (2017): 2447–54.
67. John Betjemann, J. Claude Hemphill, and Urmimala Sarkar, "Time for Neurologists to Drop the Reflex Hammer on Hypertension," *JAMA Neurology* 76, no. 11 (2019): 1277–78.
68. Séverine Sabia, Aurore Fayosse, Julien Dumurgier, Alexis Schnitzler, Jean-Philippe Empana, Klaus P. Ebmeier, Aline Dugravot, Mika Kivimäki, and Archana Singh-Manoux, "Association of Ideal Cardiovascular Health at Age 50 with Incidence of Dementia: 25 Year Follow-up of Whitehall II Cohort Study," *BMJ* 366 (2019): l4414.
69. M. J. A. P. Daemen, "The Heart and the Brain: An Intimate and Underestimated Relation," *Netherlands Heart Journal* 21, no. 2 (2013): 53–54.
70. Diarmaid Hughes, Conor Judge, Robert Murphy, Elaine Loughlin, Maria Costello, William Whiteley, Jackie Bosch, Martin J. O'Donnell, and Michelle Canavan, "Association of Blood Pressure Lowering With Incident Dementia or Cognitive Impairment: A Systematic Review and Meta-analysis," *Journal of the American Medical Association* 323, no. 19 (2020): 1934–44.
71. Schrecker and Bombra, *How Politics Makes Us Sick*.
72. Jeff D. Williamson, Nicholas M. Pajewski, Alexander P. Auchus, R. Nick Bryan, Gordon Chelune, Alfred K. Cheung, Maryjo L. Cleveland, et al., "Effect of Intensive vs. Standard Blood Pressure Control on Probable Dementia: A Randomized Clinical Trial," *Journal of the American Medical Association* 321, no. 6 (February 12, 2019): 553–61, https://doi.org/10.1001/jama.2018.21442.
73. Brent M. Egan, Yumin Zhao, and R. Neal Axon, "US Trends in Prevalence, Awareness, Treatment, and Control of Hypertension, 1988-2008," *Journal of the American Medical Association*303, no. 20 (2010): 2043–50.
74. Elena V. Kuklina, Paula W. Yoon, and Nora L. Keenan, "Trends in High Levels of Low-Density Lipoprotein Cholesterol in the United States, 1999-2006," *Journal of the American Medical Association*302, no. 19 (2009): 2104–10.

75. Yaffe, "Prevention of Cognitive Impairment," 548–49.
76. Ayodele Odutayo, Peter Gill, Shaun Shepherd, Aquila Akingbade, Sally Hopewell, Karthik Tennankore, Benjamin H. Hunn, and Connor A. Emdin, "Income Disparities in Absolute Cardiovascular Risk and Cardiovascular Risk Factors in the United States, 1999-2014," *JAMA Cardiology* 2, no. 7 (2017): 782–90.
77. D. Koller and Julie P. W. Bynum, "Dementia in the USA: State Variation in Prevalence," *Journal of Public Health* 37, no. 4 (December 1, 2015): 597–604, https://doi.org/10.1093/pubmed/fdu080.
78. "History of the Surgeon General's Reports on Smoking and Health," CDC, lastupdated, November 15, 2019, https://www.cdc.gov/tobacco/data_statistics/sgr/history/index.htm.
79. See "Current Cigarette Smoking among Adults in the United States," Centers for Disease Control and Prevention, last updated November 18, 2019, https://www.cdc.gov/tobacco/data_statistics/fact_sheets/adult_data/cig_smoking/index.htm; and US Office of the Surgeon General, *The Health Consequences of Smoking—50 Years of Progress: A Report of the Surgeon General* (Atlanta, GA: Department of Health and Human Services, National Center for Chronic Disease Prevention and Health Promotion, Office on Smoking and Health, 2014).
80. Hannah Ritchie and Max Roser, "Smoking," Our World in Data, May 2013, https://ourworldindata.org/smoking.
81. Kenneth M. Langa and Eric B. Larson, "Education, Brain Health, and Improving Life Opportunities for Women," *Journal of the Economics of Ageing* 4 (2014): 56–58.
82. See Deborah E. Barnes, Thaddeus J. Haight, Kala M. Mehta, Michelle C. Carlson, Lewis H. Kuller, and Ira B. Tager, "Secondhand Smoke, Vascular Disease, and Dementia Incidence: Findings from the Cardiovascular Health Cognition Study," *American Journal of Epidemiology* 171, no. 3 (2010): 292–302; Ruoling Chen, "Association of Environmental Tobacco Smoke with Dementia and Alzheimer's Disease among Never Smokers," *Alzheimer's and Dementia* 8, no. 6 (2012): 590–95.
83. Anne Case and Angus Deaton, *Deaths of Despair and the Future of Capitalism* (Princeton, NJ: Princeton University Press, 2020.
84. Claudia L. Satizabal, Alexa S. Beiser, Vincent Chouraki, Geneviève Chêne, Carole Dufouil, and Sudha Seshadri, "Incidence of Dementia over Three Decades in the Framingham Heart Study," *New England Journal of Medicine* 374, no. 6 (2016): 523–32.
85. Langa, Larson, and Crimmins, "Comparison of the Prevalence of Dementia."
86. Langa and Larson, "Education, Brain Health."
87. Hugh C. Hendrie, Valerie Smith-Gamble, Kathleen A. Lane, Christianna Purnell, Daniel O. Clark, and Sujuan Gao, "The Association of Early Life Factors and Declining Incidence Rates of Dementia in an Elderly Population of African Americans," *Journals of Gerontology: Series B* 73, supp. 1 (2018): S82–S89.
88. Kathleen S. Hall and Hugh C. Hendrie, "Early Childhood Environment and Dementia," *Lancet* 380, no. 9836 (July 2012): 11–12, https://doi.org/10.1016/S0140-6736(12)60767-3.
89. Martin Prince, Daisy Acosta, Cleusa P. Ferri, Mariella Guerra, Yueqin Huang, Juan J. Llibre Rodriguez, Aquiles Salas, et al., "Dementia Incidence and Mortality in Middle-Income Countries, and Associations with Indicators of Cognitive Reserve: A 10/66 Dementia Research Group Population-Based Cohort Study," *Lancet* 380, no. 9836 (2012): 50–58.
90. Robert Katzman, "Education and the Prevalence of Dementia and Alzheimer's Disease," *Neurology* 43, no. 1 (1993): 13.
91. William E. Leuchtenburg, *The FDR Years: On Roosevelt and His Legacy* (New York: Columbia University Press, 1995), 258.
92. John R. Thelin, Jason R. Edwards, Eric Moyen, Joseph B. Berger, and Maria Vita Calkins, "Higher Education in the United States—Historical Development, System," *Education Encyclopedia*, StateUniversity.com, accessed February 27, 2020, https://education.stateuniversity.com/pages/2044/Higher-Education-in-United-States.html.

93. John Bound and Sarah Turner, "Going to War and Going to College: Did World War II and the G.I. Bill Increase Educational Attainment for Returning Veterans?" *Journal of Labor Economics* 20, no. 4 (October 1, 2002): 784–815, https://doi.org/10.1086/342012.
94. Scott Carlson, "When College Was a Public Good," *Chronicle of Higher Education*, November 27, 2016, https://www.chronicle.com/article/When-College-Was-a-Public-Good/238501.
95. Margaret M. Strain, "In Defense of a Nation: The National Defense Education Act, Project English, and the Origins of Empirical Research in Composition," *JAC* 25, no. 3 (2005): 513–42, https://www.jstor.org/stable/20866703.
96. Stein, *Pivotal Decade*, 16.
97. "Student Enrollment Reports," Enrollment Services—Analysis and Reporting, The Ohio State University, accessed February 27, 2020, http://oesar.osu.edu/student_enrollment.aspx.
98. Devin Fergus, "My Students Pay Too Much for College: Blame Reagan," *Washington Post*, September 2, 2014, https://www.washingtonpost.com/posteverything/wp/2014/09/02/my-students-pay-too-much-for-college-blame-reagan/.
99. Carlson, "When College Was a Public Good."
100. Fergus, "My Students Pay Too Much for College."
101. Clay Shirky, "The End of Higher Education's Golden Age," Independent Educational Services, accessed February 27, 2020, http://www.ies-consulting.org/index.php/news-articles/184-the-end-of-higher-educations-golden-age.
102. "Tuition Costs of Colleges and Universities," National Center for Education Statistics, accessed February 27, 2020, https://nces.ed.gov/fastfacts/display.asp?id=76.
103. A full analysis of runaway costs and the decline of higher education (including the emergence of parasitic for-profit universities in the United States) is beyond the scope of this chapter, but scholars like Wendy Brown at the University of California, Berkeley, have done exceptionally interesting work in this area. For instance, see "Forum 22, Wendy Brown—The End of the Corporate University: What We Are Now," video, 1:32:43, UC Davis Forums, May 26, 2015, https://www.youtube.com/watch?v=Z5EWYohECRQ.
104. Ronald Brownstein, "American Higher Education Hits a Dangerous Milestone," *Atlantic*, May 3, 2018, https://www.theatlantic.com/politics/archive/2018/05/american-higher-education-hits-a-dangerous-milestone/559457/.
105. Judith Scott-Clayton and Jing Li, "Black-White Disparity in Student Loan Debt More than Triples after Graduation," *Brookings* (blog), October 20, 2016, https://www.brookings.edu/research/black-white-disparity-in-student-loan-debt-more-than-triples-after-gradution/.
106. Ben Miller, "New Federal Data Show a Student Loan Crisis for African American Borrowers," Center for American Progress, October 16, 2017, https://www.americanprogress.org/issues/education-postsecondary/news/2017/10/16/440711/new-federal-data-show-student-loan-crisis-african-american-borrowers/.
107. Caroline Preston, "To Pay for College, More Students Are Promising a Piece of Their Future to Investors," *Hechinger Report*, February 19, 2020, https://hechingerreport.org/income-share-agreements-to-pay-for-college-more-students-are-promising-a-piece-of-their-future-to-investors/.
108. Sparky Abraham and Nathan Robinson, "What Is Education For?" *Current Affairs*, August 11, 2018, https://www.currentaffairs.org/2018/08/what-is-education-for.
109. Nicolai Franzmeier, Emrah Düzel, Frank Jessen, Katharina Buerger, Johannes Levin, Marco Duering, Martin Dichgans, et al., "Left Frontal Hub Connectivity Delays Cognitive Impairment in Autosomal-Dominant and Sporadic Alzheimer's Disease," *Brain* 141, no. 4 (April 1, 2018): 1186–1200, https://doi.org/10.1093/brain/awy008.
110. Oliver Sacks, *Everything in Its Place: First Loves and Last Tales* (New York: Knopf, 2019), 1214.
111. Micaela Y. Chan, Jinkyung Na, Phillip F. Agres, Neil K. Savalia, Denise C. Park, and Gagan S. Wig, "Socioeconomic Status Moderates Age-Related Differences in the Brain's

Functional Network Organization and Anatomy across the Adult Lifespan," *Proceedings of the National Academy of Sciences* 115, no. 22 (May 29, 2018): E5144–53.

112. See David A. Snowdon, Susan J. Kemper, James A. Mortimer, Lydia H. Greiner, David R. Wekstein, and William R. Markesbery, "Linguistic Ability in Early Life and Cognitive Function and Alzheimer's Disease in Late Life: Findings from the Nun Study," *Journal of the American Medical Association* 275, no. 7 (1996): 528–32; Peter Nordström, Anna Nordström, Marie Eriksson, Lars-Olof Wahlund, and Yngve Gustafson, "Risk Factors in Late Adolescence for Young-Onset Dementia in Men: A Nationwide Cohort Study," *JAMA Internal Medicine* 173, no. 17 (2013): 1612–18; Merete Osler, Gunhild T. Christensen, Ellen Garde, Erik L. Mortensen, and Kaare Christensen, "Cognitive Ability in Young Adulthood and Risk of Dementia in a Cohort of Danish Men, Brothers, and Twins," *Alzheimer's and Dementia* 13, no. 12 (2017): 1355–63; Tom C. Russ, Jean Hannah, G. David Batty, Christopher C. Booth, Ian J. Deary, and John M. Starr, "Childhood Cognitive Ability and Incident Dementia: The 1932 Scottish Mental Survey Cohort into Their Tenth Decade," *Epidemiology* 28, no. 3 (2017): 361; Serhiy Dekhtyar, Hui-Xin Wang, Kirk Scott, Anna Goodman, Ilona Koupil, and Agneta Herlitz, "A Life-Course Study of Cognitive Reserve in Dementia—from Childhood to Old Age," *American Journal of Geriatric Psychiatry* 23, no. 9 (2015): 885–96; Ian J. Deary, Martha C. Whiteman, John M. Starr, Lawrence J. Whalley, and Helen C. Fox, "The Impact of Childhood Intelligence on Later Life: Following up the Scottish Mental Surveys of 1932 and 1947," *Journal of Personality and Social Psychology* 86, no. 1 (2004): 130; Alison R. Huang, Kiersten L. Strombotne, Elizabeth Mokyr Horner, and Susan J. Lapham, "Adolescent Cognitive Aptitudes and Later-in-Life Alzheimer Disease and Related Disorders," *JAMA Network Open* 1, no. 5 (2018): e181726–e181726; Prashanthi Vemuri, Timothy G. Lesnick, Scott A. Przybelski, Mary Machulda, David S. Knopman, Michelle M. Mielke, Rosebud O. Roberts, et al., "Association of Lifetime Intellectual Enrichment with Cognitive Decline in the Older Population," *JAMA Neurology* 71, no. 8 (2014): 1017–24.
113. Hsiu-Chih Liu, P. Chou, K. N. Lin, S. J. Wang, J. L. Fuh, H. C. Lin, C. Y. Liu, et al., "Assessing Cognitive Abilities and Dementia in a Predominantly Illiterate Population of Older Individuals in Kinmen," *Psychological Medicine* 24, no. 3 (1994): 763–70.
114. Randall Rothenberg, *The Neoliberals: Creating the New American Politics* (New York: Simon and Schuster, 1984), 27.
115. Edward R. Berchick, Emily Hood, and Jessica C. Barnett, *Health Insurance Coverage in the United States: 2017*, Current Population Reports (Washington DC: US GPO, 2018).
116. Sara R. Collins, Munira Z. Gunja, and Michelle M. Doty, "How Well Does Insurance Coverage Protect Consumers from Health Care Costs?" Commonwealth Fund, October 17, 2017, https://www.commonwealthfund.org/publications/issue-briefs/2017/oct/how-well-does-insurance-coverage-protect-consumers-health-care.
117. Robin Osborn, David Squires, Michelle M. Doty, Dana O. Sarnak, and Eric C. Schneider, "In New Survey of Eleven Countries, US Adults Still Struggle with Access to and Affordability of Health Care," *Health Affairs* 35, no. 12 (2016): 2327–36.
118. "2019 Employer Health Benefits Survey—Section 1: Cost of Health Insuance." *KFF* (blog), September 25, 2019, https://www.kff.org/report-section/ehbs-2019-section-1-cost-of-health-insurance/.
119. Martin Luther King Jr., speech to the Medical Committee for Human Rights, Chicago, March 25, 1966.
120. *Report on the Economic Well-Being of US Households in 2017* (Washington, DC: Board of Governors of the Federal Reserve, 2018).
121. Eric B. Larson, Kristine Yaffe, and Kenneth M. Langa, "New Insights into the Dementia Epidemic," *New England Journal of Medicine* 369, no. 24 (December 12, 2013): 2275–77, https://doi.org/10.1056/NEJMp1311405.
122. "The Haury Conversation—Noam Chomsky Talks with Toni Massaro," video, 1:42:07, collegeofsbs, November 15, 2017, https://www.youtube.com/watch?v=QkTMdox56bY.

(When we shared with Chomsky that there was a strong scientific argument to be made that the most effective "intervention" for Alzheimer's may well be abolishing fees for university tuition and adult education and training programs, he wrote back to us, "That is *extremely* interesting!")

123. Case and Deaton, *Deaths of Despair*.
124. Case and Deaton, "Rising Morbidity and Mortality in Midlife."
125. Vincent Schiraldi and Jason Ziedenberg, *Cellblocks or Classrooms?: The Funding of Higher Education and Corrections and Its Impact on African American Men* (Washington, DC: Justice Policy Institute, 2002).
126. The insurance industry alone shells out upwards of $80 million in lobbying expenditures annually and hires just under 1,000 lobbyists annually. See "Health Services/HMOs Lobbying Profile," OpenSecrets, accessed February 27, 2020, https://www.opensecrets.org/federal-lobbying/industries/summary?cycle=2017&id=H03.
127. Alex Emmons, "The Senate's Military Spending Increase Alone Is Enough to Make Public College Free," *Intercept*, September 19, 2017, https://theintercept.com/2017/09/18/the-senates-military-spending-increase-alone-is-enough-to-make-public-college-free/.
128. U.S. military spending commonly exceeds the total spending of its next 10 rivals put together. See Aude Fleurant, Sam Perlo-Freeman, Pieter D. Wezeman, Siemon T. Wezeman, and Noel Kelly, *Trends in World Military Expenditure, 2016* (Solna, Sweden: Stockholm International Research Institute, 2017), 1–8.
129. Martin Luther King Jr., "A Revolution of Values," in *Rethinking Globalization: Teaching for Justice in an Unjust World*, ed. Bill Bigelow and Bob Peterson (Milwaukee, WI: Rethinking School, 2002), 327–28. Speech available at "Martin Luther King The Three Evils of Society," video, 43:10, E. Joesph Doalmsavid, September 14, 2013, https://www.youtube.com/watch?v=j8d-IYSM-08.
130. Dwight D. Eisenhower commented similarly in his 1953 "Cross of Iron" speech: "Every gun that is made, every warship launched, every rocket fired signifies, in the final sense, a theft from those who hunger and are not fed, those who are cold and are not clothed." See "Chance for Peace Speech," *Wikipedia*, last updated December 23, 2019, https://en.wikipedia.org/w/index.php?title=Chance_for_Peace_speech&oldid=932123643.
131. Paul Lincoln, Kevin Fenton, Charles Alessi, Martin Prince, Carol Brayne, Marc Wortmann, Kiran Patel, John Deanfield, and Modi Mwatsama, "The Blackfriars Consensus on Brain Health and Dementia," *Lancet* 383, no. 9931 (2014): 1805–6.
132. Livingston et al., "Dementia Prevention, Intervention, and Care."
133. Hanan Qasim, Zubair A. Karim, Jose O. Rivera, Fadi T. Khasawneh, and Fatima Z. Alshbool, "Impact of Electronic Cigarettes on the Cardiovascular System," *Journal of the American Heart Association* 6, no. 9 (September 22, 2017), https://doi.org/10.1161/JAHA.117.006353.
134. Klodian Dhana, Denis A. Evans, Kumar B. Rajan, David A. Bennett, and Martha C. Morris,"Healthy Lifestyle and the Risk of Alzheimer Dementia: Findings from 2 Longitudinal Studies," *Neurology*, June 17, 2020, https://doi.org/10.1212/WNL.0000000000009816.
135. Yu-Tzu Wu, Laura Fratiglioni, Fiona E. Matthews, Antonio Lobo, Monique MB Breteler, Ingmar Skoog, and Carol Brayne, "Dementia in Western Europe: Epidemiological Evidence and Implications for Policy Making," *Lancet Neurology* 15, no. 1 (2016): 116–24.
136. Richard G. Wilkinson and Kate Pickett, *The Spirit Level: Why Greater Equality Makes Societies Stronger* (New York: Bloomsbury Press, 2010), 232.
137. Tatum Anderson, "Carol Brayne: A Life-Course Approach to Prevent Dementia," *Bulletin of the World Health Organization* 96, no. 3 (2018): 153–54.
138. Sam Norton, Fiona E. Matthews, Deborah E. Barnes, Kristine Yaffe, and Carol Brayne, "Potential for Primary Prevention of Alzheimer's Disease: An Analysis of Population-Based Data," *Lancet Neurology* 13, no. 8 (2014): 788–94.

139. Nick Slater, "Taking Orwell's Name in Vain," *Current Affairs*, October 11, 2017, https://www.currentaffairs.org/2017/10/taking-orwells-name-in-vain.
140. O. Dag, "George Orwell: Why Socialists Don't Believe in Fun," 1943, Orwell.ru, last modified December 29, 2019, https://orwell.ru/library/articles/socialists/english/e_fun.
141. Livingston et al., "Dementia Prevention, Intervention, and Care."

CHAPTER 5. FLINT *STILL* DOESN'T HAVE CLEAN WATER

1. "QuickFacts: Flint City, Michigan," U.S. Census Bureau, accessed February 28, 2020, https://www.census.gov/quickfacts/fact/table/flintcitymichigan/INC110218.
2. Mona Hanna-Attisha, "Opinion: I Helped Expose the Lead Crisis in Flint—Here's What Other Cities Should Do," *New York Times*, August 27, 2019, sec. Opinion, https://www.nytimes.com/2019/08/27/opinion/lead-water-flint.html.
3. Werner Troesken, *The Great Lead Water Pipe Disaster* (Cambridge, MA: MIT Press, 2006), 41.
4. Lead levels are four times higher among convicted juvenile offenders than nondelinquent high school students. See Herbert L. Needleman, Christine McFarland, Roberta B. Ness, Stephen E. Fienberg, and Michael J. Tobin, "Bone Lead Levels in Adjudicated Delinquents: A Case Control Study," *Neurotoxicology and Teratology* 24, no. 6 (2002): 711–17.
5. Robert J. Sampson and Alix S. Winter, "Poisoned Development: Assessing Childhood Lead Exposure as a Cause of Crime in a Birth Cohort Followed through Adolescence," *Criminology* 56, no. 2 (May 2018): 269–301, https://doi.org/10.1111/1745-9125.12171.
6. Herbert L. Needleman and Constantine A. Gatsonis, "Low-Level Lead Exposure and the IQ of Children: A Meta-analysis of Modern Studies," *Journal of the American Medical Association* 263, no. 5 (1990): 673–78.
7. Jessica Wolpaw Reyes, "Lead Exposure and Behavior: Effects on Antisocial and Risky Behavior among Children and Adolescents," *Economic Inquiry* 53, no. 3 (2015): 1580–1605.
8. Troesken, *Great Lead Water Pipe Disaster*.
9. Aaron Reuben, Jonathan D. Schaefer, Terrie E. Moffitt, Jonathan Broadbent, Honalee Harrington, Renate M. Houts, Sandhya Ramrakha, Richie Poulton, and Avshalom Caspi, "Association of Childhood Lead Exposure with Adult Personality Traits and Lifelong Mental Health," *JAMA Psychiatry* 76, no. 4 (April 1, 2019): 418–25, https://doi.org/10.1001/jamapsychiatry.2018.4192.
10. Mark G. A. Opler, Stephen L. Buka, Justina Groeger, Ian McKeague, Catherine Wei, Pam Factor-Litvak, Michaeline Bresnahan, et al., "Prenatal Exposure to Lead, δ-Aminolevulinic Acid, and Schizophrenia: Further Evidence." *Environmental Health Perspectives* 116, no. 11 (2008): 1586–90.
11. Alexander C. McFarlane, Amelia K. Searle, Miranda Van Hooff, Peter A. Baghurst, Michael G. Sawyer, Cherrie Galletly, Malcolm R. Sim, and Levina S. Clark, "Prospective Associations between Childhood Low-Level Lead Exposure and Adult Mental Health Problems: The Port Pirie Cohort Study," *Neurotoxicology* 39 (2013): 11–17.
12. David K. Marcus, Jessica J. Fulton, and Erin J. Clarke, "Lead and Conduct Problems: A Meta-Analysis," *Journal of Clinical Child and Adolescent Psychology* 39, no. 2 (2010): 234–41.
13. John Paul Wright, Kim N. Dietrich, M. Douglas Ris, Richard W. Hornung, Stephanie D. Wessel, Bruce P. Lanphear, Mona Ho, and Mary N. Rae, "Association of Prenatal and Childhood Blood Lead Concentrations with Criminal Arrests in Early Adulthood," *PLoS Medicine* 5, no. 5 (2008): e101.
14. Amber L. Beckley, Avshalom Caspi, Jonathan Broadbent, Honalee Harrington, Renate M. Houts, Richie Poulton, Sandhya Ramrakha, Aaron Reuben, and Terrie E. Moffitt,

"Association of Childhood Blood Lead Levels with Criminal Offending," *JAMA Pediatrics* 172, no. 2 (2018): 166–73.

15. David M. Fergusson, Joseph M. Boden, and L. John Horwood, "Dentine Lead Levels in Childhood and Criminal Behaviour in Late Adolescence and Early Adulthood," *Journal of Epidemiology and Community Health* 62, no. 12 (2008): 1045–50.
16. John Paul Wright, Danielle Boisvert, and Jamie Vaske, "Blood Lead Levels in Early Childhood Predict Adulthood Psychopathy," *Youth Violence and Juvenile Justice* 7, no. 3 (2009): 208–22.
17. David C. Bellinger, "Very Low Lead Exposures and Children's Neurodevelopment," *Current Opinion in Pediatrics* 20, no. 2 (2008): 172–77.
18. Theodore I. Lidsky and Jay S. Schneider, "Lead Neurotoxicity in Children: Basic Mechanisms and Clinical Correlates," *Brain* 126, no. 1 (2003): 5–19.
19. Abby Goodnough, "Flint Weighs Scope of Harm to Children Caused by Lead in Water," *New York Times*, January 29, 2016.
20. Sarah Hulett, "Flint Pediatricians Raise Alarm about Lead Levels in City Water," Michigan Radio NPR, September 24, 2015, https://www.michiganradio.org/post/flint-pediatricians-raise-alarm-about-lead-levels-city-water.
21. "Hurley Doctor Recommends Switching Away from Flint River Water," video, 1:03, *MLive*, September 24, 2015, https://www.youtube.com/watch?v=6tELb594WTw.
22. L. Leopold, "Have Democrats Abandoned Ohio Auto Workers to Trump?" *Truthdig*, June 4, 2019, https://www.truthdig.com/articles/have-democrats-abandoned-ohio-auto-workers-to-trump/.
23. Chris Arnade, *Dignity: Seeking Respect in Back Row America* (New York: Penguin, 2019), 50.
24. Thom Hartmann, "Reaganomics Killed America's Middle Class," *Salon*, April 19, 2014, https://www.salon.com/2014/04/19/reaganomics_killed_americas_middle_class_partner/.
25. Andrew R. Highsmith, *Demolition Means Progress: Flint, Michigan, and the Fate of the American Metropolis* (Chicago: University of Chicago Press, 2015).
26. Bill Vlasic and Nick Bunkley, "The Last Holdouts Cast Their Lot with G.M.," *New York Times*, May 20, 2009, sec. Business, https://www.nytimes.com/2009/05/21/business/21holdouts.html.
27. Terressa A. Benz, "Toxic Cities: Neoliberalism and Environmental Racism in Flint and Detroit Michigan," *Critical Sociology* 45, no. 1 (2019): 49–62.
28. Jonathan Oosting, "How Michigan's Revenue Sharing 'Raid' Cost Communities Billions for Local Services," *MLive*, March 30, 2014, https://www.mlive.com/lansing-news/2014/03/michigan_revenue_sharing_strug.html.
29. David Fasenfest, "A Neoliberal Response to an Urban Crisis: Emergency Management in Flint, MI," *Critical Sociology* 45, no. 1 (2019): 33–47.
30. Cadmus Group, *U.S. Environmental Protection Agency Public Water System Supervision Program Final Report: Program Review for the Michigan Department of Environmental Quality Water Bureau* (Washington, DC: EPA Office of Ground Water and Drinking Water, August 30, 2010), https://www.epa.gov/sites/production/files/2015-11/documents/program-review-mdeq-water-bureau-20100830-76pp_0.pdf.
31. "Democracy, Disposability, and the Flint Water Crisis," *Third Coast Conspiracy* (blog), January 18, 2016, https://thirdcoastconspiracy.wordpress.com/2016/01/18/democracy-disposability-and-the-flint-water-crisis/.
32. Michigan Civil Rights Commission, *The Flint Water Crisis: Systemic Racism through the Lens of Flint* (Lansing: Michigan Department of Civil Rights, February 17, 2017), https://www.michigan.gov/documents/mdcr/VFlintCrisisRep-F-Edited3-13-17_554317_7.pdf.
33. Naomi Klein, "The Worst of Donald Trump's Toxic Agenda Is Lying in Wait—A Major U.S. Crisis Will Unleash It," *Intercept*, June 10, 2017, https://theintercept.com/2017/06/10

/the-worst-of-donald-trumps-toxic-agenda-is-lying-in-wait-a-major-u-s-crisis-will-unleash-it/.

34. Lindsey Smith, "After Ignoring and Trying to Discredit People in Flint, the State Was Forced to Face the Problem," Michigan Radio NPR, December 16, 2015, https://www.michiganradio.org/post/after-ignoring-and-trying-discredit-people-flint-state-was-forced-face-problem.
35. Julia Craven and Tyler Tynes, "The Racist Roots of Flint's Water Crisis," *Huffington Post*, February 3, 2016.
36. Ana Aceves, "Flint Water Tied to Fetal Death and Lower Fertility Rates," *NOVA*, September 22, 2017, https://www.pbs.org/wgbh/nova/article/flint-water-tied-to-fetal-death-and-lower-fertility-rates/.
37. Ron Fonger, "General Motors Shutting off Flint River Water at Engine Plant over Corrosion Worries," *MLive*, January 20, 2019, https://www.mlive.com/news/flint/2014/10/general_motors_wont_use_flint.html.
38. Brian Manzullo, "Michael Moore Calls Barack Obama Drinking Flint Water 'Disappointing,'" *Detroit Free Press*, May 4, 2016, https://www.freep.com/story/news/local/michigan/flint-water-crisis/2016/05/04/flint-water-crisis-michael-moore-barack-obama/83940370/.
39. Ron Fonger, "Army Calls Cease Fire on Military Exercises that Rattled Flint," *MLive*, June 11, 2015, https://www.mlive.com/news/flint/2015/06/military_exercises_over_in_fli.html.
40. Elisha Anderson, "People of Flint Speak: 'Nobody Should . . . Be Living like This,'" *Detroit Free Press*, January 17, 2016, https://www.freep.com/story/news/local/michigan/flint-water-crisis/2016/01/17/people-live-with-flint-water-crisis/78860228/.
41. Andrew R. Highsmith, "Epilogue: 'America Is a Thousand Flints,'" in *Demolition Means Progress: Flint, Michigan, and the Fate of the American Metropolis* (Chicago: University of Chicago Press, 2015), 268–86.
42. M. B. Pell and Joshua Schneyer, "Reuters Finds Lead Levels Higher than Flint's in Thousands of Locales," *Reuters*, December 19, 2016, http://www.reuters.com/investigates/special-report/usa-lead-testing/.
43. "Looking for Lead." *Reuters*, December 19, 2016, http://www.reuters.com/investigates/special-report/usa-lead-testing/#interactive-lead.
44. Michael Wines, "Flint Is in the News, but Lead Poisoning Is Even Worse in Cleveland," *New York Times*, March 3, 2016, sec. U.S., https://www.nytimes.com/2016/03/04/us/lead-paint-contamination-persists-in-many-cities-as-cleanup-falters.html.
45. Peter A. Baghurst, Shilu Tong, Michael G. Sawyer, Jane Burns, and Anthony J. McMichael, "Sociodemographic and Behavioural Determinants of Blood Lead Concentrations in Children Aged 11-13 Years: The Port Pirie Cohort Study," *Medical Journal of Australia* 170, no. 2 (1999): 63–67.
46. Sampson and Winter, "Poisoned Development."
47. Vann R. Newkirk II, "Environmental Racism Is the New Jim Crow," *Atlantic*, June 5, 2017, https://www.theatlantic.com/video/index/529137/environmental-racism-is-the-new-jim-crow/.
48. Delese Wear, Joseph Zarconi, Julie M. Aultman, Michelle R. Chyatte, and Arno K. Kumagai, "Remembering Freddie Gray: Medical Education for Social Justice," *Academic Medicine: Journal of the Association of American Medical Colleges* 92, no. 3 (2017): 312–17, https://doi.org/10.1097/ACM.0000000000001355.
49. Terrence McCoy, "Freddie Gray's Life a Study on the Effects of Lead Paint on Poor Blacks," *Washington Post*, April 29, 2015, sec. Local, https://www.washingtonpost.com/local/freddie-grays-life-a-study-in-the-sad-effects-of-lead-paint-on-poor-blacks/2015/04/29/0be898e6-eea8-11e4-8abc-d6aa3bad79dd_story.html.
50. Ibid.
51. Ibid.
52. Baghurst et al., "Sociodemographic and Behavioural Determinants."

53. Aaron Reuben, Avshalom Caspi, Daniel W. Belsky, Jonathan Broadbent, Honalee Harrington, Karen Sugden, Renate M. Houts, Sandhya Ramrakha, Richie Poulton, and Terrie E. Moffitt, "Association of Childhood Blood Lead Levels with Cognitive Function and Socioeconomic Status at Age 38 Years and with IQ Change and Socioeconomic Mobility between Childhood and Adulthood," *Journal of the American Medical Association* 317, no. 12 (2017): 1244–51, https://doi.org/10.1001/jama.2017.1712.
54. Marc G. Weisskopf, Susan P. Proctor, Robert O. Wright, Joel Schwartz, Avron Spiro III, David Sparrow, Huiling Nie, and Howard Hu, "Cumulative Lead Exposure and Cognitive Performance among Elderly Men," *Epidemiology* 18, no. 1 (2007): 59–66.
55. Marc G. Weisskopf, Robert O. Wright, Joel Schwartz, Avron Spiro III, David Sparrow, Antonio Aro, and Howard Hu, "Cumulative Lead Exposure and Prospective Change in Cognition among Elderly Men: The VA Normative Aging Study," *American Journal of Epidemiology* 160, no. 12 (2004): 1184–93.
56. R. A. Shih, T. A. Glass, K. Bandeen-Roche, M. C. Carlson, K. I. Bolla, A. C. Todd, and B. S. Schwartz, "Environmental Lead Exposure and Cognitive Function in Community-Dwelling Older Adults," *Neurology* 67, no. 9 (November 14, 2006): 1556–62, https://doi.org/10.1212/01.wnl.0000239836.26142.c5.
57. Edwin van Wijngaarden, James R. Campbell, and Deborah A. Cory-Slechta, "Bone Lead Levels Are Associated with Measures of Memory Impairment in Older Adults," *Neurotoxicology* 30, no. 4 (2009): 572–80.
58. Nosratola D. Vaziri, "Mechanisms of Lead-Induced Hypertension and Cardiovascular Disease," *American Journal of Physiology-Heart and Circulatory Physiology* 295, no. 2 (2008): H454–H465.
59. Joel Schwartz, "Lead, Blood Pressure, and Cardiovascular Disease in Men and Women," *Environmental Health Perspectives* 91 (1991): 71–75.
60. Bruce P. Lanphear, Stephen Rauch, Peggy Auinger, Ryan W. Allen, and Richard W. Hornung, "Low-Level Lead Exposure and Mortality in US Adults: A Population-Based Cohort Study," *Lancet Public Health* 3, no. 4 (2018): e177–e184.
61. Emily Atkin, "Did Flint's Water Crisis Damage Kids' Brains?" *New Republic*, February 14, 2018, https://newrepublic.com/article/147066/flints-water-crisis-damage-kids-brains.
62. Ibid.
63. Russell Flegal and Donald Smith, "Lead Levels in Preindustrial Humans," *New England Journal of Medicine* 326, no. 19 (1992): 1293–94.
64. "Double Up in Flint," Fair Food Network, accessed February 28, 2020, https://fairfoodnetwork.org/projects/double-up-flint/.
65. Mona Hanna-Attisha, "Opinion: I'm Sick of Asking Children to Be Resilient," *New York Times*, May 12, 2020, sec. Opinion, https://www.nytimes.com/2020/05/12/opinion/sunday/flint-inequality-race-coronavirus.html.
66. Fredrik deBoer, "Lead Exposure Continues to Needlessly Destroy Lives," People's Policy Project, October 5, 2017, https://www.peoplespolicyproject.org/2017/10/05/lead-exposure-continues-to-needlessly-destroy-lives/.
67. Keith Ellison and Wenonah Hauter, "Lead Is a National Crisis: We Need to Fight for Clean, Publicly Owned Water Before It Is Too Late," *In These Times*, April 27, 2018, http://inthesetimes.com/article/21095/lead_water_flint_keith_ellison_infrastructure.
68. *Base Nation* official book website, accessed February 28, 2020, https://www.basenation.us/.
69. David Vine, "Where in the World Is the U.S. Military?" *Politico*, July/August 2015, https://www.politico.com/magazine/story/2015/06/us-military-bases-around-the-world-119321.html.
70. Lead Service Line Replacement Collaborative website, accessed February 28, 2020, https://www.lslr-collaborative.org/.
71. Amanda Macias, "America Has Spent $6.4 Trillion on Wars in the Middle East and Asia since 2001, a New Study Says," CNBC, November 20, 2019, https://www.cnbc.com/2019/11/20/us-spent-6point4-trillion-on-middle-east-wars-since-2001-study.html.

72. This interactive *Living New Deal Map* allows users to examine the lasting effects of the New Deal in communities across the United States, accessed May 27, 2020, https://livingnewdeal.org/map/.
73. Gary Ridley, "15 Years and $60M Needed to Replace Flint's Lead Water Lines, Emails Show," *MLive*, January 21, 2016, https://www.mlive.com/news/flint/2016/01/15_years_and_60m_needed_to_rep.html.
74. "10 Policies to Prevent and Respond to Childhood Lead Exposure," Pew Research, August 30, 2017, http://pew.org/2wEsGHv.
75. James L. Pirkle, Debra J. Brody, Elaine W. Gunter, Rachel A. Kramer, Daniel C. Paschal, Katherine M. Flegal, and Thomas D. Matte, "The Decline in Blood Lead Levels in the United States: The National Health and Nutrition Examination Surveys (NHANES)," *Journal of the American Medical Association* 272, no. 4 (1994): 284–91.
76. Herbert L. Needleman, "The Removal of Lead from Gasoline: Historical and Personal Reflections," *Environmental Research* 84, no. 1 (September 1, 2000): 20–35, https://doi.org/10.1006/enrs.2000.4069.
77. Pirkle et al., "The Decline in Blood Lead Levels."
78. Jessica Wolpaw Reyes, *Environmental Policy as Social Policy? The Impact of Childhood Lead Exposure on Crime* (Cambridge, MA: National Bureau of Economic Research, 2007).
79. Alan S. Kaufman, Xiaobin Zhou, Matthew R. Reynolds, Nadeen L. Kaufman, Garo P. Green, and Lawrence G. Weiss, "The Possible Societal Impact of the Decrease in US Blood Lead Levels on Adult IQ," *Environmental Research* 132 (2014): 413–20.
80. Esme Fuller-Thomson and Sydney A. Jopling, "Could the Adoption of Unleaded Gasoline in the 1970s Play a Role in the Precipitous Decline in Dementia Prevalence?" *JAMA Internal Medicine* 177, no. 6 (June 1, 2017): 892–93, https://doi.org/10.1001/jamainternmed.2017.1074.
81. Troesken, *Great Lead Water Pipe Disaster*, 22.
82. Nadja Popovich, Livia Albeck-Ripka, and Kendra Pierre-Louis, "95 Environmental Rules Being Rolled Back under Trump," *New York Times*, June 2, 2019, sec. Climate, https://www.nytimes.com/interactive/2019/climate/trump-environment-rollbacks.html.
83. Coral Davenport, "Trump Rule Would Limit E.P.A.'s Control over Water Pollution," *New York Times*, December 6, 2018, sec. Climate, https://www.nytimes.com/2018/12/06/climate/trump-water-pollution-wotus-replacement.html.
84. Ledyard King and Richard Wolf, "Supreme Court Will Consider Letting Groundwater Pollution Escape Regulation under Clean Water Act," *USA Today*, February 19, 2019, https://www.usatoday.com/story/news/politics/2019/02/19/supreme-court-rule-regulation-polluted-groundwater-epa-clean-water-act/2915360002/.
85. Albert Camus, *The Plague*, (London: Penguin, 2002), 195.

CHAPTER 6. #POORLIVESMATTER

1. Peter Rugh, "Hurricane Sandy Relief Turns to Protest," *Waging Nonviolence* (blog), December 17, 2012, https://wagingnonviolence.org/2012/12/hurricane-sandy-relief-turns-to-protest/.
2. Sarah Jaffe, *Necessary Trouble: Americans in Revolt* (New York: Nation Books, 2017), 203.
3. Steven Greenhouse, "With Day of Protests, Fast-Food Workers Seek More Pay," *New York Times*, November 29, 2012, sec. New York, https://www.nytimes.com/2012/11/30/nyregion/fast-food-workers-in-new-york-city-rally-for-higher-wages.html.
4. "Fast Food Industry Analysis 2020—Cost and Trends," Franchise Help, accessed March 3, 2020, https://www.franchisehelp.com/industry-reports/fast-food-industry-analysis-2020-cost-trends/.
5. "May 2019 National Occupational Employment and Wage Estimates," US Bureau of Labor Statistics, accessed March 3, 2020, https://www.bls.gov/oes/current/oes_nat.htm.
6. Ned Renikoff, "Historic Fast Food Strike Draws Lessons from MLK's Last Campaign," MSNBC, April 4, 2013, http://www.msnbc.com/all-in/historic-fast-food-strike-draws-lessons.

7. Lisa De Bode, "Poverty Wages Pose Risk to Fast-Food Industry's Profits, Experts Say," *Al Jazeera America*, April 22, 2014, http://america.aljazeera.com/articles/2014/4/22/fast-food-workersmcdonaldspovertywageminimum.html.
8. "Occupational Employment by Race and Ethnicity, 2011," *TED: The Economics Daily*, US Bureau of Labor Statistics, October 26, 2012, https://www.bls.gov/opub/ted/2012/ted_20121026.htm.
9. Sylvia A. Allegretto, Marc Doussard, Dave Graham-Squire, Ken Jacobs, Dan Thompson, and Jeremy Thompson, "Fast Food, Poverty Wages: The Public Cost of Low-Wage Jobs in the Fast-Food Industry," *Center for Labor Research and Education* (blog), October 15, 2013, http://laborcenter.berkeley.edu/fast-food-poverty-wages-the-public-cost-of-low-wage-jobs-in-the-fast-food-industry/.
10. Eric B. Larson and Joan DeClaire, *Enlightened Aging: Building Resilience for a Long, Active Life* (Lanham, MD: Rowman and Littlefield, 2017), 89.
11. Paola Gilsanz, Elizabeth Rose Mayeda, Maria Glymour, Charles P. Quesenberry, Dan Mungas, Charles S. DeCarli, and Rachel A. Whitmer, "Birth in a High Infant Mortality State: Race and Risk of Dementia," *Alzheimer's and Dementia: The Journal of the Alzheimer's Association* 13, no. 7 (2017): P210–11.
12. Sarah Whittle, Nandita Vijayakumar, Julian G. Simmons, Meg Dennison, Orli Schwartz, Christos Pantelis, Lisa Sheeber, Michelle L. Byrne, and Nicholas B. Allen, "Role of Positive Parenting in the Association between Neighborhood Social Disadvantage and Brain Development across Adolescence," *JAMA Psychiatry* 74, no. 8 (2017): 824–32.
13. W. Ryan Powell, William R. Buckingham, Jamie L Larson, et al., "Association of Neighborhood-Level Disadvantage with Alzheimer Disease Neuropathology," *JAMA Network Open* 3, no. 6 (2020): e207559.
14. Julie Turkewitz, "Fast-Food Union Organizers Get Some Historical Perspective," *City Room* (blog), March 29, 2013, https://cityroom.blogs.nytimes.com/2013/03/29/fast-food-union-organizers-get-some-historical-perspective/.
15. Dave Jamieson, "Workers Across U.S. 'Fight For $15' in Strikes for Wage Hikes," *HuffPost*, November 29, 2016, https://www.huffpost.com/entry/minimum-wage-protests-fight-for-15_n_583df76ee4b0ae0e7cda8333.
16. USDA ERS, "Key Statistics and Graphics," USDA Economic Research Service, last updated September 4, 2019, https://www.ers.usda.gov/topics/food-nutrition-assistance/food-security-in-the-us/key-statistics-graphics.aspx.
17. Natalie DiBlasio, "Hunger in America: 1 in 7 Rely on Food Banks," *USA Today*, August 17, 2014, https://www.usatoday.com/story/news/nation/2014/08/17/hunger-study-food/14195585/.
18. Emily Jane Fox, "McDonald's Helps Workers Get Food Stamps," *CNNMoney*, October 23, 2013, https://money.cnn.com/2013/10/23/news/companies/mcdonalds-help-line-workers/index.html.
19. Alina Selyukh, "McDonald's Fired CEO Is Getting Millions, Putting Spotlight On Pay Gap," November 5, 2019, https://www.npr.org/2019/11/05/776305627/mcdonalds-fired-ceo-is-getting-millions-putting-spotlight-on-pay-gap.
20. Lei Cao, Lan Tan, Hui-Fu Wang, Teng Jiang, Xi-Chen Zhu, Huan Lu, Meng-Shan Tan, and Jin-Tai Yu, "Dietary Patterns and Risk of Dementia: A Systematic Review and Meta-analysis of Cohort Studies," *Molecular Neurobiology* 53, no. 9 (2016): 6144–54.
21. David Vauzour, Maria Camprubi-Robles, Sophie Miquel-Kergoat, Cristina Andres-Lacueva, Diána Bánáti, Pascale Barberger-Gateau, Gene L. Bowman, et al., "Nutrition for the Ageing Brain: Towards Evidence for an Optimal Diet," *Ageing Research Reviews* 35 (May 1, 2017): 222–40, https://doi.org/10.1016/j.arr.2016.09.010.
22. Ondine Van De Rest, Lenneke W. A. Van Hooijdonk, Esmée Doets, Olga J. G. Schiepers, Ans Eilander, and Lisette C. P. G. M. De Groot, "B Vitamins and n-3 Fatty Acids for Brain Development and Function: Review of Human Studies," *Annals of Nutrition and Metabolism* 60, no. 4 (2012): 272–92.

23. Ilianna Lourida, Maya Soni, Joanna Thompson-Coon, Nitin Purandare, Iain A. Lang, Obioha C. Ukoumunne, and David J. Llewellyn, "Mediterranean Diet, Cognitive Function, and Dementia: A Systematic Review," *Epidemiology* (2013): 479–89.
24. Singh, Balwinder, Ajay K. Parsaik, Michelle M. Mielke, Patricia J. Erwin, David S. Knopman, Ronald C. Petersen, and Rosebud O. Roberts, "Association of Mediterranean Diet with Mild Cognitive Impairment and Alzheimer's Disease: A Systematic Review and Meta-analysis," *Journal of Alzheimer's Disease* 39, no. 2 (2014): 271–82.
25. Nikolaos Scarmeas, Yaakov Stern, Ming-Xin Tang, Richard Mayeux, and Jose A. Luchsinger, "Mediterranean Diet and Risk for Alzheimer's Disease," *Annals of Neurology: Official Journal of the American Neurological Association and the Child Neurology Society* 59, no. 6 (2006): 912–21.
26. Samantha Gardener, Yian Gu, Stephanie R. Rainey-Smith, Jennifer B. Keogh, Peter Marshall Clifton, S. L. Mathieson, Kevin Taddei, et al. "Adherence to a Mediterranean Diet and Alzheimer's Disease Risk in an Australian Population," *Translational Psychiatry* 2, no. 10 (2012): e164.
27. Nikolaos Scarmeas, Yaakov Stern, Richard Mayeux, Jennifer J. Manly, Nicole Schupf, and Jose A. Luchsinger, "Mediterranean Diet and Mild Cognitive Impairment," *Archives of neurology* 66, no. 2 (2009): 216–25.
28. Costas A. Anastasiou, Mary Yannakoulia, Mary H. Kosmidis, Efthimios Dardiotis, Giorgos M. Hadjigeorgiou, Paraskevi Sakka, Xanthi Arampatzi, Anastasia Bougea, Ioannis Labropoulos, and Nikolaos Scarmeas, "Mediterranean Diet and Cognitive Health: Initial Results from the Hellenic Longitudinal Investigation of Ageing and Diet," *PloS One* 12, no. 8 (2017): e0182048.
29. Ilianna Lourida, Eilis Hannon, Thomas J. Littlejohns, Kenneth M. Langa, Elina Hyppönen, Elżbieta Kuźma, and David J. Llewellyn, "Association of Lifestyle and Genetic Risk with Incidence of Dementia," *Journal of the American Medical Association* 322, no. 5 (2019): 430–37.
30. Stephanie R. Rainey-Smith, Yian Gu, Samantha L. Gardener, James D. Doecke, Victor L. Villemagne, Belinda M. Brown, Kevin Taddei, et al., "Mediterranean Diet Adherence and Rate of Cerebral Aβ-Amyloid Accumulation: Data from the Australian Imaging, Biomarkers and Lifestyle Study of Ageing," *Translational Psychiatry* 8, no. 1 (October 30, 2018): 1–7, https://doi.org/10.1038/s41398-018-0293-5.
31. Francesco Sofi, Rosanna Abbate, Gian Franco Gensini, and Alessandro Casini, "Accruing Evidence on Benefits of Adherence to the Mediterranean Diet on Health: An Updated Systematic Review and Meta-analysis," *American Journal of Clinical Nutrition* 92, no. 5 (2010): 1189–96.
32. Frank Qian, Gang Liu, Frank B. Hu, Shilpa N. Bhupathiraju, and Qi Sun, "Association between Plant-Based Dietary Patterns and Risk of Type 2 Diabetes: A Systematic Review and Meta-analysis," *JAMA Internal Medicine* 179, no. 10 (2019): 1335–44.
33. Gotaro Kojima, Christina Avgerinou, Steve Iliffe, and Kate Walters, "Adherence to Mediterranean Diet Reduces Incident Frailty Risk: Systematic Review and Meta-analysis," *Journal of the American Geriatrics Society* 66, no. 4 (2018): 783–88.
34. Claire T. McEvoy, Heidi Guyer, Kenneth M. Langa, and Kristine Yaffe, "Neuroprotective Diets Are Associated with Better Cognitive Function: The Health and Retirement Study," *Journal of the American Geriatrics Society* 65, no. 8 (2017): 1857–62.
35. Kathleen M. Hayden, Yamin Wang, Daniel Beavers, Jiu-Chiuan Chen, Mark A. Espeland, Christopher N. Ford, Laura B. Harrington, et al., "The MIND Diet and Incident Dementia: Findings from the Women's Health Initiative Memory Study," *Alzheimer's and Dementia: The Journal of the Alzheimer's Association* 13, no. 7 (2017): P858.
36. Amy Jennings, Stephen C. Cunnane, and Anne Marie Minihane, "Can Nutrition Support Healthy Cognitive Ageing and Reduce Dementia Risk?" *BMJ* 369 (June 26, 2020), https://doi.org/10.1136/bmj.m2269.
37. Schrecker and Bambra, *How Politics Makes Us Sick*, 35.

38. Benjamin T. Crookston, Kirk A. Dearden, Stephen C. Alder, Christina A. Porucznik, Joseph B. Stanford, Ray M. Merrill, Ty T. Dickerson, and Mary E. Penny, "Impact of Early and Concurrent Stunting on Cognition," *Maternal and Child Nutrition* 7, no. 4 (2011): 397–409.
39. Sandra E. Black, Paul J. Devereux, and Kjell G. Salvanes, "From the Cradle to the Labor Market? The Effect of Birth Weight on Adult Outcomes," *Quarterly Journal of Economics* 122, no. 1 (2007): 409–39.
40. Philip Oreopoulos, Mark Stabile, Randy Walld, and Leslie L. Roos, "Short-, Medium-, and Long-Term Consequences of Poor Infant Health an Analysis Using Siblings and Twins," *Journal of Human Resources* 43, no. 1 (2008): 88–138.
41. David J. P. Barker, "The Developmental Origins of Chronic Adult Disease," *Acta Paediatrica* 93 (2004): 26–33.
42. Kelli A. Komro, Melvin D. Livingston, Sara Markowitz, and Alexander C. Wagenaar, "The Effect of an Increased Minimum Wage on Infant Mortality and Birth Weight," *American Journal of Public Health* 106, no. 8 (2016): 1514–16, https://doi.org/10.2105/AJPH.2016.303268.
43. John P. Haran, Shakti K. Bhattarai, Sage E. Foley, Protiva Dutta, Doyle V. Ward, Vanni Bucci, and Beth A. McCormick, "Alzheimer's Disease Microbiome Is Associated with Dysregulation of the Anti-inflammatory P-glycoprotein Pathway," *MBio* 10, no. 3 (2019): e00632–19.
44. Chunmei Jiang, Guangning Li, Pengru Huang, Zhou Liu, and Bin Zhao, "The Gut Microbiota and Alzheimer's Disease," *Journal of Alzheimer's Disease* 58, no. 1 (2017): 1–15, https://doi.org/10.3233/JAD-161141.
45. Nicholas M. Vogt, Robert L. Kerby, Kimberly A. Dill-McFarland, Sandra J. Harding, Andrew P. Merluzzi, Sterling C. Johnson, Cynthia M. Carlsson, et al., "Gut Microbiome Alterations in Alzheimer's Disease," *Scientific Reports* 7, no. 1 (2017): 1–11, https://doi.org/10.1038/s41598-017-13601-y.
46. Rong Xu and QuanQiu Wang, "Towards Understanding Brain-Gut-Microbiome Connections in Alzheimer's Disease," *BMC Systems Biology* 10, no. 3 (2016): 63.
47. Francesca Pistollato, Sandra Sumalla Cano, Iñaki Elio, Manuel Masias Vergara, Francesca Giampieri, and Maurizio Battino, "Role of Gut Microbiota and Nutrients in Amyloid Formation and Pathogenesis of Alzheimer Disease," *Nutrition Reviews* 74, no. 10 (2016): 624–34.
48. Helen Tremlett, Kylynda C. Bauer, Silke Appel-Cresswell, Brett B. Finlay, and Emmanuelle Waubant, "The Gut Microbiome in Human Neurological Disease: A Review," *Annals of Neurology* 81, no. 3 (2017): 369–82.
49. Izaskun Garcia-Mantrana, Marta Selma-Royo, Cristina Alcantara, and María C. Collado, "Shifts on Gut Microbiota Associated to Mediterranean Diet Adherence and Specific Dietary Intakes on General Adult Population," *Frontiers in Microbiology* 9 (2018): 890.
50. Kevin A. Matthews, Wei Xu, Anne H. Gaglioti, James B. Holt, Janet B. Croft, Dominic Mack, and Lisa C. McGuire, "Racial and Ethnic Estimates of Alzheimer's Disease and Related Dementias in the United States (2015-2060) in Adults Aged ≥ 65 Years," *Alzheimer's and Dementia* 15, no. 1 (2019): 17–24.
51. Dominic Rushe and Tom Silverstone, "Fran Works Six Days a Week in Fast Food, and yet She's Homeless: 'It's Economic Slavery,'" *Guardian*, August 21, 2017, sec. US News, https://www.theguardian.com/us-news/2017/aug/21/missouri-fast-food-workers-better-pay-popeyes-economics.
52. Adam Gabbatt, "US Fast-Food Workers Strike over Low Wages in Nationwide Protests," *Guardian*, December 5, 2013, sec. World News, https://www.theguardian.com/world/2013/dec/05/fast-food-workers-strike-minimum-wage.
53. "Occupational Employment by Race and Ethnicity."
54. Megan Zuelsdorff, Carey E. Gleason, Amy J. Kind, Rebecca L. Koscik, Sterling C. Johnson, and Ozioma C. Okonkwo, "Lifetime Stressful Experiences, Racial Disparities, and

Cognitive Performance: Findings from the Wisconsin Registry for Alzheimer's Prevention (WRAP) Study," *Alzheimer's and Dementia: The Journal of the Alzheimer's Association* 13, no. 7 (2017): P212.

55. Sheldon Cohen and Denise Janicki-Deverts, "Who's Stressed? Distributions of Psychological Stress in the United States in Probability Samples from 1983, 2006, and 2009," *Journal of Applied Social Psychology* 42, no. 6 (2012): 1320–34.
56. Amy Bernstein, Linda T. Bilheimer, and Diane M. Makuc, *Health, United States, 2010: With Special Feature on Death and Dying* (Hyattsville, MD: National Center for Health Statistics, 2011).
57. Schrecker and Bambra, *How Politics Makes Us Sick*, 65.
58. Research from the 2019 Alzheimer's Association International Conference (AAIC) showed that LGBTQ Americans were 29% more likely to report memory loss and confusion, likely due to higher rates of depression, separate health concerns such as PTSD, inability to work, high stress, and lack of access to regular health care.
59. Al Hazzouri, Adina Zeki, Tali Elfassy, Stephen Sidney, David Jacobs, and Kristine Yaffe, "Sustained Economic Hardship and Cognitive Function: The Coronary Artery Risk Development in Young Adults Study," *American Journal of Preventive Medicine* 52, no. 1 (2017): 1–9.
60. Micaela Y. Chan, Jinkyung Na, Phillip F. Agres, Neil K. Savalia, Denise C. Park, and Gagan S. Wig, "Socioeconomic Status Moderates Age-Related Differences in the Brain's Functional Network Organization and Anatomy across the Adult Lifespan," *Proceedings of the National Academy of Sciences* 115, no. 22 (May 29, 2018): E5144–53, https://doi.org/10.1073/pnas.1714021115.
61. Teresa Seeman, Duncan Thomas, Sharon Stein Merkin, Kari Moore, Karol Watson, and Arun Karlamangla, "The Great Recession Worsened Blood Pressure and Blood Glucose Levels in American Adults," *Proceedings of the National Academy of Sciences* 115, no. 13 (March 27, 2018): 3296–3301, https://doi.org/10.1073/pnas.1710502115.
62. A. Mani, S. Mullainathan, E. Shafir, and J. Zhao, "Poverty Impedes Cognitive Function," *Science* 341 (2013): 976–80.
63. Guy Standing, "The Precariat: The New Dangerous Class," *Amalgam* 6, nos. 6-7 (2014): 115–19.
64. Schrecker and Bambra, *How Politics Makes Us Sick*, 56.
65. Roberto De Vogli, Jane E. Ferrie, Tarani Chandola, Mika Kivimäki, and Michael G. Marmot, "Unfairness and Health: Evidence from the Whitehall II Study," *Journal of Epidemiology and Community Health* 61, no. 6 (2007): 513–18.
66. Schrecker and Bambra, *How Politics Makes Us Sick*, 53–56.
67. Nina E. Fultz, Giorgio Bonmassar, Kawin Setsompop, Robert A. Stickgold, Bruce R. Rosen, Jonathan R. Polimeni, and Laura D. Lewis, "Coupled Electrophysiological, Hemodynamic, and Cerebrospinal Fluid Oscillations in Human Sleep," *Science* 366, no. 6465 (2019): 628–31.
68. Amanda Shim, Megan Hogan, Kathryn Halldin, Hannah Clark, Beka Behrens, Cassidy Griffith, Ogie Queen Umasabor-Bubu, and Omonigho Michael Bubu, "Sleep Disordered Breathing, ApoE4 and β-Amyloid Deposition in Cognitively Normal Elderly," *Alzheimer's and Dementia: The Journal of the Alzheimer's Association* 13, no. 7 (2017): P1124–25.
69. Robert T. Muller, "Fast Food Industry Demands 'Emotional Labour' from Employees," *Psychology Today*, October 5, 2016, https://www.psychologytoday.com/blog/talking-about-trauma/201610/fast-food-industry-demands-emotional-labour-employees.
70. Case and Deaton, *Deaths of Despair*.
71. Steven H. Woolf and Heidi Schoomaker, "Life Expectancy and Mortality Rates in the United States, 1959-2017," *Journal of the American Medical Association* 322, no. 20 (2019): 1996–2016.
72. Case and Deaton, "Mortality and Morbidity in the 21st Century."

73. Elizabeth M. Stein, Keith P. Gennuso, Donna C. Ugboaja, and Patrick L. Remington, "The Epidemic of Despair among White Americans: Trends in the Leading Causes of Premature Death, 1999-2015," *American Journal of Public Health* 107, no. 10 (2017): 1541–47.
74. Nathan Robinson, *Trump: Anatomy of a Monstrosity* (Somerville, MA: Current Affairs Press, 2017), 664.
75. Jennifer Miller, "Which Profession Has the Highest Rate Of Drug Abuse?" *Fast Company*, September 3, 2014, https://www.fastcompany.com/3034936/which-profession-has-the-highest-rate-of-drug-abuse.
76. Michaël Schwarzinger, Bruce G. Pollock, Omer SM Hasan, Carole Dufouil, Jürgen Rehm, S. Baillot, Quentin Guibert, F. Planchet, and S. Luchini, "Contribution of Alcohol Use Disorders to the Burden of Dementia in France 2008-13: A Nationwide Retrospective Cohort Study," *Lancet Public Health* 3, no. 3 (2018): e124–32.
77. Guochao Zhong, Yi Wang, Yong Zhang, Jeff Jianfei Guo, and Yong Zhao, "Smoking Is Associated with an Increased Risk of Dementia: A Meta-analysis of Prospective Cohort Studies with Investigation of Potential Effect Modifiers," *PloS one* 10, no. 3 (2015): e0118333.
78. J. Paul Leigh, Wesley A. Leigh, and Juan Du, "Minimum Wages and Public Health: A Literature Review," *Preventive Medicine* 118 (2019): 122–34.
79. Ayodele Odutayo, Peter Gill, Shaun Shepherd, Aquila Akingbade, Sally Hopewell, Karthik Tennankore, Benjamin H. Hunn, and Connor A. Emdin, "Income Disparities in Absolute Cardiovascular Risk and Cardiovascular Risk Factors in the United States, 1999-2014," *JAMA Cardiology* 2, no. 7 (July 1, 2017): 782–90, https://doi.org/10.1001/jamacardio.2017.1658.
80. Cody Delistraty, "How Each Generation Gets the Drugs It Deserves," *Aeon* January 4, 2017, https://aeon.co/essays/how-each-generation-gets-the-drugs-it-deserves.
81. Jared S Hopkins and Andrew Scurria, "Sacklers Received as Much as $13 Billion in Profits from Purdue Pharma," *Wall Street Journal,* October 5, 2019, sec: Business, www.wsj.com/articles/sacklers-received-12-billion-to-13-billion-in-profits-from-oxycontin-maker-purdue-pharma-11570221797.
82. Josh Eidelson, "Fast Food Walkout Planned in Chicago," *Salon*, April 24, 2013, https://www.salon.com/2013/04/24/fast_food_walkout_planned_in_chicago/.
83. Odutayo et al., "Income Disparities in Absolute Cardiovascular Risk."
84. Gregory A. Panza, Beth A. Taylor, Hayley V. MacDonald, Blair T. Johnson, Amanda L. Zaleski, Jill Livingston, Paul D. Thompson, and Linda S. Pescatello, "Can Exercise Improve Cognitive Symptoms of Alzheimer's Disease?" *Journal of the American Geriatrics Society* 66, no. 3 (2018): 487–95, https://doi.org/10.1111/jgs.15241.
85. Chun Liang Hsu, John R. Best, Jennifer C. Davis, Lindsay S. Nagamatsu, Shirley Wang, Lara A. Boyd, G. Y. Robin Hsiung, Michelle W. Voss, Janice Jennifer Eng, and Teresa Liu-Ambrose, "Aerobic Exercise Promotes Executive Functions and Impacts Functional Neural Activity among Older Adults with Vascular Cognitive Impairment," *British Journal of Sports Medicine* 52, no. 3 (2018): 184–91.
86. Prabha Siddarth, Berna Rahi, Natacha D. Emerson, Alison C. Burggren, Karen J. Miller, Susan Bookheimer, Helen Lavretsky, Bruce Dobkin, Gary Small, and David A. Merrill, "Physical Activity and Hippocampal Sub-region Structure in Older Adults with Memory Complaints," *Journal of Alzheimer's Disease* 61, no. 3 (2018): 1089–96.
87. Kan Ding, Takashi Tarumi, David C. Zhu, Benjamin Y. Tseng, Binu P. Thomas, Marcel Turner, Justin Repshas, et al., "Cardiorespiratory Fitness and White Matter Neuronal Fiber Integrity in Mild Cognitive Impairment," *Journal of Alzheimer's Disease* 61, no. 2 (2018): 729–39.
88. Panza et al., "Can Exercise Improve Cognitive Symptoms of Alzheimer's Disease?"
89. Junyeon Won, Alfonso J. Alfini, Lauren R. Weiss, Corey S. Michelson, Daniel D. Callow, Sushant M. Ranadive, Rodolphe J. Gentili, and J. Carson Smith, "Semantic Memory

Activation after Acute Exercise in Healthy Older Adults," *Journal of the International Neuropsychological Society* 25, no. 6 (2019): 557–68.

90. Kevin Loria, "The Healing Power of Nature," *Consumer Reports*, July 15, 2019, https://www.consumerreports.org/health-wellness/healing-power-nature-outdoors/.
91. Howard Frumkin, Gregory N. Bratman, Sara Jo Breslow, Bobby Cochran, Peter H. Kahn Jr., Joshua J. Lawler, Phillip S. Levin, et al., "Nature Contact and Human Health: A Research Agenda," *Environmental Health Perspectives* 125, no. 7 (2017): 075001.
92. Lauren Effron, Christina Ng, and Lauren Pearle, "When Working 2 Fast Food Jobs, 16 Hours a Day Still Isn't Enough," *ABC News*, January 13, 2017, https://abcnews.go.com/US/working-fast-food-jobs-16-hours-day/story?id=44707695.
93. Emma García and Elaine Weiss, *Education Inequalities at the School Starting Gate: Gaps, Trends, and Strategies to Address Them* (Washington, DC: Economic Policy Institute, 2017).
94. Nicholas Kristof and Sheryl WuDunn, "Who Killed the Knapp Family?" *New York Times*, January 9, 2020, https://www.nytimes.com/2020/01/09/opinion/sunday/deaths-despair-poverty.html?smid=nytcore-ios-share.
95. Bryce Covert, "McDonald's Employee Received a Severe Burn, Manager Told Her to Put Mustard on It," *Think Progress*, March 16, 2015, https://archive.thinkprogress.org/mcdonalds-employee-received-a-severe-burn-manager-told-her-to-put-mustard-on-it-baeb1c67d91d/.
96. "Burned at McDonald's, Treated with Mustard," video, 2:55, Fight for 15, March 16, 2015, https://www.youtube.com/watch?v=xN9TdrYeZzU.
97. Isabelle Baldi, Anne Gruber, Virginie Rondeau, Pierre Lebailly, Patrick Brochard, and Colette Fabrigoule, "Neurobehavioral Effects of Long-Term Exposure to Pesticides: Results from the 4-Year Follow-up of the PHYTONER Study," *Occupational and Environmental Medicine* 68, no. 2 (2011): 108–15.
98. Fabien Dutheil, Philippe Beaune, Christophe Tzourio, Marie-Anne Loriot, and Alexis Elbaz, "Interaction between ABCB1 and Professional Exposure to Organochlorine Insecticides in Parkinson Disease," *Archives of Neurology* 67, no. 6 (2010): 739–45.
99. Maryse F. Bouchard, Jonathan Chevrier, Kim G. Harley, Katherine Kogut, Michelle Vedar, Norma Calderon, Celina Trujillo, et al., "Prenatal Exposure to Organophosphate Pesticides and IQ in 7-Year-Old Children," *Environmental Health Perspectives* 119, no. 8 (2011): 1189–95.
100. Jose G. Salazar, Diana Ribes, Maria Cabre, Jose L Domingo, Fernando Sanchez-Santed, and Maria Teresa Colomina, "Amyloid β Peptide Levels Increase in Brain of AβPP Swedish Mice after Exposure to Chlorpyrifos," *Current Alzheimer Research* 8, no. 7 (2011): 732–40.
101. Stephanie M. Engel, James Wetmur, Jia Chen, Chenbo Zhu, Dana Boyd Barr, Richard L. Canfield, and Mary S. Wolff, "Prenatal Exposure to Organophosphates, Paraoxonase 1, and Cognitive Development in Childhood," *Environmental Health Perspectives* 119, no. 8 (2011): 1182–88.
102. Jason R. Richardson, Ananya Roy, Stuart L. Shalat, Richard T. Von Stein, Muhammad M. Hossain, Brian Buckley, Marla Gearing, Allan I. Levey, and Dwight C. German, "Elevated Serum Pesticide Levels and Risk for Alzheimer Disease," *JAMA Neurology* 71, no. 3 (2014): 284–90.
103. Yelena Ogneva-Himmelberger and Liyao Huang, "Spatial Distribution of Unconventional Gas Wells and Human Populations in the Marcellus Shale in the United States: Vulnerability Analysis," *Applied Geography* 60 (June 1, 2015): 165–74, https://doi.org/10.1016/j.apgeog.2015.03.011.
104. Jill E. Johnston, Emily Werder, and Daniel Sebastian, "Wastewater Disposal Wells, Fracking, and Environmental Injustice in Southern Texas," *American Journal of Public Health* 106, no. 3 (2016): 550–56.

105. United Church of Christ, Commission for Racial Justice, *Toxic Wastes and Race in the United States: A National Report on the Racial and Socio-economic Characteristics of Communities with Hazardous Waste Sites* (New York: Public Data Access, 1987).
106. Lawrence Wright, "The Dark Bounty of Texas Oil," *New Yorker*, December 25, 2017, https://www.newyorker.com/magazine/2018/01/01/the-dark-bounty-of-texas-oil.
107. Sara G. Rasmussen, Elizabeth L. Ogburn, Meredith McCormack, Joan A. Casey, Karen Bandeen-Roche, Dione G. Mercer, and Brian S. Schwartz, "Association between Unconventional Natural Gas Development in the Marcellus Shale and Asthma Exacerbations," *JAMA Internal Medicine* 176, no. 9 (2016): 1334–43.
108. Aaron W. Tustin, Annemarie G. Hirsch, Sara G. Rasmussen, Joan A. Casey, Karen Bandeen-Roche, and Brian S. Schwartz, "Associations between Unconventional Natural Gas Development and Nasal and Sinus, Migraine Headache, and Fatigue Symptoms in Pennsylvania," *Environmental Health Perspectives* 125, no. 2 (February 1, 2017): 189–97, https://doi.org/10.1289/EHP281.
109. M. L. Finkel, "Shale Gas Development and Cancer Incidence in Southwest Pennsylvania," *Public Health* 141 (December 1, 2016): 198–206, https://doi.org/10.1016/j.puhe.2016.09.008.
110. Lisa M. McKenzie, William B. Allshouse, Tim E. Byers, Edward J. Bedrick, Berrin Serdar, and John L. Adgate, "Childhood Hematologic Cancer and Residential Proximity to Oil and Gas Development," *PLoS ONE* 12, no. 2 (February 15, 2017): e0170423, https://doi.org/10.1371/journal.pone.0170423.
111. Janet Currie, Michael Greenstone, and Katherine Meckel, "Hydraulic Fracturing and Infant Health: New Evidence from Pennsylvania," *Science Advances* 3, no. 12 (December 1, 2017): e1603021, https://doi.org/10.1126/sciadv.1603021.
112. Russell A. Wilke and Jerome W. Freeman, "Potential Health Implications Related to Fracking," *Journal of the American Medical Association* 318, no. 17 (2017): 1645–46.
113. Amanda Gillooly, "Fracking Injuries: What You Need to Know and Why You Need a Gas Drilling Accident Lawyer," Pribanic and Pribanic, October 5, 2015, https://pribanic.com/marcellus-shale-drilling-fracking-injuries-what-you-need-to-know/.
114. Ihab Mikati, Adam F. Benson, Thomas J. Luben, Jason D. Sacks, and Jennifer Richmond-Bryant, "Disparities in Distribution of Particulate Matter Emission Sources by Race and Poverty Status," *American Journal of Public Health* 108, no. 4 (2018): 480–85.
115. Ellen Ruppel Shell, "The New Alzheimer's–Air Pollution Link," *Scientific American*, May 1, 2020, https://doi.org/10.1038/scientificamerican0520-42.
116. Yaohua Tian, Hui Liu, Yiqun Wu, Yaqin Si, Jing Song, Yaying Cao, Man Li, et al., "Association between Ambient Fine Particulate Pollution and Hospital Admissions for Cause Specific Cardiovascular Disease: Time Series Study in 184 Major Chinese Cities," *BMJ* 367 (December 30, 2019): 16572, https://doi.org/10.1136/bmj.l6572.
117. "Babies' Brains 'Damaged by Pollution,'" *BBC News*, December 6, 2017, sec. Health, https://www.bbc.com/news/health-42250558.
118. Laura K. Fonken, Xiaohua Xu, Zachary M. Weil, Guohua Chen, Qinghua Sun, Sanjay Rajagopalan, and Randy J. Nelson, "Air Pollution Impairs Cognition, Provokes Depressive-like Behaviors and Alters Hippocampal Cytokine Expression and Morphology," *Molecular Psychiatry* 16, no. 10 (2011): 987–95.
119. Mafalda Cacciottolo, Xinhui Wang, Ira Driscoll, Nicholas Woodward, Arian Saffari, Jeanette Reyes, Mark L. Serre, et al., "Particulate Air Pollutants, APOE Alleles and Their Contributions to Cognitive Impairment in Older Women and to Amyloidogenesis in Experimental Models," *Translational Psychiatry* 7, no. 1 (2017): e1022.
120. Marianthi-Anna Kioumourtzoglou, Joel D. Schwartz, Marc G. Weisskopf, Steven J. Melly, Yun Wang, Francesca Dominici, and Antonella Zanobetti, "Long-Term PM2.5 Exposure and Neurological Hospital Admissions in the Northeastern United States," *Environmental Health Perspectives* 124, no. 1 (2016): 23–29.

121. Michelle L. Block and Lilian Calderón-Garcidueñas, "Air Pollution: Mechanisms of Neuroinflammation and CNS Disease," *Trends in Neurosciences* 32, no. 9 (2009): 506–16.
122. Hong Chen, Jeffrey C. Kwong, Ray Copes, Karen Tu, Paul J. Villeneuve, Aaron Van Donkelaar, Perry Hystad, et al., "Living Near Major Roads and the Incidence of Dementia, Parkinson's Disease, and Multiple Sclerosis: A Population-Based Cohort Study," *Lancet* 389, no. 10070 (2017): 718–26.
123. Chau-Ren Jung, Yu-Ting Lin, and Bing-Fang Hwang, "Ozone, Particulate Matter, and Newly Diagnosed Alzheimer's Disease: A Population-Based Cohort Study in Taiwan," *Journal of Alzheimer's Disease* 44, no. 2 (2015): 573–84.
124. Diana Younan, Andrew J. Petkus, Keith F. Widaman, Xinhui Wang, Ramon Casanova, Mark A. Espeland, Margaret Gatz, et al., "Particulate Matter and Episodic Memory Decline Mediated by Early Neuroanatomic Biomarkers of Alzheimer's Disease," *Brain* 143, no. 1 (January 1, 2020): 289–302, https://doi.org/10.1093/brain/awz348.
125. Kelly C. Bishop, Jonathan D. Ketcham, and Nicolai V. Kuminoff, *Hazed and Confused: The Effect of Air Pollution on Dementia*, no. w24970 (Cambridge, MA: National Bureau of Economic Research, 2018).
126. Dana Loomis, Margarita Castillejos, Diane R. Gold, William McDonnell, and Victor Hugo Borja-Aburto, "Air Pollution and Infant Mortality in Mexico City," *Epidemiology* 10, no. 2 (1999): 118–23.
127. Janet Raloff, "Destination Brain," *Science News* 177, no. 11 (2010): 16–20.
128. Sarah J. Stock and Tom Clemens. "Traffic Pollution Is Linked to Poor Pregnancy Outcomes," *BMJ* 359 (December 5, 2017): j5511, https://doi.org/10.1136/bmj.j5511.
129. "Regulatory Rollbacks," Environmental Integrity Project, accessed March 3, 2020, https://environmentalintegrity.org/trump-watch-epa/regulatory-rollbacks/.
130. Susan Okie, "Traumatic Brain Injury in the War Zone," *New England Journal of Medicine* 352, no. 20 (2005): 2043–47.
131. Terri L. Tanielian and Lisa Jaycox, *Invisible Wounds of War: Psychological and Cognitive Injuries, Their Consequences, and Services to Assist Recovery*, vol. 1. (Santa Monica, CA: Rand, 2008).
132. Benjamin B. Trotter, Meghan E. Robinson, William P. Milberg, Regina E. McGlinchey, and David H. Salat, "Military Blast Exposure, Ageing and White Matter Integrity," *Brain* 138, no. 8 (2015): 2278–92.
133. Sharon Shively, Ann I. Scher, Daniel P. Perl, and Ramon Diaz-Arrastia, "Dementia Resulting from Traumatic Brain Injury: What Is the Pathology?" *Archives of Neurology* 69, no. 10 (2012): 1245–51.
134. S. Fleminger, D. L. Oliver, S. Lovestone, S. Rabe-Hesketh, and A. Giora, "Head Injury as a Risk Factor for Alzheimer's Disease: The Evidence 10 Years on; a Partial Replication," *Journal of Neurology, Neurosurgery and Psychiatry* 74, no. 7 (2003): 857–62.
135. J. A. Mortimer, C. M. Van Duijn, V. Chandra, Laura Fratiglioni, A. B. Graves, A. Heyman, A. F. Jorm, et al., "Head Trauma as a Risk Factor for Alzheimer's Disease: A Collaborative Re-analysis of Case-Control Studies," *International Journal of Epidemiology* 20, suppl. 2 (1991): S28–S35.
136. Z. Guo, L. A. Cupples, A. Kurz, S. H. Auerbach, L. Volicer, H. Chui, R. C. Green, et al., "Head Injury and the Risk of AD in the MIRAGE Study," *Neurology* 54, no. 6 (2000): 1316–23.
137. Peter Nordström, Karl Michaëlsson, Yngve Gustafson, and Anna Nordström, "Traumatic Brain Injury and Young Onset Dementia: A Nationwide Cohort Study," *Annals of Neurology* 75, no. 3 (2014): 374–81.
138. Wei Li, Shannon L. Risacher, Thomas W. McAllister, and Andrew J. Saykin, "Traumatic Brain Injury and Age at Onset of Cognitive Impairment in Older Adults," *Journal of neurology* 263, no. 7 (2016): 1280–85.

139. Anna Nordström and Peter Nordström, "Traumatic Brain Injury and the Risk of Dementia Diagnosis: A Nationwide Cohort Study," *PLoS Medicine* 15, no. 1 (2018), https://doi.org/10.1371/journal.pmed.1002496.
140. Rahul Raj, Jaakko Kaprio, Miikka Korja, Era D. Mikkonen, Pekka Jousilahti, and Jari Siironen, "Risk of Hospitalization with Neurodegenerative Disease after Moderate-to-Severe Traumatic Brain Injury in the Working-Age Population: A Retrospective Cohort Study Using the Finnish National Health Registries," *PLoS Medicine* 14, no. 7 (2017): e1002316.
141. Jeff Schaffert, Christian LoBue, Charles L. White III, Hsueh-Sheng Chiang, Nyaz Didehbani, Laura Lacritz, Heidi Rossetti, Marisara Dieppa, John Hart Jr, and C. Munro Cullum, "Traumatic Brain Injury History Is Associated with an Earlier Age of Dementia Onset in Autopsy-Confirmed Alzheimer's Disease," *Neuropsychology* 32, no. 4 (2018): 410.
142. Deborah E. Barnes, Amy L. Byers, Raquel C. Gardner, Karen H. Seal, W. John Boscardin, and Kristine Yaffe, "Association of Mild Traumatic Brain Injury with and without Loss of Consciousness with Dementia in US Military Veterans," *JAMA Neurology* 75, no. 9 (2018): 1055–61.
143. Suzanne Corkin, T. John Rosen, Edith V. Sullivan, and Rae Ann Clegg, "Penetrating Head Injury in Young Adulthood Exacerbates Cognitive Decline in Later Years," *Journal of Neuroscience* 9, no. 11 (1989): 3876–83.
144. Vanessa Raymont, Amanda Greathouse, Katherine Reding, Robert Lipsky, Andres Salazar, and Jordan Grafman, "Demographic, Structural and Genetic Predictors of Late Cognitive Decline after Penetrating Head Injury," *Brain* 131, no. 2 (2008): 543–58.
145. Deborah E. Barnes, Allison Kaup, Katharine A. Kirby, Amy L. Byers, Ramon Diaz-Arrastia, and Kristine Yaffe, "Traumatic Brain Injury and Risk of Dementia in Older Veterans," *Neurology* 83, no. 4 (2014): 312–19.
146. M. Critchley, "Punch-Drunk Syndromes: The Chronic Traumatic Encephalopathy of Boxers," in *Hommage a Clovis Vincent* (Paris: Maloine, 1949).
147. A. C. McKee, N. J. Cairns, D. W. Dickson, R. D. Folkerth, C. Dirk Keene, I. Litvan, et al., "The First NINDS/NIBIB Consensus Meeting to Define Neuropathological Criteria for the Diagnosis of Chronic Traumatic Encephalopathy," *Acta Neuropathologica* 131, no. 1 (2015): 75–86.
148. Jonathan D. Cherry, Thor D. Stein, Yorghos Tripodis, Victor E. Alvarez, Bertrand R. Huber, Rhoda Au, Patrick T. Kiernan, et al., "CCL11 Is Increased in the CNS in Chronic Traumatic Encephalopathy but Not in Alzheimer's Disease," *PloS ONE* 12, no. 9 (2017): e0185541, http://journals.plos.org/plosone/article/file?id=10.1371/journal.pone.0185541&type=printable.
149. Robert A. Stern, Charles H. Adler, Kewei Chen, Michael Navitsky, Ji Luo, David W. Dodick, Michael L. Alosco, et al., "Tau Positron-Emission Tomography in Former National Football League Players," *New England Journal of Medicine* 380 (2019): 1716–25, https://www.nejm.org/doi/full/10.1056/NEJMoa1900757?query=featured_home.
150. Joe Ward, Josh Williams, and Sam Manchester, "111 N.F.L. Brains: All but One Had C.T.E.," *New York Times*, July 25, 2017, sec. Sports, https://www.nytimes.com/interactive/2017/07/25/sports/football/nfl-cte.html.
151. "Study Suggests Link between Youth Football and Later-Life Emotional, Behavioral Impairment," EurekAlert!, press release, September 19, 2017, https://www.eurekalert.org/pub_releases/2017-09/buso-ssl091417.php.
152. Naeim Bahrami, Dev Sharma, Scott Rosenthal, Elizabeth M. Davenport, Jillian E. Urban, Benjamin Wagner, Youngkyoo Jung, et al., "Subconcussive Head Impact Exposure and White Matter Tract Changes over a Single Season of Youth Football," *Radiology* 281, no. 3 (2016): 919–26.
153. Scooby Axson, "'Concussion' Doc: Kids Playing Football Is Abuse," *Sports Illustrated*, August 8, 2017, https://www.si.com/nfl/2017/08/08/bennet-omalu-cte-football.

154. Amy Lutz, "Who Joins the Military? A Look at Race, Class, and Immigration Status," *Journal of Political and Military Sociology* 36, no. 2 (2008): 167–88.
155. Adam Dean, "Free Trade Doesn't Just Lead to Job Loss: It Means More Deaths from Drug Overdoses and Increased Military Recruitment," *Washington Post*, July 15, 2019, https://www.washingtonpost.com/politics/2019/07/15/free-trade-doesnt-just-lead-job-loss-it-means-higher-deaths-drug-overdoses-more-military-recruitment/.
156. Adam Dean, "NAFTA's Army: Free Trade and US Military Enlistment," *International Studies Quarterly* 62, no. 4 (2018): 845–56.
157. Richard Lapchick, Philip Costa, Tamara Sherrod, and Rahman Anjorin, "The 2012 Racial and Gender Report Card: National Football League," UCF Institute for Diversity and Ethics in Sport, September 13, 2012, http://www.tidesport.org/RGRC/2012/2012_NFL_RGRC.pdf.
158. "Burkmont Resources and Information," Burkmont.com, accessed March 4, 2020, http://www.burkmont.com/2015/10/the-nfl-might-have-growing-poverty.html.
159. Matt Kawahara, "Why Fewer Kids Are Playing Football: A Study in Decline," *San Francisco Chronicle*, October 25, 2018, https://www.sfchronicle.com/sports/article/Why-fewer-kids-are-playing-football-A-study-in-13319241.php.
160. "Making the Economic Case for a $15 Minimum Wage," the Century Foundation, January 28, 2019, https://tcf.org/content/commentary/making-economic-case-15-minimum-wage/.
161. "The Fight for $15 Is Winning for Women and Families," National Women's Law Center, April 26, 2017, https://nwlc.org/resources/the-fight-for-15-is-winning-for-women-and-families/.
162. Robert Reich, "On Labor, Tragically, Trump Was Right," *Newsweek*, August 28, 2017, https://www.yahoo.com/news/robert-reich-labor-tragically-trump-143003799.html.
163. Brian Rahmer (@brianrahmer), "The disheartening percentage of Americans living in extreme poverty—that is, living on less than half the poverty threshold—has increased since the 1970s. #SOH @HiAP," Twitter, March 3, 2018, 5:14 p.m., https://twitter.com/brianrahmer/status/970075031060537344.
164. John A. Kaufman, Leslie K. Salas-Hernández, Kelli A. Komro, and Melvin D. Livingston, "Effects of Increased Minimum Wages by Unemployment Rate on Suicide in the USA," *Journal of Epidemiology and Community Health* 74, no. 3 (March 1, 2020): 219–24, https://doi.org/10.1136/jech-2019-212981.
165. Noam Chomsky, *Who Rules the World?* (New York: Picador, 2017), 262.
166. "Top Charts of 2017: 12 Charts That Show the Real Problems Policies Must Tackle, Not the Made-up Ones," Economic Policy Institute, December 21, 2017, https://www.epi.org/publication/top-charts-of-2017-12-charts-that-show-the-real-problems-policies-must-tackle-not-the-made-up-ones/.
167. "Future of Work," McKinsey and Company, last updated July 11, 2019, https://www.mckinsey.com/featured-insights/future-of-work.
168. Réka Nagy, "AI Can Identify Alzheimer's a Decade before Symptoms Show," *Student Newspaper*, September 30, 2017, https://studentnewspaper.org/ai-can-identify-alzheimers-a-decade-before-symptoms-show/.
169. Ned Resnikoff, "Nearly Half of All Americans Support Job Guarantee," MSNBC, January 13, 2014, http://www.msnbc.com/all/guaranteed-job-everyone.
170. Mark Paul, William Darity Jr., and Darrick Hamilton, "Why We Need a Federal Job Guarantee,"*Jacobin*, February 2017, https://jacobinmag.com/2017/02/federal-job-guarantee-universal-basic-income-investment-jobs-unemployment/.
171. Leslie Davis and Hannah Hartig, "Two-Thirds of Americans Favor Raising Federal Minimum Wage to $15 an Hour," *Pew Research Center*, July 30, 2019, https://www.pewresearch.org/fact-tank/2019/07/30/two-thirds-of-americans-favor-raising-federal-minimum-wage-to-15-an-hour/.

172. "State Minimum Wages: 2020 Minimum Wage by State," National Conference of State Legislatures, January 6, 2020, https://www.ncsl.org/research/labor-and-employment/state-minimum-wage-chart.aspx.
173. Paul Davidson, "Minimum Wage Hikes: 18 States, 20 Cities to Lift Pay Floors Jan. 1," *Milwaukee Journal Sentinel*, December 19, 2017, https://www.jsonline.com/story/money/2017/12/19/minimum-wage-hikes-18-states-20-cities-lift-pay-floors-jan-1/961213001/.
174. Jordan Weissmann, "Target Says It Will Raise Its Minimum Wage to $15 by 2020," *Slate*, September 25, 2017, https://slate.com/business/2017/09/target-says-it-will-move-to-a-usd15-minimum-wage-by-2020.html.
175. Todd Carmichael, "La Colombe Founder: If You Can't Pay Employees a Living Wage, You Don't Deserve to Be in Business," *Philadelphia Inquirer*, September 19, 2017, https://www.inquirer.com/philly/opinion/commentary/la-colombe-todd-carmichael-minimum-wage-increase-20170919.html.
176. Quoctrung Bui, "50 Years of Shrinking Union Membership, in One Map," NPR, February 23, 2015, https://www.npr.org/sections/money/2015/02/23/385843576/50-years-of-shrinking-union-membership-in-one-map.
177. "Union Members Summary," US Bureau of Labor Statistics, Economic News Release, January 22, 2020, https://www.bls.gov/news.release/union2.nr0.htm.
178. Matt Bruenig, "Nordic Socialism Is Realer Than You Think," MattBruenig.com, July 28, 2017, http://mattbruenig.com/2017/07/28/nordic-socialism-is-realer-than-you-think/.
179. "Union Members Summary."
180. Barry Ritholtz, "Ronald Reagan: 'Where Free Unions and Collective Bargaining Are Forbidden, Freedom Is Lost,' " *Big Picture*, March 7, 2011, https://ritholtz.com/2011/03/ronald-reagan-where-free-unions-and-collective-bargaining-are-forbidden-freedom-is-lost/.
181. In Germany, workers have between one-third and one-half of seats on a company's supervisory board, which brings some parity in power between labor and management, albeit imperfectly.
182. Matthew Desmond, "The $15 Minimum Wage Doesn't Just Improve Lives: It Saves Them," *New York Times*, February 21, 2019, sec. Magazine, https://www.nytimes.com/interactive/2019/02/21/magazine/minimum-wage-saving-lives.html.
183. Daniel R. George, Wilbert Beachy, John Chan, Forbes Cameron, Jane Trinkkeller, and Jed D. Gonzalo, "Teaching Population Health: Using the Classroom as a Bridge to the Community," *Med Teach* 38 (2016): 1182–83.
184. Daniel R. George, Monica Manglani, Kaitlin Minnehan, Alexander Chacon, Alexandra Gundersen, Cheryl Dellasega, and Jennifer L. Kraschnewski, "Examining Feasibility of Mentoring Families at a Farmers' Market and Community Garden," *American Journal of Health Education* 47, no. 2 (2016): 94–98.
185. Houda Bouhmam, David Boothe, and Daniel R. George, "Hosting Syrian Refugees: Resources Exist in Our Communities," *American Journal of Public Health* 107, no. 7 (2017): 1013.
186. Marco Canevelli, Flaminia Lucchini, Federica Quarata, Giuseppe Bruno, and Matteo Cesari, "Nutrition and Dementia: Evidence for Preventive Approaches?" *Nutrients* 8, no. 3 (2016): 144.
187. Douglas J. Wiebe, Bernadette A. D'Alonzo, Robin Harris, Margot Putukian, and Carolyn Campbell-McGovern, "Association between the Experimental Kickoff Rule and Concussion Rates in Ivy League Football," *Journal of the American Medical Association* 320, no. 19 (November 20, 2018): 2035–36, https://doi.org/10.1001/jama.2018.14165.
188. "Injury Data," NFL Player Health and Safety, accessed January 23, 2020, https://www.playsmartplaysafe.com/newsroom/reports/injury-data.
189. Jeffrey M. Jones, "Pro Football Losing Fans; Other Sports Holding Steady," Gallup, October 13, 2017, https://news.gallup.com/poll/220562/pro-football-losing-fans-sports-holding-steady.aspx.

190. Adam Kilgore and Scott Clement, "Poll: Nine in 10 Sports Fans Say NFL Brain Injuries Are a Problem, but 74 Percent Are Still Football Fans," *Washington Post*, September 6, 2017, https://www.washingtonpost.com/sports/poll-nfl-remains-as-popular-as-ever-despite-head-injuries-other-concerns/2017/09/06/238bef8a-9265-11e7-8754-d478688d23b4_story.html.
191. Jay Cassano, "Defense Department: The War on Terror Has Cost $250 Million a Day for 16 Years," *International Business Times*, October 31, 2017, https://www.ibtimes.com/political-capital/defense-department-war-terror-has-cost-250-million-day-16-years-2608639.
192. Andrew Keshner, "Here's How Much the War on Terror Contributed to America's Opioid Crisis," *MarketWatch*, September 22, 2019, https://www.marketwatch.com/story/heres-how-much-the-war-on-terror-contributed-to-americas-opioid-crisis-2019-09-18.
193. Jake Johnson, "'We Will Not Be Complicit': Protesting Assault on Yemen, Italian Dock Workers Refuse to Load Saudi Weapons Vessel," Common Dreams, May 21, 2019, https://www.commondreams.org/news/2019/05/21/we-will-not-be-complicit-protesting-assault-yemen-italian-dock-workers-refuse-load.
194. Elena Holodny, "One Group Would Greatly Benefit from Raising the Minimum Wage—and It Shows How America Has Failed Them," *Business Insider*, November 10, 2017, https://www.businessinsider.com/veterans-day-minimum-wage-2017-11.
195. Amy Nathan Wright, "Civil Rights 'Unfinished Business': Poverty, Race, and the 1968 Poor People's Campaign" (PhD diss., University of Texas, Austin, 2007), 156.
196. Marian Wright Edelman, "Revisiting Marks, Mississippi," *HuffPost*, March 25, 2011, https://www.huffpost.com/entry/revisiting-marks-mississi_b_840786.
197. Paul Steckler, interview with Ralph Abernathy, October 22, 1988, Eyes on the Prize II Interviews, Washington University Digital Gateway Texts, http://digital.wustl.edu/e/eii/eiiweb/abe5427.0819.003marc_record_interviewee_process.html.
198. "Statement on Visit to the USA, by Professor Philip Alston, United Nations Special Rapporteur on Extreme Poverty and Human Rights," UN Human Rights Office of the High Commissioner, December 15, 2017, https://www.ohchr.org/EN/NewsEvents/Pages/DisplayNews.aspx?NewsID=22533.
199. Tim Smeeding, "Cash Matters and Place Matters: A Child Poverty Plan that Capitalizes on New Evidence," *Pathways*, Spring 2017, 14–20.
200. Martin Luther King Jr., May 1965 speech to the Negro American Labor Council, in T. Jackson, *From Civil Rights to Human Rights* (Philadelphia: University of Pennsylvania Press, 2009), 230.

CHAPTER 7. TURNING UP THE HEAT ON GLOBAL WARMING

1. Joan Brunkard, Gonza Namulanda, and Raoult Ratard, "Hurricane Katrina Deaths, Louisiana, 2005," *Disaster Medicine and Public Health Preparedness* 2, no. 4 (December 2008): 215–23, https://doi.org/10.1097/DMP.0b013e31818aaf55.
2. Kacie Seil, Ariel Spira-Cohen, and Jennifer Marcum, "Injury Deaths Related to Hurricane Sandy, New York City, 2012," *Disaster Medicine and Public Health Preparedness* 10, no. 3 (2016): 378–85, https://doi.org/10.1017/dmp.2016.36.
3. Energy Policy Institute, "Is the Public Willing to Pay to Help Fix Climate Change?" Energy Policy Institute at the University of Chicago and the AP-NORC Center for Public Affairs Research, January 2019, http://www.apnorc.org/projects/Documents/EPIC%20fact%20sheet_v4_DTP.pdf.
4. Steven Perlberg, "The Climate Is Changing: How Often Climate Is Covered On TV Networks? Not So Much," *BuzzFeed News*, December 3, 2018, https://www.buzzfeednews.com/article/stevenperlberg/climate-change-cable-news-coverage.
5. "The Truth about Big Oil and Climate Change," *Economist*, February 9, 2019, https://www.economist.com/leaders/2019/02/09/the-truth-about-big-oil-and-climate-change.
6. Nathan Robinson, "The Choice We Face," *Current Affairs*, February 9, 2019, https://www.currentaffairs.org/2019/02/the-choice-we-face.

7. "Climate Change," ExxonMobil, accessed February 28, 2020, https://corporate.exxonmobil.com:443/Energy-and-environment/Environmental-protection/Climate-change.
8. US Global Change Research Program, *Fourth National Climate Assessment*, vol. 2, *Impacts Risks, and Adaptation in the United States* (Washington, DC: USGCRP, 2018), https://nca2018.globalchange.gov.
9. Cynthia McPherson Frantz and F. Stephan Mayer, "The Importance of Connection to Nature in Assessing Environmental Education Programs," in "Evaluating Environmental Education," special issue, *Studies in Educational Evaluation* 41 (June 1, 2014): 85–89, https://doi.org/10.1016/j.stueduc.2013.10.001.
10. *World Happiness Report 2019*, accessed February 28, 2020, http://worldhappiness.report/.
11. Robert Rohde, "Global Temperature Report for 2018," Berkeley Earth, January 24, 2019, http://berkeleyearth.org/2018-temperatures/.
12. In 2019, Secretary of State Mike Pompeo put a rather "interesting" neoliberal spin on melting ice sheets: "Steady reductions in sea ice are opening new passageways and new opportunities for trade, that can potentially slash the time it takes for ships to travel between Asia and the West by as much as 20 days." See Justin Wise, "Pompeo Says Shrinking Arctic Sea Ice Presents 'New Opportunities for Trade,'" *Hill*, May 6, 2019, https://thehill.com/policy/energy-environment/442413-pompeo-says-shrinking-arctic-sea-ice-presents-new-opportunities-for.
13. "Summary for Policymakers of IPCC Special Report on Global Warming of 1.5°C Approved by Governments," IPCC, October 8, 2018, https://www.ipcc.ch/2018/10/08/summary-for-policymakers-of-ipcc-special-report-on-global-warming-of-1-5c-approved-by-governments/.
14. David Wallace-Wells, *The Uninhabitable Earth: A Story of the Future* (London: Penguin UK, 2019).
15. Tyler Stone, "Obama: Suddenly America Is the Biggest Oil Producer, That Was Me, People," *Real Clear Politics*, November 28, 2017, https://www.realclearpolitics.com/video/2018/11/28/obama_suddenly_america_is_the_biggest_oil_producer_that_was_me_people.html.
16. Steve Horn, "Obama Admin Quietly Enables Oil and Gas Drilling on Public Lands and Waters, Weakens Endangered Species Act," *DeSmog* (blog), September 29, 2016, https://www.desmogblog.com/2016/09/29/obama-admin-oil-gas-public-lands-waters-endangered-species-act.
17. Bill McKibben, "Why We Should Name Hurricanes after Fossil Fuel Corporations," *Guardian*, November 6, 2012, sec. Opinion, https://www.theguardian.com/commentisfree/2012/nov/06/hurricanes-climate-change-fossil-fuels.
18. Thomas F. Stocker, Dahe Qin, Gian-Kasper Plattner, Melinda Tignor, Simon K. Allen, Judith Boschung, Alexander Nauels, Yu Xia, Vincent Bex, and Pauline M. Midgley, *Climate Change 2013: The Physical Science Basis* (Cambridge: Cambridge University Press, 2014).
19. US EPA, Office of Air and Radiation, "Causes of Climate Change," accessed February 28, 2020, https://19january2017snapshot.epa.gov/climate-change-science/causes-climate-change_.html.
20. US EPA, *Climate Change Indicators in the United States 2016* (Washington, DC: EPA, 2016).
21. Wallace-Wells, *Uninhabitable Earth.*
22. Paul Griffin, Richard Heede, and Ian van Der Vlugt, *The Carbon Majors Database: CDP Carbon Majors Report* (London: CDP, 2017).
23. "Mercury and Health," World Health Organization, March 31, 2017, https://www.who.int/news-room/fact-sheets/detail/mercury-and-health.
24. Lisa Friedman and Coral Davenport, "E.P.A. Weakens Controls on Mercury," *New York Times*, April 16, 2020, sec. Climate, https://www.nytimes.com/2020/04/16/climate/epa-mercury-coal.html.

25. Andrea Thompson, "From Fish to Humans, A Microplastic Invasion May Be Taking a Toll," *Scientific American*, September 4, 2018, https://www.scientificamerican.com/article/from-fish-to-humans-a-microplastic-invasion-may-be-taking-a-toll/.
26. Ed Yong, "A Troubling Discovery in the Deepest Ocean Trenches," *Atlantic*, February 27, 2019, https://www.theatlantic.com/science/archive/2019/02/deepest-ocean-trenches-animals-eat-plastic/583657/.
27. "Plastic Bottles Release Potentially Harmful Chemicals (Bisphenol A) after Contact with Hot Liquids," *ScienceDaily*, February 4, 2008, https://www.sciencedaily.com/releases/2008/01/080130092108.htm.
28. Ashley Fetters, "Sperm Counts Continue to Fall," *Atlantic*, October 12, 2018, https://www.theatlantic.com/family/archive/2018/10/sperm-counts-continue-to-fall/572794/.
29. Stephen Leahy, "Fracking Boom Tied to Methane Spike in Earth's Atmosphere," *National Geographic*, August 15, 2019, https://www.nationalgeographic.com/environment/2019/08/fracking-boom-tied-to-methane-spike-in-earths-atmosphere/.
30. Robert W. Howarth, "Ideas and Perspectives: Is Shale Gas a Major Driver of Recent Increase in Global Atmospheric Methane?" *Biogeosciences* 16, no. 15 (2019): 3033–46.
31. "Regulatory Rollback Tracker," Environmental and Energy Law Program, Harvard Law School, accessed February 28, 2020, https://eelp.law.harvard.edu/regulatory-rollback-tracker/.
32. Justin Farrell, "Corporate Funding and Ideological Polarization about Climate Change," *Proceedings of the National Academy of Sciences* 113, no. 1 (January 5, 2016): 92–97, https://doi.org/10.1073/pnas.1509433112.
33. Naomi Klein, *This Changes Everything: Capitalism vs. the Climate* (New York: Simon and Schuster, 2014).
34. Klein, *Shock Doctrine*.
35. I'm Not a Robot? *Bloomberg*, accessed February 28, 2020, https://www.bloomberg.com/tosv2.html.
36. John Zeisel, Barry Reisberg, Peter Whitehouse, Robert Woods, and Ad Verheul, "Ecopsychosocial Interventions in Cognitive Decline and Dementia: A New Terminology and a New Paradigm," *American Journal of Alzheimer's Disease and Other Dementias* 31, no. 6 (2016): 502–7.
37. Richard Horton and Selina Lo, "Planetary Health: A New Science for Exceptional Action," *Lancet* 386, no. 10007 (2015): 1921–22, https://doi.org/10.1016/S0140-6736(15)61038-8.
38. US Global Change Research Program, *Fourth National Climate Assessment*.
39. Helen L. Berry, Thomas D. Waite, Keith BG Dear, Anthony G. Capon, and Virginia Murray, "The Case for Systems Thinking about Climate Change and Mental Health," *Nature Climate Change* 8, no. 4 (2018): 282–90.
40. Jean Rhodes, Christian Chan, Christina Paxson, Cecilia Elena Rouse, Mary Waters, and Elizabeth Fussell, "The Impact of Hurricane Katrina on the Mental and Physical Health of Low-Income Parents in New Orleans," *American Journal of Orthopsychiatry* 80, no. 2 (April 2010): 237–47, https://doi.org/10.1111/j.1939-0025.2010.01027.x.
41. Tamma A. Carleton, "Reply to Plewis, Murari et al., and Das: The Suicide-Temperature Link in India and the Evidence of an Agricultural Channel Are Robust," *Proceedings of the National Academy of Sciences* 115, no. 2 (January 9, 2018): E118–21, https://doi.org/10.1073/pnas.1715454115.
42. Ivan C. Hanigan, Colin D. Butler, Philip N. Kokic, and Michael F. Hutchinson, "Suicide and Drought in New South Wales, Australia, 1970–2007," *Proceedings of the National Academy of Sciences* 109, no. 35 (August 28, 2012): 13950–55, https://doi.org/10.1073/pnas.1112965109.
43. Marshall Burke, Felipe González, Patrick Baylis, Sam Heft-Neal, Ceren Baysan, Sanjay Basu, and Solomon Hsiang, "Higher Temperatures Increase Suicide Rates in the United

States and Mexico," *Nature Climate Change* 8, no. 8 (August 2018): 723–29, https://doi.org/10.1038/s41558-018-0222-x.

44. Phan Minh Trang, Joacim Rocklöv, Kim Bao Giang, Gunnar Kullgren, and Maria Nilsson, "Heatwaves and Hospital Admissions for Mental Disorders in Northern Vietnam," *PLoS ONE* 11, no. 5 (May 19, 2016): e0155609. https://doi.org/10.1371/journal.pone.0155609.
45. Nick Obradovich, Robyn Migliorini, Sara C. Mednick, and James H. Fowler, "Nighttime Temperature and Human Sleep Loss in a Changing Climate," *Science Advances* 3, no. 5 (May 1, 2017): e1601555, https://doi.org/10.1126/sciadv.1601555.
46. Kenichi Azuma, Koichi Ikeda, Naoki Kagi, U. Yanagi, Kenichi Hasegawa, and Haruki Osawa, "Effects of Water-Damaged Homes after Flooding: Health Status of the Residents and the Environmental Risk Factors," *International Journal of Environmental Health Research* 24, no. 2 (2014): 158–75.
47. J. Swim, S. Clayton, T. Doherty, R. Gifford, G. Howard, J. Reser, P. Stern, and K. Weber, *Psychology and Global Climate Change: Addressing a Multifaceted Phenomenon and Set of Challenges*, Report of the American Psychological Association Task Force on the Interface between Psychology and Global Climate Change (Washington, DC: APA, 2010).
48. United States Department of Defense, *Quadrennial Defense Review Report* (Washington, DC: DOD, February 2010), https://archive.defense.gov/qdr/QDR%20as%20of%2029JAN10%201600.pdf.
49. Ibid, 85.
50. Ben Ehrenreich, "Climate Change Is Here—and It Looks Like Starvation," *Nation*, March 1, 2019, https://www.thenation.com/article/archive/climate-change-media-humanitarian-crises/.
51. Wesley Langat, "As Water Falls Short, Conflict between Herders and Farmers Sharpens," *Reuters*, November 23, 2015, https://www.reuters.com/article/kenya-climatechange-conflict-idUSL8N13D4G420151123.
52. Emmanuel Akinwotu, "Nigeria's Farmers and Herders Fight a Deadly Battle for Scarce Resources," *New York Times*, June 25, 2018, sec. World, https://www.nytimes.com/2018/06/25/world/africa/nigeria-herders-farmers.html.
53. OECD, "Herders vs Farmers: Resolving Deadly Conflict in the Sahel and West Africa," *Medium*, April 18, 2018, https://medium.com/@OECD/herders-vs-farmers-resolving-deadly-conflict-in-the-sahel-and-west-africa-e096702b5055.
54. C-F. Schleussner, Tabea K. Lissner, Erich M. Fischer, Jan Wohland, Mahé Perrette, Antonius Golly, Joeri Rogelj, et al., "Differential Climate Impacts for Policy-Relevant Limits to Global Warming: The Case of 1.5 C and 2 C," *Earth System Dynamics* 7 (2016): 327–51.
55. "The richest 0.54%, or 42 million people across the world, are responsible for more emissions than the poorest half of the global population, or 3.8 billion people"; Chris Hedges, "Saving the Planet Means Overthrowing the Ruling Elites," *Truthdig*, September 23, 2019, https://www.truthdig.com/articles/saving-the-planet-means-overthrowing-the-ruling-elites/.
56. Joanna A. Ruszkiewicz, Alexey A. Tinkov, Anatoly V. Skalny, Vasileios Siokas, Efthimios Dardiotis, Aristidis Tsatsakis, Aaron B. Bowman, João BT da Rocha, and Michael Aschner, "Brain Diseases in Changing Climate," *Environmental Research* 177 (2019): 108637.
57. Imen Belhadj Slimen, Taha Najar, Abdeljelil Ghram, Hajer Dabbebi, Moncef Ben Mrad, and Manef Abdrabbah, "Reactive Oxygen Species, Heat Stress and Oxidative-Induced Mitochondrial Damage: A Review," *International Journal of Hyperthermia* 30, no. 7 (2014): 513–23.
58. Meg Anderson and Sean McMinn, "As Rising Heat Bakes U.S. Cities, the Poor Often Feel It Most," NPR, September 3, 2019, https://www.npr.org/2019/09/03/754044732/as-rising-heat-bakes-u-s-cities-the-poor-often-feel-it-most.
59. Davide Mattei and Angelo Pietrobelli, "Micronutrients and Brain Development," *Current Nutrition Reports* 8, no. 2 (2019): 99–107.

60. USGCRP, *Fourth National Climate Assessment.*
61. E. Marie Muehe, Tianmei Wang, Carolin F. Kerl, Britta Planer-Friedrich, and Scott Fendorf, "Rice Production Threatened by Coupled Stresses of Climate and Soil Arsenic," *Nature Communications* 10, no. 1 (2019): 1–10.
62. Ruszkiewicz et al., "Brain Diseases in Changing Climate," 177.
63. Ibid.
64. Ibid.
65. Intergovernmental Panel on Climate Change, "Summary for Policymakers of IPCC Special Report on Global Warming of 1.5° C Approved by Governments," IPCC, October 8, 2018, https://www.ipcc.ch/2018/10/08/summary-for-policymakers-of-ipcc-special-report-on-global-warming-of-1-5c-approved-by-governments/
66. Alexandria Ocasio-Cortez, "Recognizing the Duty of the Federal Government to Create a Green New Deal," H.R. 109, 116th Cong., 1st sess. (2019).
67. Ibid.
68. Peter Wade, "Alexandria Ocasio-Cortez Criticizes Capitalism, Political Moderates at SXSW," *Rolling Stone* (blog), March 10, 2019, https://www.rollingstone.com/politics/politics-news/alexandria-ocasio-cortez-sxsw-806323/.
69. Of course, an ecopsychosocial perspective also must guide us in evaluating how our adaptation strategies to climate change (such as increasing industrial production of renewables) may also create new challenges for brain health and the environment.
70. Alex Morris, "Alexandria Ocasio-Cortez Wants the Country to Think Big," *Rolling Stone* (blog), February 27, 2019, https://www.rollingstone.com/politics/politics-features/alexandria-ocasio-cortez-congress-interview-797214/.
71. Abel Gustafson, Seth Rosenthal, Anthony Leiserowitz, Edward Maibach, John Kotcher, Matthew Ballew, and Matthew Goldberg, "The Green New Deal Has Strong Bipartisan Support," Yale Program on Climate Change Communication, December 14, 2018, https://climatecommunication.yale.edu/publications/the-green-new-deal-has-strong-bipartisan-support/.
72. Christina Wilkie, "Donald Trump Attacks Alexandria Ocasio-Cortez's Green New Deal at a Campaign Rally in a Preview of Things to Come for the 2020 Election," CNBC, February 12, 2019, https://www.cnbc.com/2019/02/12/trump-targets-alexandria-ocasio-cortez-green-new-deal-in-campaign-speech.html.
73. Sunrise Movement (@sunrisemvmt), "This is how @SenFeinstein reacted to children asking her to support the #GreenNewDeal resolution—with smugness + disrespect. This is a fight for our generation's survival. Her reaction is why young people desperately want new leadership in Congress," Twitter, February 22, 2019, 4:36 p.m., https://twitter.com/sunrisemvmt/status/1099075460649107458.
74. "OK Boomer," *Wikipedia*, last updated February 28, 2020, https://en.wikipedia.org/w/index.php?title=OK_Boomer&oldid=943014033.
75. Felix Biederman, Matt Christman, Brendan James, and Will Menaker, *The Chapo Guide to Revolution: A Manifesto against Logic, Facts, and Reason* (New York: Touchstone, 2018), 280.
76. Naomi Klein, *On Fire: The (Burning) Case for a Green New Deal* (New York: Simon and Schuster, 2019).
77. "Ursula K. Le Guin Quotes," Goodreads, accessed February 28, 2020, https://www.goodreads.com/quotes/3238058-we-live-in-capitalism-its-power-seems-inescapable-so-did.
78. Danielle F. Lawson, Kathryn T. Stevenson, M. Nils Peterson, Sarah J. Carrier, Renee L. Strnad, and Erin Seekamp, "Children Can Foster Climate Change Concern among Their Parents," *Nature Climate Change* 9, no. 6 (June 2019): 458-62, https://doi.org/10.1038/s41558-019-0463-3.
79. Robert Hackett, "Noam Chomsky: 'In a Couple of Generations, Organized Human Society May Not Survive,'" *Canada's National Observer*, February 12, 2019,

https://www.nationalobserver.com/2019/02/12/features/noam-chomsky-couple-generations-organized-human-society-may-not-survive-has-be.

80. Rebecca Beitsch, "Sanders: Instead of Weapons Funding We Should Pool Resources to Fight Climate Change," *Hill*, December 19, 2019, https://thehill.com/policy/energy-environment/475421-sanders-instead-of-weapons-funding-we-should-pool-resources-to.
81. MintPress News, "U.S. Military Is World's Biggest Polluter," EcoWatch, May 15, 2017, https://www.ecowatch.com/military-largest-polluter-2408760609.html.
82. Alexander Nazaryan, "The US Department of Defense Is One of the World's Biggest Polluters," *Newsweek*, July 17, 2014, https://www.newsweek.com/2014/07/25/us-department-defence-one-worlds-biggest-polluters-259456.html.
83. Paula Span, "Older People Are Contributing to Climate Change, and Suffering from It," *New York Times*, May 24, 2019, sec. Health, https://www.nytimes.com/2019/05/24/health/climate-change-elderly.html.
84. As Ronald Reagan said in his 1984 State of the Union address: "Preservation of our environment is not a liberal or conservative challenge, it's common sense." Reagan would unfortunately go on to cut the EPA budget during his presidency.
85. Caitlin Johnstone, "Only Enlightened Collectivism Can Save Us," *Consortium News*, July 24, 2019, https://consortiumnews.com/2019/07/24/only-enlightened-collectivism-can-save-us/.

CHAPTER 8. OCCUPY THE NURSING HOME!

1. Kelly McEvers, "Theater Artist Anne Basting Named MacArthur Fellow," *All Things Considered*, September 22, 2016, https://www.npr.org/2016/09/22/495069555/theater-artist-anne-basting-named-macarthur-fellow.
2. Anne Basting, *Creative Care: A Revolutionary Approach to Dementia and Elder Care* (New York: HarperCollins, 2020).
3. "Family Fears Grandmother Aware of Her Surroundings," *Onion*, September 30, 2014, https://local.theonion.com/family-fears-grandmother-aware-of-her-surroundings-1819576982.
4. Elisa Kawam, "The Rise of Neoliberal Rhetoric and the Intersection of Modern Day Medicaid Priority: A Population Study of Young People in Nursing Homes," *Disability Studies Quarterly* 32, no. 1 (January 5, 2012), https://doi.org/10.18061/dsq.v32i1.1643.
5. Oliver Sacks, "The Healing Power of Gardens," *New York Times*, April 18, 2019, sec. Opinion, https://www.nytimes.com/2019/04/18/opinion/sunday/oliver-sacks-gardens.html.
6. Tom Kitwood, "Person and Process in Dementia," *International Journal of Geriatric Psychiatry* 8 (1993): 545.
7. Tom Kitwood, "Positive Long-Term Changes in Dementia: Some Preliminary Observations," *Journal of Mental Health* 4 (1995): 134.
8. A particularly poignant example of Naomi Feil working with a nursing home resident named Gladys Wilson can be viewed here: "Gladys Wilson and Naomi Feil," video, 5:46, memorybridge, May 26, 2009, https://www.youtube.com/watch?v=CrZXz10FcVM
9. "Best Life," the Green House Project, accessed February 29, 2020, https://www.thegreenhouseproject.org/solutions/Best_Life_Memory_Care.
10. Lauren Harris-Kojetin, Manisha Sengupta, Jessica Penn Lendon, Vincent Rome, Roberto Valverde, and Christine Caffrey, *Long-Term Care Providers and Services Users in the United States, 2015–2016*, Vital and Health Statistics series 3, no. 43 (Washington, DC: National Center for Health Statistics, 2019).
11. Julien Mercille, "Neoliberalism and Health Care: The Case of the Irish Nursing Home Sector," *Critical Public Health* 28, no. 5 (October 20, 2018): 546–59, https://doi.org/10.1080/09581596.2017.1371277.

12. Charlene Harrington, Brian Olney, Helen Carillo, and Taewoon Kang, "Nurse Staffing and Deficiencies in the Largest For-Profit Nursing Home Chains and Chains Owned by Private Equity Companies," *Health Services Research* 47, no. 1 (2012): 106–28, https://doi.org/10.1111/j.1475-6773.2011.01311.x.
13. "Non-Profit vs. For-Profit Nursing Homes: Is There a Difference in Care?," Center for Medicare Advocacy, March 15, 2012, https://medicareadvocacy.org/non-profit-vs-for-profit-nursing-homes-is-there-a-difference-in-care/.
14. Stewart Bell and Andrew Russell, "Coronavirus: Ontario's Worst Hit Nursing Homes and Who Owns Them," *Global News*, June 16, 2020, https://globalnews.ca/news/7059683/coronavirus-ontarios-worst-hit-nursing-homes/.
15. Meagan Day, "The Coming Long-Term Care Crisis," *Jacobin*, October 23, 2019, https://jacobinmag.com/2019/10/long-term-care-crisis-seniors-medicare-aging.
16. Caroline F. Pearson, Charlene C. Quinn, Sai Loganathan, A. Rupa Datta, Beth Burnham Mace, and David C. Grabowski, "The Forgotten Middle: Many Middle-Income Seniors Will Have Insufficient Resources for Housing and Health Care," *Health Affairs* 38, no. 5 (April 24, 2019), https://doi.org/10.1377/hlthaff.2018.05233.
17. "How Much Can a Home Health Aide Expect to Get Paid?" *US News and World Report*, accessed June 17, 2020, https://money.usnews.com/careers/best-jobs/home-health-aide/salary.
18. "Stimulus Check Warning: Nursing Homes Are Stealing Residents' Checks, FTC Report Says." CNN, May 19, 2020, https://www.cnn.com/2020/05/19/us/stimulus-checks-nursing-home-theft-trnd/index.html.
19. Libby Watson, "The Intolerable Cruelty of Our Eldercare System," *New Republic*, May 26, 2020, https://newrepublic.com/article/157801/intolerable-cruelty-eldercare-system.
20. Jessica Silver-Greenberg and Amy Julia Harris, "'They Just Dumped Him Like Trash': Nursing Homes Evict Vulnerable Residents," *New York Times*, June 21, 2020, sec. Business, https://www.nytimes.com/2020/06/21/business/nursing-homes-evictions-discharges-coronavirus.html.
21. Laura Strickler, Stephanie Gosk, and Shelby Hanssen, "A Nursing Home Chain Collapses, and Elderly Residents Pay the Price," *NBC News*, July 19, 2019, https://www.nbcnews.com/health/aging/nursing-home-chain-grows-too-fast-collapses-elderly-disabled-residents-n1025381.
22. Matthew Goldstein, "$146 Million Default by Nursing Home Chain Leaves U.S. on the Hook," *New York Times*, May 31, 2019, sec. Business, https://www.nytimes.com/2019/05/31/business/nursing-homes-mortgage-hud.html.
23. Jennifer Gollan, "Investigating Labor Abuse of Caregivers," *Reveal*, accessed February 29, 2020, https://www.revealnews.org/article/caregivers/.
24. Geeta Anand, "How Not to Grow Old in America," *New York Times*, August 29, 2019, sec. Opinion, https://www.nytimes.com/2019/08/29/opinion/sunday/dementia-assisted-living.html.
25. Anand, "How Not to Grow Old in America."
26. When physicians recommend such activities, especially in writing, they become part of the growing movement called *social prescribing*. One of the characteristics of the American dementia (even when evident in other countries) is its limited view of evidence. We all enjoy music, art, dance, and being outdoors to varying degrees and in various ways. Yet when it comes to people with dementia, somehow we now need to provide evidence that these activities benefit and improve quality of life.
27. "Meet Me," MoMA, accessed February 29, 2020, https://www.moma.org/visit/accessibility/meetme/.
28. Carolyn Halpin-Healy, "Well-Chosen Objects Support Well-Being for People with Dementia and Their Care Partners," *Journal of Museum Education* 42, no. 3 (2017): 224–35.

29. Girija Kaimal, Kendra Ray, and Juan Muniz, "Reduction of Cortisol Levels and Participants' Responses Following Art Making," *Art Therapy* 33, no. 2 (2016): 74–80.
30. Paul M. Camic, Erin L. Baker, and Victoria Tischler, "Theorizing How Art Gallery Interventions Impact People with Dementia and Their Caregivers," *Gerontologist* 56, no. 6 (2016): 1033–41.
31. Carys Jones, Gill Windle, and Rhiannon Tudor Edwards, "Dementia and Imagination: A Social Return on Investment Analysis Framework for Art Activities for People Living with Dementia," *Gerontologist* 60, no. 1 (2020): 112–23.
32. AliveInside.org home page, accessed February 29, 2020, https://www.aliveinside.org/.
33. John Blacking, *How Musical Is Man?* The John Danz Lectures (Seattle: University of Washington Press, 1973), 116.
34. John Bufalini and Daniel R. George, "Power of Music," *Journal of the American Geriatrics Society*, forthcoming.
35. Julene K. Johnson, Anita L. Stewart, Michael Acree, Anna M. Nápoles, Jason D. Flatt, Wendy B. Max, and Steven E. Gregorich, "A Community Choir Intervention to Promote Well-Being among Diverse Older Adults: Results from the Community of Voices Trial," *Journals of Gerontology: Series B* 75, no. 3 (February 14, 2020): 549–59, https://doi.org/10.1093/geronb/gby132.
36. Julene K. Johnson, Martha Rodriquez-Salazar, Sylvia Sherman, Jennifer Peringer, Anna M. Nápoles, Shireen McSpadden, and Anita L. Stewart, *Community of Voices Study Choir Program Manual* (San Francisco: Regents of the University of California, 2018), https://cov.ucsf.edu/sites/g/files/tkssra1901/f/wysiwyg/Community%20of%20Voices%20Program%20Manual.pdf.
37. Giving Voice website, accessed May 31, 2020, https://givingvoicechorus.org/join-a-chorus/. To see the Giving Voice Chorus in action, "Giving Voice Chorus Overpowers Alzheimer's," video, 2:09, WCCO CBS Minnesota, December 3, 2014, https://www.youtube.com/watch?v=QGHCKsHGNGs
38. See Elizabeth Lokon, Yue Li, and Suzanne Kunkel, "Allophilia: Increasing College Students' 'Liking' of Older Adults with Dementia through Arts-Based Intergenerational Experiences," *Gerontology and Geriatrics Education*, September 10, 2018, 1–14; Elizabeth Lokon, Yue Li, and Jyotsana Parajuli, "Using Art in an Intergenerational Program to Improve Students' Attitudes toward People with Dementia," *Gerontology and Geriatrics Education* 38, no. 4 (2017): 407–24; Elizabeth Lokon, Jennifer M. Kinney, and Suzanne Kunkel, "Building Bridges across Age and Cognitive Barriers through Art: College Students' Reflections on an Intergenerational Program with Elders Who Have Dementia," *Journal of Intergenerational Relationships* 10, no. 4 (2012): 337–54; Takashi Yamashita, Jennifer M. Kinney, and Elizabeth J. Lokon, "The Impact of a Gerontology Course and a Service-Learning Program on College Students' Attitudes toward People with Dementia," *Journal of Applied Gerontology* 32, no. 2 (2013): 139–63.
39. Philip E. Sauer, Joan Fopma-Loy, Jennifer M. Kinney, and Elizabeth Lokon, " 'It Makes Me Feel Like Myself': Person-Centered versus Traditional Visual Arts Activities for People with Dementia," *Dementia* 15, no. 5 (2016): 895–912.
40. Kate Levenberg, Elizabeth Lokon, and Daniel R. George, "Opening Minds through Art: A Preliminary Study Evaluating the Effects of a Creative Expression Program on Persons Living with Dementia and their Primary Caregivers." Forthcoming.
41. Alzheimer's Poetry Project home page, accessed February 29, 2020, http://www.alzpoetry.com.
42. Dementia Positive home page, accessed February 29, 2020, http://www.dementiapositive.co.uk/.
43. Gary Glazner and Daniel B. Kaplan, "The Alzheimer's Poetry Project," *Journal of the American Medical Association* 320, no. 22 (December 11, 2018): 2294–95, https://doi.org/10.1001/jama.2018.16340.

44. Aagje M. C. Swinnen, "Healing Words: A Study of Poetry Interventions in Dementia Care," *Dementia* 15, no. 6 (2016): 1377–1404.
45. Alaina J. Garrie, Shruti Goel, and Martin M. Forsberg, "Medical Students' Perceptions of Dementia after Participation in Poetry Workshop with People with Dementia," *International Journal of Alzheimer's Disease* 2016 (2016): 1–7, https://doi.org/10.1155/2016/2785105.
46. Kathrin Rehfeld, Patrick Müller, Norman Aye, Marlen Schmicker, Milos Dordevic, Jörn Kaufmann, Anita Hökelmann, and Notger G. Müller, "Dancing or Fitness Sport? The Effects of Two Training Programs on Hippocampal Plasticity and Balance Abilities in Healthy Seniors," *Frontiers in Human Neuroscience* 11 (June 15, 2017): 305, https://doi.org/10.3389/fnhum.2017.00305.
47. Dance for PD website, accessed May 31, 2020, https://danceforparkinsons.org/.
48. Kairos Alive! website, accessed May 31, 2020, https://kairosalive.org/; Dance Exchange website, accessed May 31, 2020, http://danceexchange.org/.
49. Bernie Warren and Peter Spitzer, "Laughing to Longevity—the Work of Elder Clowns," *Lancet* 378, no. 9791 (August 13, 2011): 562–63, https://doi.org/10.1016/S0140-6736(11)61280-4.
50. Pia Kontos, Karen-Lee Miller, Romeo Colobong, Luis I. Palma Lazgare, Malcolm Binns, Lee-Fay Low, Claire Surr, and Gary Naglie, "Elder-Clowning in Long-Term Dementia Care: Results of a Pilot Study," *Journal of the American Geriatrics Society* 64, no. 2 (February 2016): 347–53, https://doi.org/10.1111/jgs.13941.
51. Cathy Free, "Comedians Are Being Hired by the Hour to Help Dementia Patients Their Goal? 'A Full Belly Laugh,'" *Washington Post*, September 17, 2019, https://www.washingtonpost.com/lifestyle/2019/09/17/comedians-are-being-hired-by-hour-help-dementia-patients-their-goal-full-belly-laugh/.
52. Anne Cleary, Anne Roiko, Nicola W. Burton, Kelly S. Fielding, Zoe Murray, and Gavin Turrell, "Changes in Perceptions of Urban Green Space Are Related to Changes in Psychological Well-Being: Cross-Sectional and Longitudinal Study of Mid-Aged Urban Residents," *Health and Place* 59 (September 2019): 102201, https://doi.org/10.1016/j.healthplace.2019.102201.
53. Caoimhe Twohig-Bennett and Andy Jones, "The Health Benefits of the Great Outdoors: A Systematic Review and Meta-Analysis of Greenspace Exposure and Health Outcomes," *Environmental Research* 166 (2018): 628–37, https://doi.org/10.1016/j.envres.2018.06.030.
54. Colin A. Capaldi, Raelyne L. Dopko, and John M. Zelenski, "The Relationship between Nature Connectedness and Happiness: A Meta-Analysis," *Frontiers in Psychology* 5 (September 8, 2014): 976, https://doi.org/10.3389/fpsyg.2014.00976.
55. A. C. Miller, L. C. Hickman, and G. K. Lemasters, "A Distraction Technique for Control of Burn Pain," *Journal of Burn Care and Rehabilitation* 13, no. 5 (1992): 576–80.
56. Gregory B. Diette, Noah Lechtzin, Edward Haponik, Aline Devrotes, and Haya R. Rubin, "Distraction Therapy with Nature Sights and Sounds Reduces Pain during Flexible Bronchoscopy: A Complementary Approach to Routine Analgesia," *Chest* 123, no. 3 (2003): 941–49.
57. M. M. Tse, J. K. Ng, J. W. Chung, and T. K. Wong, "The Effect of Visual Stimuli on Pain Threshold and Tolerance," *Journal of Clinical Nursing* 11, no. 4 (2002): 462–69.
58. Rosalia Lelchuk Staricoff, "Arts in Health: The Value of Evaluation," *Journal of the Royal Society for the Promotion of Health* 126, no. 3 (2006): 116–20.
59. Ellen Vincent, Dina Battisto, Larry Grimes, and James McCubbin, "The Effects of Nature Images on Pain in a Simulated Hospital Patient Room," *HERD: Health Environments Research and Design Journal* 3, no. 3 (2010): 42–55.
60. Upali Nanda, Cheryl Chanaud, Michael Nelson, Xi Zhu, Robyn Bajema, and Ben H. Jansen, "Impact of Visual Art on Patient Behavior in the Emergency Department Waiting Room," *Journal of Emergency Medicine* 43, no. 1 (2012): 172–81.

61. Mark B. Detweiler, Pamela F. Murphy, Kye Y. Kim, Laura C. Myers, and Afshan Ashai, "Scheduled Medications and Falls in Dementia Patients Utilizing a Wander Garden," *American Journal of Alzheimer's Disease and Other Dementias* 24, no. 4 (2009): 322–32.
62. Man-Li Liao, Sheng-Jung Ou, Chung Heng Hsieh, Zhelin Li, and Chia-Chun Ko, "Effects of Garden Visits on People with Dementia: A Pilot Study," *Dementia* 19, no. 4 (2018): 1009–28.
63. Marianne Blake and Gary Mitchell, "Horticultural Therapy in Dementia Care: A Literature Review," *Nursing Standard (2014+)* 30, no. 21 (2016): 41.
64. Iosief Abraha, Joseph M. Rimland, Fabiana Mirella Trotta, Giuseppina Dell'Aquila, Alfonso Cruz-Jentoft, Mirko Petrovic, Adalsteinn Gudmundsson, et al., "Systematic Review of Systematic Reviews of Non-pharmacological Interventions to Treat Behavioural Disturbances in Older Patients with Dementia," *BMJ Open* 7, no. 3 (2017): e012759.
65. Mark B. Detweiler, Taral Sharma, Jonna G. Detweiler, Pamela F. Murphy, Sandra Lane, Jack Carman, Amara S. Chudhary, Mary H. Halling, and Kye Y. Kim, "What Is the Evidence to Support the Use of Therapeutic Gardens for the Elderly?" *Psychiatry Investigation* 9, no. 2 (2012): 100.
66. Rebecca Whear, Jo Thompson Coon, Alison Bethel, Rebecca Abbott, Ken Stein, and Ruth Garside, "What Is the Impact of Using Outdoor Spaces such as Gardens on the Physical and Mental Well-Being of Those with Dementia? A Systematic Review of Quantitative and Qualitative Evidence," *Journal of the American Medical Directors Association* 15, no. 10 (2014): 697–705.
67. Jogé Boumans, Leonieke C. van Boekel, Caroline A. Baan, and Katrien G. Luijkx, "How Can Autonomy Be Maintained and Informal Care Improved for People with Dementia Living in Residential Care Facilities: A Systematic Literature Review," *Gerontologist* 59, no. 6 (2019): e709–30.
68. Margaret Calkins, Joseph G. Szmerekovsky, and Stacey Biddle, "Effect of Increased Time Spent Outdoors on Individuals with Dementia Residing in Nursing Homes," *Journal of Housing for the Elderly* 21, no. 3-4 (2007): 211–28.
69. Erja Rappe and Päivi Topo, "Contact with Outdoor Greenery Can Support Competence among People with Dementia," *Journal of Housing for the Elderly* 21, no. 3-4 (2007): 229–48.
70. Christina M. Gigliotti and Shannon E. Jarrott, "Effects of Horticulture Therapy on Engagement and Affect," *Canadian Journal on Aging/La Revue canadienne duvieillissement* 24, no. 4 (2005): 367–77.
71. Sarah Noone and Nicholas Jenkins, "Digging for Dementia: Exploring the Experience of Community Gardening from the Perspectives of People with Dementia," *Aging and Mental Health* 22, no. 7 (2018): 881–88.
72. Y. Lee and S. Kim, "Effects of Indoor Gardening on Sleep, Agitation, and Cognition in Dementia Patients—A Pilot Study," *International Journal of Geriatric Psychiatry* 23, no. 5 (2008): 485–89.
73. Piran C. L. White, Jonathan Wyatt, Garuth Chalfont, J. Martin Bland, Christopher Neale, Dominic Trepel, and Hilary Graham, "Exposure to Nature Gardens Has Time-Dependent Associations with Mood Improvements for People with Mid- and Late-Stage Dementia: Innovative Practice," *Dementia* 17, no. 5 (2018): 627–34.
74. Seiko Goto, Xuting Shen, Minkai Sun, Yutaka Hamano, and Karl Herrup, "The Positive Effects of Viewing Gardens for Persons with Dementia," *Journal of Alzheimer's Disease* 66, no. 4 (2018): 1705–20.
75. Detweiler et al., "Scheduled Medications and Falls," 322–32.
76. Liao et al., "Effects of Garden Visits on People with Dementia."
77. Abraha et al., "Systematic Review of Systematic Reviews."
78. Gigliotti and Jarrott, "Effects of Horticulture Therapy."
79. White et al., "Exposure to Nature Gardens."

80. Ibid.
81. Whear et al., "What Is the Impact of Using Outdoor Spaces?"
82. Sacks, "Healing Power of Gardens."
83. Ibid.
84. I. Khan, "Convention on Psychotropic Substances, 1971: The Role and Responsibilities of the World Health Organization," *Progress in Neuro-psychopharmacology* 3, nos. 1–3 (1979): 11–14.
85. Robin L. Carhart-Harris and Guy M. Goodwin, "The Therapeutic Potential of Psychedelic Drugs: Past, Present, and Future," *Neuropsychopharmacology* 42, no. 11 (2017): 2105–13.
86. Stephen Ross, "Therapeutic Use of Classic Psychedelics to Treat Cancer-Related Psychiatric Distress," *International Review of Psychiatry* 30, no. 4 (2018): 317–30.
87. Roland Griffiths, "A Single Dose of Psilocybin Produces Substantial and Enduring Decreases in Anxiety and Depression in Patients with a Life-Threatening Cancer Diagnosis: A Randomized Double-Blind Trial," *Neuropsychopharmacology* 40 (2015): S90–S91.
88. Daniel R. George and Ryan Hanson, "Imagining a Role for Psychedelics in Dementia Care," *American Journal of Geriatric Psychiatry* 27, no. 9 (2019): 1028–30.
89. Ibid.
90. Abbie Rosner, "Are Investors Ready to Change Their Minds about Psychedelic Drugs?" *Forbes*, January 27, 2020, https://www.forbes.com/sites/abbierosner/2020/01/27/are-investors-ready-to-change-their-minds-about-psychedelic-drugs/.
91. Nick Wells, "Canada's First 'Dementia Village' Set to Open Its Doors," *CTV News*, May 28, 2019, https://bc.ctvnews.ca/canada-s-first-dementia-village-set-to-open-its-doors-1.4441535.
92. "Senior Helpers Launches Town Square Franchising," CISION, press release, July 12, 2018, https://www.prnewswire.com/news-releases/senior-helpers-launches-town-square-franchising-300679836.html.
93. Kate Johnson, "'Dementia Village' Creates Artificial Reality," *Medscape*, September 11, 2019, http://www.medscape.com/viewarticle/918026.
94. Stacey Burling, "Assisted Living Too Costly by 2029," *Philadelphia Inquirer*, April 25, 2019, http://digital.olivesoftware.com/olive/ODN/PhiladelphiaInquirerNJ/shared/ShowArticle.aspx?doc=PHQN%2F2019%2F04%2F25&entity=Ar01300&sk=DBC9F708&mode=text.
95. Anand, "How Not to Grow Old in America."
96. Meagan Day, "The Coming Long-Term Care Crisis," *Jacobin*, October 23, 2019, https://jacobinmag.com/2019/10/long-term-care-crisis-seniors-medicare-aging.

CHAPTER 9. A BRIDGE BEYOND LONELINESS

1. Susan J. Douglas, "Still Living with Sexism (after All These Years): How Neoliberalism Operates at the Intersections of Sexism and Ageism," *Soundings: A Journal of Politics and Culture* 58, no. 1 (2014): 34–43.
2. Gingrich, *Winning the Future*.
3. Paula Span, "Many Americans Will Need Long-Term Care: Most Won't Be Able to Afford It," *New York Times*, May 10, 2019, sec. Health, https://www.nytimes.com/2019/05/10/health/assisted-living-costs-elderly.html.
4. Watson, "Intolerable Cruelty."
5. Tine Buffel and Chris Phillipson, "A Manifesto for the Age-Friendly Movement: Developing a New Urban Agenda," *Journal of Aging and Social Policy* 30, no. 2 (2018): 173–92.
6. Christopher Phillipson, "Developing Age-Friendly Work in the Twenty-First Century: NewChallenges and Agendas," *Working with Older People* 22, no. 1 (2018): 3–8.
7. Andrew Gamble, *Can the Welfare State Survive?* (New York: Wiley, 2016).
8. Stephen McBride and Bryan M. Evans, eds., *The Austerity State* (Toronto, ON: University of Toronto Press, 2017).

9. Katherine S. Newman, *Downhill from Here: Retirement Insecurity in the Age of Inequality* (New York: Metropolitan Books, 2019).
10. Ibid.
11. Miller McPherson, Lynn Smith-Lovin, and Matthew E. Brashears, "Social Isolation in America: Changes in Core Discussion Networks over Two Decades," *American Sociological Review* 71, no. 3 (2006): 353–75.
12. Amanda Grenier, Liz Lloyd, and Chris Phillipson, "Precarity in Late Life: Rethinking Dementia as a 'Frailed' Old Age," *Sociology of Health and Illness* 39, no. 2 (2017): 318–30.
13. Katie Hafner, "Researchers Confront an Epidemic of Loneliness," *New York Times*, September 5, 2016, sec. Health, https://www.nytimes.com/2016/09/06/health/lonliness-aging-health-effects.html.
14. Ellen E. Lee, Colin Depp, Barton W. Palmer, Danielle Glorioso, Rebecca Daly, Jinyuan Liu, Xin M. Tu, et al., "High Prevalence and Adverse Health Effects of Loneliness in Community-Dwelling Adults across the Lifespan: Role of Wisdom as a Protective Factor," *International Psychogeriatrics* 31, no. 10 (2018): 1–16.
15. Ceylan Yeginsu, "U.K. Appoints a Minister for Loneliness," *New York Times*, January 17, 2018, sec. World, https://www.nytimes.com/2018/01/17/world/europe/uk-britain-loneliness.html.
16. "UK Must Tackle Loneliness, Says Report," *BBC News*, December 14, 2017, sec. UK, https://www.bbc.com/news/uk-42354807.
17. Shiho Fukada, "Japan's Prisons Are a Haven for Elderly Women: Lonely Seniors are Shoplifting in Search of the Community and Stability of Jail," *Bloomberg Businessweek*, March 16, 2018, https://www.bloomberg.com/news/features/2018-03-16/japan-s-prisons-are-a-haven-for-elderly-women.
18. Kay Hymowitz, "A Nation Dying in Despair, and Family Breakdown Is Part of the Problem," *Washington Examiner*, September 26, 2019, https://www.washingtonexaminer.com/opinion/a-nation-dying-in-despair-and-family-breakdown-is-part-of-the-problem.
19. Ed Butler, "Why Some Japanese Pensioners Want to Go to Jail," *BBC News*, January 31, 2019, sec. Stories, https://www.bbc.com/news/stories-47033704.
20. Louise C. Hawkley and John T. Cacioppo, "Aging and Loneliness: Downhill Quickly?" *Current Directions in Psychological Science* 16, no. 4 (2007): 187–91.
21. Vivek Murthy, *Together: The Healing Power of Human Connection* (New York: Harper Wave, 2020).
22. Vivek Murthy, "Work and the Loneliness Epidemic," *Harvard Business Review*, September 26, 2017, https://hbr.org/2017/09/work-and-the-loneliness-epidemic.
23. Louise C. Hawkley, Ronald A. Thisted, Christopher M. Masi, and John T. Cacioppo, "Loneliness Predicts Increased Blood Pressure: 5-Year Cross-Lagged Analyses in Middle-Aged and Older Adults," *Psychology and Aging* 25, no. 1 (2010): 132.
24. Yadollah Abolfathi Momtaz, Tengku Aizan Hamid, Suraya Yusoff, Rahimah Ibrahim, Sen Tyng Chai, Nurizan Yahaya, and Siti Suhailah Abdullah, "Loneliness as a Risk Factor for Hypertension in Later Life," *Journal of Aging and Health* 24, no. 4 (2012): 696–710.
25. Mark S. Kaplan, Nathalie Huguet, David H. Feeny, and Bentson H. McFarland, "Self-Reported Hypertension Prevalence and Income among Older Adults in Canada and the United States," *Social Science and Medicine* 70, no. 6 (2010): 844–49.
26. Sarah S. Knox and Kerstin Uvnäs-Moberg, "Social Isolation and Cardiovascular Disease: An Atherosclerotic Pathway?" *Psychoneuroendocrinology* 23, no. 8 (1998): 877–90.
27. Nicole K. Valtorta, Mona Kanaan, Simon Gilbody, Sara Ronzi, and Barbara Hanratty, "Loneliness and Social Isolation as Risk Factors for Coronary Heart Disease and Stroke: Systematic Review and Meta-Analysis of Longitudinal Observational Studies," *Heart* 102, no. 13 (July 1, 2016): 1009–16, https://doi.org/10.1136/heartjnl-2015-308790.
28. Sheila M. Manemann, Alanna M. Chamberlain, Véronique L. Roger, Joan M. Griffin, Cynthia M. Boyd, Thomas K. M. Cudjoe, Daniel Jensen, et al., "Perceived Social Isolation and Outcomes in Patients with Heart Failure," *Journal of the American Heart Association* 7, no. 11 (2018): e008069.

29. John T. Cacioppo, Louise C. Hawkley, L. Elizabeth Crawford, John M. Ernst, Mary H. Burleson, Ray B. Kowalewski, William B. Malarkey, Eve Van Cauter, and Gary G. Berntson, "Loneliness and Health: Potential Mechanisms," *Psychosomatic Medicine* 64, no. 3 (2002): 407–17.
30. Julianne Holt-Lunstad, Timothy B. Smith, and J. Bradley Layton, "Social Relationships and Mortality Risk: A Meta-Analytic Review," *PLoS Medicine* 7, no. 7 (July 27, 2010): e1000316, https://doi.org/10.1371/journal.pmed.1000316.
31. See Nancy J. Donovan, Qiong Wu, Dorene M. Rentz, Reisa A. Sperling, Gad A. Marshall, and M. Maria Glymour, "Loneliness, Depression and Cognitive Function in Older U.S. Adults," *International Journal of Geriatric Psychiatry* 32, no. 5 (2017): 564–73, https://doi.org/10.1002/gps.4495.
32. Robert S. Wilson, Kristin R. Krueger, Steven E. Arnold, Julie A. Schneider, Jeremiah F. Kelly, Lisa L. Barnes, Yuxiao Tang, and David A. Bennett, "Loneliness and Risk of Alzheimer Disease," *Archives of General Psychiatry* 64, no. 2 (2007): 234–40.
33. Caitlin E. Coyle and Elizabeth Dugan, "Social Isolation, Loneliness and Health among Older Adults," *Journal of Aging and Health* 24, no. 8 (2012): 1346–63.
34. See Laura Fratiglioni and Hui-Xin Wang, "Brain Reserve Hypothesis in Dementia," *Journal of Alzheimer's Disease* 12, no. 1 (2007): 11–22; Laura Fratiglioni, Stephanie Paillard-Borg, and Bengt Winblad, "An Active and Socially Integrated Lifestyle in Late Life Might Protect against Dementia," *Lancet Neurology* 3, no. 6 (2004): 343–53.
35. See Karen A. Ertel, M. Maria Glymour, and Lisa F. Berkman, "Effects of Social Integration on Preserving Memory Function in a Nationally Representative US Elderly Population," *American Journal of Public Health* 98, no. 7 (2008): 1215–20; Dana A. Glei, David A. Landau, Noreen Goldman, Yi-Li Chuang, Germán Rodríguez, and Maxine Weinstein, "Participating in Social Activities Helps Preserve Cognitive Function: An Analysis of a Longitudinal, Population-Based Study of the Elderly," *International Journal of Epidemiology* 34, no. 4 (2005): 864–71; François Béland, Maria-Victoria Zunzunegui, Beatriz Alvarado, Angel Otero, and Teodoro del Ser, "Trajectories of Cognitive Decline and Social Relations," *Journals of Gerontology Series B: Psychological Sciences and Social Sciences* 60, no. 6 (2005): P320–30.
36. See Lisa F. Berkman and S. Leonard Syme, "Social Networks, Host Resistance, and Mortality: A Nine-Year Follow-Up Study of Alameda County Residents," *American Journal of Epidemiology* 109, no. 2 (1979): 186–204; Alex H. S. Harris and Carl E. Thoresen, "Volunteering Is Associated with Delayed Mortality in Older People: Analysis of the Longitudinal Study of Aging," *Journal of Health Psychology* 10, no. 6 (2005): 739–52; Bertil S. Hanson, Sven-Olof Isacsson, Lars Janzon, and Sven-Eric Lindell, "Social Network and Social Support Influence Mortality in Elderly Men: Prospective Population Study of 'Men Born in 1914,' Malmö, Sweden," *American Journal of Epidemiology* 130, no. 1 (1989): 100–111; James S. House, Cynthia Robbins, and Helen L. Metzner, "The Association of Social Relationships and Activities with Mortality: Prospective Evidence from the Tecumseh Community Health Study," *American Journal of Epidemiology* 116, no. 1 (1982): 123–40; Ichiro Kawachi, Graham A. Colditz, Alberto Ascherio, Eric B. Rimm, Edward Giovannucci, Meir J. Stampfer, and Walter C. Willett, "A Prospective Study of Social Networksin Relation to Total Mortality and Cardiovascular Disease in Men in the USA," *Journal of Epidemiology and Community Health* 50, no. 3 (1996): 245–51; Teresa E. Seeman, George A. Kaplan, Lisa Knudsen, Richard Cohen, and Jack Guralnik, "Social Network Ties and Mortality among Tile Elderly in the Alameda County Study," *American Journal of Epidemiology* 126, no. 4 (1987): 714–23; Thomas M. Vogt, John P. Mullooly, Denise Ernst, Clyde R. Pope, and Jack F. Hollis, "Social Networks as Predictors of Ischemic Heart Disease, Cancer, Stroke and Hypertension: Incidence, Survival and Mortality," *Journal of Clinical Epidemiology* 45, no. 6 (1992): 659–66.
37. See Lennart Welin, K. Svärdsudd, Suzanne Ander-Peciva, Gosta Tibblin, Bodil Tibblin, Bo Larsson, and Lars Wilhelmsen, "Prospective Study of Social Influences on Mortality: The Study of Men Born in 1913 and 1923," *Lancet* 325, no. 8434 (1985): 915–18; Brenda W. J. H.

Penninx, Theo Van Tilburg, Didi M. W. Kriegsman, Dorly J. H. Deeg, A. Joan P. Boeke, and Jacques Th. M. Van Eijk, "Effects of Social Support and Personal Coping Resources on Mortality in Older Age: The Longitudinal Aging Study Amsterdam," *American Journal of Epidemiology* 146, no. 6 (1997): 510–19; George A. Kaplan, Jukka T. Salonen, Richard D. Cohen, Richard J. Brand, S. Leonard Syme, and Pekka Puska, "Social Connections and Mortality from All Causes and from Cardiovascular Disease: Prospective Evidence from Eastern Finland," *American Journal of Epidemiology* 128, no. 2 (1988): 370–80; Lisa F. Berkman, Maria Melchior, Jean-François Chastang, Isabelle Niedhammer, Annette Leclerc, and Marcel Goldberg, "Social Integration and Mortality: A Prospective Study of French Employees of Electricity of France–Gas of France: The GAZEL Cohort," *American Journal of Epidemiology* 159, no. 2 (2004): 167–74.

38. See Suzanne C. Ho, "Health and Social Predictors of Mortality in an Elderly Chinese Cohort," *American Journal of Epidemiology* 133, no. 9 (1991): 907–21; Hidehiro Sugisawa, Jersey Liang, and Xian Liu, "Social Networks, Social Support, and Mortality among Older People in Japan," *Journal of Gerontology* 49, no. 1 (1994): S3–S13.
39. Lynne C. Giles, Gary F. V. Glonek, Mary A. Luszcz, and Gary R. Andrews, "Effect of Social Networks on 10 Year Survival in Very Old Australians: The Australian Longitudinal Study of Aging," *Journal of Epidemiology and Community Health* 59, no. 7 (2005): 574–79.
40. Tara L. Gruenewald, Arun S. Karlamangla, Gail A. Greendale, Burton H. Singer, and Teresa E. Seeman, "Feelings of Usefulness to Others, Disability, and Mortality in Older Adults: The MacArthur Study of Successful Aging," *Journals of Gerontology Series B: Psychological Sciences and Social Sciences* 62, no. 1 (2007): P28–P37.
41. Aliya Alimujiang, Ashley Wiensch, Jonathan Boss, Nancy L. Fleischer, Alison M. Mondul, Karen McLean, Bhramar Mukherjee, and Celeste Leigh Pearce, "Association between Life Purpose and Mortality among US Adults Older than 50 Years," *JAMA Network Open* 2, no. 5 (2019): e194270.
42. Kazushi Okamoto and Yuko Tanaka, "Subjective Usefulness and 6-Year Mortality Risks among Elderly Persons in Japan," *Journals of Gerontology Series B: Psychological Sciences and Social Sciences* 59, no. 5 (2004): P246–49.
43. Toshimasa Sone, Naoki Nakaya, Kaori Ohmori, Taichi Shimazu, Mizuka Higashiguchi, Masako Kakizaki, Nobutaka Kikuchi, Shinichi Kuriyama, and Ichiro Tsuji, "Sense of Life Worth Living (Ikigai) and Mortality in Japan: Ohsaki Study," *Psychosomatic Medicine* 70, no. 6 (2008): 709–15.
44. K. H. Pitkala, Marja-Liisa Laakkonen, Timo E. Strandberg, and Reijo S. Tilvis, "Positive Life Orientation as a Predictor of 10-Year Outcome in an Aged Population," *Journal of Clinical Epidemiology* 57, no. 4 (2004): 409–14.
45. A. Grand, P. Grosclaude, H. Bocquet, J. Pous, and J. L. Albarede, "Predictive Value of Life Events, Psychosocial Factors and Self-Rated Health on Disability in an Elderly Rural French Population," *Social Science and Medicine* 27, no. 12 (1988): 1337–42.
46. Joe Tomaka, Sharon Thompson, and Rebecca Palacios, "The Relation of Social Isolation, Loneliness, and Social Support to Disease Outcomes among the Elderly," *Journal of Aging and Health* 18, no. 3 (2006): 359–84.
47. Dan Buettner, *The Blue Zones Solution: Eating and Living Like the World's Healthiest People* (Washington, DC: National Geographic Books, 2015).
48. Christine M. Proulx, Angela L. Curl, and Ashley E. Ermer, "Longitudinal Associations between Formal Volunteering and Cognitive Functioning," *Journals of Gerontology: Series B* 73, no. 3 (2018): 522–31.
49. See Phyllis Moen, Donna Dempster-McClain, and Robin M. Williams Jr., "Successful Aging: A Life-Course Perspective on Women's Multiple Roles and Health," *American Journal of Sociology* 97, no. 6 (1992): 1612–38; Marc A. Musick, A. Regula Herzog, and James S. House, "Volunteering and Mortality among Older Adults: Findings from a National Sample," *Journals of Gerontology Series B: Psychological Sciences and Social Sciences* 54, no. 3 (1999): S173–80; Doug Oman, Carl E. Thoresen, and Kay McMahon, "Volunteerism and

Mortality among the Community-Dwelling Elderly," *Journal of Health Psychology* 4, no. 3 (1999): 301–16.

50. "Social Determinants of Health," WHO, accessed March 1, 2020, https://www.who.int/so cial_determinants/en/.
51. Tad Friend, "Why Ageism Never Gets Old," *New Yorker*, November 20, 2017.
52. Dawn Alley, Phoebe Liebig, Jon Pynoos, Tridib Banerjee, and In Hee Choi, "Creating Elder-Friendly Communities: Preparations for an Aging Society," *Journal of Gerontological Social Work* 49, nos. 1-2 (2007): 1–18.
53. Phillipson, "Developing Age-Friendly Work."
54. World Health Organization, *Measuring the Age-Friendliness of Cities: A Guide to Using Core Indicators* (Geneva: WHO, 2015), 16.
55. "How to Create a Livable Community," AARP Livable Communities Publications and Resources, accessed May 31, 2020, https://www.aarp.org/livable-communities/tool-kits -resources.
56. Lock, *Alzheimer Conundrum*.
57. Buffel and Phillipson, "Manifesto for the Age-Friendly Movement."
58. Phillipson, "Developing Age-Friendly Work."
59. Buffel and Phillipson, "Manifesto for the Age-Friendly Movement."
60. Aagje Swinnen and Mark Schweda, eds., *Popularizing Dementia: Public Expressions and Representations of Forgetfulness*, vol. 6 (New York: Transcript Verlag, 2015), 12.
61. See Dementia Friendly America website, accessed March 1, 2020, https://www.dfamerica.org.
62. "Getting Started in Your Community," Dementia Friendly America, accessed May 31, 2020, https://www.dfamerica.org/toolkit-getting-started.
63. Peter J. Whitehouse, Kathy Sykes, and Daniel R. George, "Ecological Change and Aging: A Need to Think Deeply and Act Quickly," *International Journal of Aging and Human Development* 80, no. 1 (2014): 3–9.
64. Andy Smith, "Bill Thomas Believes Modular Homes Are Solution to Middle Market Challenge," Senior Living Innovation Forum, March 13, 2019, https://info.seniorlivinginnova tionforum.com/blog/bill-thomas-believes-small-modular-homes-are-solution-to-middle -market-challenge.
65. Ibid.
66. Joyce Famakinwa, "Bill Thomas: Home Care Providers Need to Get into the Real Estate Game," *Home Health Care News*, June 17, 2019, https://homehealthcarenewscom/2019 /06/bill-thomas-home-care-providers-need-to-get-into-the-real-estate-game/.
67. Chuck Sudo, "Intergenerational Model for Dementia Care Taking Shape around Bill Thomas' Minka Homes," *Senior Housing News*, January 16, 2019, https://seniorhousing news.com/2019/01/16/intergenerational-model-for-dementia-care-taking-shape-around -bill-thomas-minka-homes/.
68. See Tiffany R. Jansen, "The Nursing Home That's Also a Dorm," *City Lab*, October 5, 2015, https://www.citylab.com/equity/2015/10/the-nursing-home-thats-also-a-dorm/408424/.
69. Anemona Hartocollis, "At Colleges, What's Old Is New: Retirees Living on Campus," *New York Times*, September 10, 2019, sec. U.S., https://www.nytimes.com/2019/09/10/us/col lege-university-retirement-communities.html.
70. Paula Span, "'We Need Each Other': Seniors Are Drawn to New Housing Arrangements," *New York Times*, September 27, 2019, sec. Health, https://www.nytimes.com/2019/09/27 /health/seniors-housing-sharing-villages.html.
71. Daniel R. George, and Grace Wagler, "Social Learning and Innovation: Developing Two Shared-Site Intergenerational Reading Programs in Hershey, Pennsylvania," *Journal of Intergenerational Relationships* 12, no. 1 (2014): 69–74.
72. See Kerry Hannon, "Why We Need to Get Rid of Senior Centers," *Forbes*, March 19, 2015, https://www.forbes.com/sites/nextavenue/2015/03/19/why-we-need-to-get-rid-of-senior -centers/.

73. Meagan Day, "Bernie Sanders Wants to Alleviate Senior Loneliness," *Jacobin*, September 17, 2019, https://jacobinmag.com/2019/09/senior-loneliness-sanders-healthcare.
74. Tomi D. Dreibelbis and Daniel R. George, "An Intergenerational Teaching Kitchen: Reimagining a Senior Center as a Shared Site for Medical Students and Elders Enrolled in a Culinary Medicine Course," *Journal of Intergenerational Relationships* 15, no. 2 (2017): 174–80.
75. Tomi Danielle Dreibelbis and Daniel R. George, "Integrating Intergenerational Mentoring into a Culinary Medicine Curriculum," *Medical Science Educator* 27, no. 4 (2017): 575–76.
76. Dreibelbis and George, "An Intergenerational Teaching Kitchen."
77. Fairhill Partners website, accessed May 31, 2020, https://fairhillpartners.org/.
78. Day, "Bernie Sanders Wants to Alleviate Senior Loneliness."
79. Gray Is Green website, accessed May 31, 2020, http://www.grayisgreen.org.
80. Elders Climate Action website, accessed May 31, 2020, https://www.eldersclimateaction.org.
81. Sam Levin and Mark Harris, "The Road Ahead: Self-Driving Cars on the Brink of a Revolution in California," *Guardian*, March 17, 2017, sec. Technology, https://www.theguardian.com/technology/2017/mar/17/self-driving-cars-california-regulation-google-uber-tesla.
82. You can check the availability in your state of Dementia Friends programs at "Dementia Friends Programs by State," Dementia Friends USA, accessed May 31, 2020, https://dementiafriendsusa.org/sessions-your-state-territory.
83. Memory Cafe website, accessed June 7, 2020, https://www.memorycafedirectory.com/.
84. To learn more, visit the Momentia website, accessed May 31, 2020, http://www.momentiaseattle.org/.
85. Meals on Wheels America website, accessed May 31, 2020, https://www.mealsonwheelsamerica.org.
86. "Delivering So Much More than Just a Meal," Meals on Wheels, August 2018, https://www.mealsonwheelsamerica.org/docs/default-source/fact-sheets/2018/2018-national/what-we-deliver_2018-fact-sheets_forpublication.pdf?sfvrsn=1410bc3b_2.
87. Ted Knutson, "Senior Hunger Surges as Boomers Swell the Ranks of the Nation's Elderly," *Forbes*, May 29, 2019, https://www.forbes.com/sites/tedknutson/2019/05/29/senior-hunger-surge-looming-as-boomers-swell-the-ranks-of-americas-elderly/.
88. Huichen Zhu and Ruopeng An, "Impact of Home-Delivered Meal Programs on Diet and Nutrition among Older Adults: A Review," *Nutrition and Health* 22, no. 2 (2013): 89–103.
89. Christopher Ingraham, "Meals on Wheels Is 'Not Showing Any Results' Only if You Ignore All These Results," *Washington Post*, March 16, 2017, https:/www.washingtonpost.com/news/wonk/wp/2017/03/16/trump-budget-chief-says-meals-on-wheels-is-not-showing-any-results-hes-wrong/.
90. Tracie Williams, "Photos: Who Actually Benefits From Meals on Wheels?" *Nation*, March 30, 2018, https://www.thenation.com/article/archive/photos-who-actually-benefits-from-meals-on-wheels/.
91. "Delivering So Much More than Just a Meal."
92. Ibid.
93. Ingraham, "Meals on Wheels."
94. Day, "Bernie Sanders Wants to Alleviate Senior Loneliness."

CHAPTER 10. THE INTERGENERATIONAL SCHOOLS

1. Daniel R. George, "Season of Mists and Mellow Fruitfulness," *Journal of the American Geriatrics Society* 58, no. 4 (2010): 788.
2. Daniel R. George, "Overcoming the Social Death of Dementia through Language," *Lancet* 376 (2010): 586–87.
3. In 2014, TIS received the Eisner Prize for Intergenerational Advocacy.
4. Albert Speer, *Inside the Third Reich* (New York: Simon and Schuster, 1970), 73.

5. These quotations also appeared in Daniel R. George, "Handing Down Memories of Jesse Owens," *Journal of the American Geriatrics Society* 59, no. 10 (2011): 1960–61.
6. Daniel R. George and Mendel E. Singer, "Intergenerational Volunteering and Quality of Life for Persons with Mild to Moderate Dementia: Results from a 5-Month Intervention Study in the United States," *American Journal of Geriatric Psychiatry* 19, no. 4 (2011): 392–96.
7. Daniel R. George, "Intergenerational Volunteering and Quality of Life: Mixed Methods Evaluation of a Randomized Control Trial Involving Persons with Mild to Moderate Dementia," *Quality of Life Research* 20, no. 7 (2011): 987–95.
8. Michelle C. Carlson, Kirk I. Erickson, Arthur F. Kramer, Michelle W. Voss, Natalie Bolea, Michelle Mielke, Sylvia McGill, George W. Rebok, Teresa Seeman, and Linda P. Fried, "Evidence for Neurocognitive Plasticity in At-Risk Older Adults: The Experience Corps Program," *Journals of Gerontology Series A: Biomedical Sciences and Medical Sciences* 64, no. 12 (2009): 1275–82.
9. Cameron J. Camp, Silvia Orsulic-Jeras, Michelle M. Lee, and Katherine S. Judge, "Effects of a Montessori-Based Intergenerational Program on Engagement and Affect for Adult Day Care Clients with Dementia," in *Successful Aging through the Life Span: Intergenerational Issues in Health*, edited by May L. Wykle, Peter J. Whitehouse, and Diana L. Morris (New York: Springer, 2004), 159–76.
10. Elza Maria de Souza, "Intergenerational Interaction in Health Promotion: A Qualitative Study in Brazil," *Revista de Saúde Pública* 37 (2003): 463–69.
11. Christopher L. Hayes, "An Observational Study in Developing an Intergenerational Shared Site Program: Challenges and Insights," *Journal of Intergenerational Relationships* 1, no. 1 (2003): 113–32.
12. Linda P. Fried, Michelle C. Carlson, Marc Freedman, Kevin D. Frick, Thomas A. Glass, Joel Hill, Sylvia McGill, et al., "A Social Model for Health Promotion for an Aging Population: Initial Evidence on the Experience Corps Model," *Journal of Urban Health* 81, no. 1 (2004): 64–78.
13. Christina Gigliotti, Matt Morris, Sara Smock, Shannon E. Jarrott, and Bonnie Graham, "An Intergenerational Summer Program Involving Persons with Dementia and Preschool Children," *Educational Gerontology* 31, no. 6 (2005): 425–41.
14. Shannon E. Jarrott and Kelly Bruno, "Intergenerational Activities Involving Persons with Dementia: An Observational Assessment," *American Journal of Alzheimer's Disease and Other Dementias* 18, no. 1 (2003): 31–37.
15. Michelle M. Lee, Cameron J. Camp, and Megan L. Malone, "Effects of Intergenerational Montessori-Based Activities Programming on Engagement of Nursing Home Residents with Dementia," *Clinical Interventions in Aging* 2, no. 3 (2007): 477.
16. Katherine S. Judge, Cameron J. Camp, and Silvia Orsulic-Jeras, "Use of Montessori-Based Activities for Clients with Dementia in Adult Day Care: Effects on Engagement," *American Journal of Alzheimer's Disease* 15, no. 1 (2000): 42–46.
17. Elza Maria de Souza and Emily Grundy, "Intergenerational Interaction, Social Capital and Health: Results from a Randomised Controlled Trial in Brazil," *Social Science and Medicine* 65, no. 7 (2007): 1397–1409.
18. Jenny C. C. Chung, "An Intergenerational Reminiscence Programme for Older Adults with Early Dementia and Youth Volunteers: Values and Challenges," *Scandinavian Journal of Caring Sciences* 23, no. 2 (2009): 259–64.
19. Eamon O'Shea, Declan Devane, Adeline Cooney, Dympna Casey, Fionnuala Jordan, AndrewHunter, Edel Murphy, John Newell, Sheelah Connolly, and Kathy Murphy, "The Impact of Reminiscence on the Quality of Life of Residents with Dementia in Long-Stay Care," *International Journal of Geriatric Psychiatry* 29, no. 10 (2014): 1062–70.
20. Yoh Murayama, Hiroshi Murayama, Masami Hasebe, Jun Yamaguchi, and Yoshinori Fujiwara, "The Impact of Intergenerational Programs on Social Capital in Japan: A Randomized Population-Based Cross-Sectional Study," *BMC Public Health* 19, no. 1 (2019): 156.

21. Christopher R. Ward, Lenore Los Kamp, and Sally Newman, "The Effects of Participation in an Intergenerational Program on the Behavior of Residents with Dementia," *Activities, Adaptation and Aging* 20, no. 4 (1996): 61–76.
22. Tetsuya Yamagami, Makoto Oosawa, Sinichi Ito, and Haruyasu Yamaguchi, "Effect of Activity Reminiscence Therapy as Brain-Activating Rehabilitation for Elderly People with and without Dementia," *Psychogeriatrics* 7, no. 2 (2007): 69–75.
23. Margaret A. Short-DeGraff and Karen Diamond, "Intergenerational Program Effects on ocial Responses of Elderly Adult Day Care Members," *Educational Gerontology: An International Quarterly* 22, no. 5 (1996): 467–82.
24. George and Singer, "Intergenerational Volunteering and Quality of Life."
25. Catherine A. Brownell, "An Intergenerational Art Program as a Means to Decrease Passive Behaviors in Patients with Dementia," *American Journal of Recreation Therapy* 7, no. 3 (2008): 5–12.
26. Kathleen Ann O'Rourke, "Intergenerational Programming: Yesterday's Memories, Today's Moments, and Tomorrow's Hopes" (PhD diss., University of Tennessee, 1999).
27. J. Lewis, "Intergenerational Programs in Skilled Nursing Facilities," *Activities Directors' Quarterly for Alzheimer's and Other Dementia Patients* 7, no. 4 (2008): 9–18.
28. Christopher R. Ward, Lenore Los Kamp, and Sally Newman, "The Effects of Participation in an Intergenerational Program on the Behavior of Residents with Dementia," *Activities, Adaptation and Aging* 20, no. 4 (1996): 61–76.
29. David J. Wren, "Reaching Out, Reaching In," *Principal Leadership* 5, no. 1 (2004): 28-33.
30. Gwen Waggoner, "Adopt an Elder: Linking Youth and the Elderly," *Activities, Adaptation and Aging* 20, no. 1 (1996): 41–52.
31. Merle Griff, Donna Lambert, Mary Dellmann-Jenkins, and Dorothy Fruit, "Intergenerational Activity Analysis with Three Groups of Older Adults," *Educational Gerontology: An International Quarterly* 22, no. 6 (1996): 601–12.
32. Daniel George, Catherine Whitehouse, and Peter Whitehouse, "A Model of Intergenerativity: How the Intergenerational School Is Bringing the Generations Together to Foster Collective Wisdom and Community Health," *Journal of Intergenerational Relationships* 9, no. 4 (2011): 389–404.
33. Emi Isaki and Mary Towle Harmon, "Children and Adults Reading Interactively: The So-cial Benefits of an Exploratory Intergenerational Program," *Communication Disorders Quarterly* 36, no. 2 (2015): 90–101.
34. Eileen Schwalbach and Sharon Kiernan, "Effects of an Intergenerational Friendly Visit Program on the Attitudes of Fourth Graders toward Elders," *Educational Gerontology* 28, no. 3 (2002): 175–87.
35. Takashi Yamashita, Jennifer M. Kinney, and Elizabeth J. Lokon, "The Impact of a Gerontology Course and a Service-Learning Program on College Students' Attitudes toward People with Dementia," *Journal of Applied Gerontology* 32, no. 2 (2013): 139–63.
36. Elizabeth Lokon, Jennifer M. Kinney, and Suzanne Kunkel, "Building Bridges across Age and Cognitive Barriers through Art: College Students' Reflections on an Intergenerational Program with Elders Who Have Dementia," *Journal of Intergenerational Relationships* 10, no. 4 (2012): 337–54.
37. Daniel R. George, Heather L. Stuckey, and Megan M. Whitehead, "An Arts-Based Intervention at a Nursing Home to Improve Medical Students' Attitudes toward Persons with Dementia," *Academic Medicine* 88, no. 6 (2013): 837–42.
38. Charles L. Slater, "Generativity versus Stagnation: An Elaboration of Erikson's Adult Stage of Human Development," *Journal of Adult Development* 10, no. 1 (2003): 53–65.
39. Joseph Shapiro, "Back to School May Help Those with Alzheimer's," NPR *Morning Edition*, June 12, 2008, https://www.npr.org/templates/story/story.php?storyId=91402614.
40. To launch ISI and celebrate the 15th anniversary of our first school, we worked with StoryBridge, a community-based theater process that blends the collected stories of the community to make a play, performed by those who shared their stories as well as other

community members, to imagine the future of the community. Richard Geer (a director), Qinghong Wei (a visual artist), Iega Jeff (a choreographer), and Jules Corriere (a playwright) created *Moments and Memories*. On one night in May, the whole school was transformed into a series of classroom-based stage productions. The culminating performance occurred on a dance floor in the gym. Original music composed by my (Peter's) friend Bob Cohen celebrated "the beauty of life," and I began referring to the initiative as the Intergenerativity Project. It illustrated the power of story, the visual arts, music, dance, and theater to create cross-platform intergenerative energy for the future.

41. Daniel R. George and Grace Wagler, "Social Learning and Innovation: Developing Two Shared-Site Intergenerational Reading Programs in Hershey, Pennsylvania," *Journal of Intergenerational Relationships* 12, no. 1 (2014): 69–74.

APPENDIX

1. U.S. Department of Health and Human Services, Health Resources and Services Administration, National Center for Health Workforce Analysis, *National and Regional Projections of Supply and Demand for Geriatricians: 2013-2025* (Rockville, MD: U.S. Department of Health and Human Services, April 2017), https://bhw.hrsa.gov/sites/default/files/bhw/health-workforce-analysis/research/projections/GeriatricsReport51817.pdf.

Index

Page numbers in *italics* refer to illustrations.